ROBERT BURTON AND THE TRANSFORMATIVE POWERS OF MELANCHOLY

Literary and Scientific Cultures
of Early Modernity

Series editors:

Mary Thomas Crane, Department of English, Boston College, USA
Henry S. Turner, Department of English, Rutgers University, USA

This series provides a forum for groundbreaking work on the relations between literary and scientific discourses in Europe, during a period when both fields were in a crucial moment of historical formation. We welcome proposals for books that address the many overlaps between modes of imaginative writing typical of the sixteenth and seventeenth centuries – poetics, rhetoric, prose narrative, dramatic production, utopia – and the vocabularies, conceptual models, and intellectual methods of newly emergent "scientific" fields such as medicine, astronomy, astrology, alchemy, psychology, mapping, mathematics, or natural history. In order to reflect the nature of intellectual inquiry during the period, the series is interdisciplinary in orientation and publishes monographs, edited collections, and selected critical editions of primary texts relevant to an understanding of the mutual implication of literary and scientific epistemologies.

Robert Burton and the Transformative Powers of Melancholy

STEPHANIE SHIRILAN
Syracuse University, USA

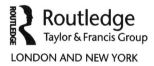

Routledge
Taylor & Francis Group

LONDON AND NEW YORK

First published 2015 by Ashgate Publishing

2 Park Square, Milton Park, Abingdon, Oxfordshire OX14 4RN
52 Vanderbilt Avenue, New York, NY 10017

Routledge is an imprint of the Taylor & Francis Group, an informa business

First issued in paperback 2019

British Library Cataloguing in Publication Data
A catalogue record for this book is available from the British Library

The Library of Congress has cataloged the printed edition as follows:
Shirilan, Stephanie.
  Robert Burton and the transformative powers of melancholy / by Stephanie Shirilan.
    pages cm. — (Literary and scientific cultures of early modernity)
  Includes bibliographical references and index.
  ISBN 978-1-4724-1701-5 (hardcover)

  1. Burton, Robert, 1577–1640—Criticism and interpretation. 2. Burton, Robert, 1577–1640. Anatomy of melancholy. 3. Melancholy in literature. 4. Mind and body therapies—England—History—17th century. 5. Bibliotherapy—England—History—17th century. 6. Depression, Mental, in literature. 7. Melancholy. I. Title.
  PR2224.S47 2015
  828'.309—dc23

                                                                           2015014046

ISBN 978-1-4724-1701-5 (hbk)
ISBN 978-0-367-87998-3 (pbk)

For Ryan, Alethea, Eden, and Lyra
In memory of Eduard Ben Tzion
(1947–2014)

Contents

List of Illustrations

Acknowledgments

Writing about the *Anatomy of Melancholy* reminds one that if all good books are *centos* any real appreciation of their efforts demands an account of their sources, not only of the ideas and arguments contained therein but the vital, if less visible, familiar spirits that animate them.

This book began as a dissertation written at Brandeis University under the direction of Mary Baine Campbell and Thomas King. A more perspicacious reader than Mary is not to be found. Whatever shines here is but a glimmer to her incandescence. Tom's mark is to be felt throughout, but without his suggestion that I read the "whole thing" rather than simply parts of the *Anatomy* for my oral exams, the love of Burton that impelled this book would never have been born.

More people have played a part in the making of this book than I can mention, but a few in particular have loaned their expertise and support at critical junctures: Carla Mazzio, Elizabeth Harvey, Clare Preston, Julia Staykova, Leen Spruit, Koen Vermeir, Rebecca Olson, Vanita Neelakanta, and members of the Syracuse English Faculty Writing Group, especially Patty Roylance, Susan Edmunds, Carol Fadda-Conrey, Mike Goode, Kevin Morrison, Roger Hallas, and Chris Hanson. Wholly unknown to him, Reid Barbour responded to a query I sent him in graduate school with a generosity that I have since come to learn is his signature. This book is deeply indebted to his kindness and mentorship. The few and proud Burtonists and would-be Burtonists I've met along my way share a resemblance with the man himself: generous, learned, and wickedly funny. I am especially grateful to Kathryn Murphy, Jonathan Sawday, Liliana Barczyk-Barakonska, and Ronald Corthell for sharing their work and thoughts.

Colleagues in the English Department and in Medieval and Renaissance Studies at Syracuse University have been strong allies since my arrival six years ago. I am most grateful to Erin Mackie and Dympna Callaghan for their mentorship, Crystal Bartolovitch for her invaluable professional advice and support, and to Susan Edmunds, Carol Fadda-Conrey, Claudia Klaver, Kevin Morrison, Patty Roylance, and Sanford Sternlicht for their good humor and generosity during times of calamity and celebration alike.

Shayna Skarf's friendship has sustained me over the years and daily proven the wisdom of Burton's words about the cure of good company. Susan Edmunds's lessons in academic survival have had the happy theme (most germane to this book) of delightfully confusing trash and treasure. Carol Fadda-Conrey kept vigil through the long, cold nights of writing and revising. Andrew Griffin loaned his incomparable critical eye to each chapter and gave the book his blessing and his heart.

Students in undergraduate courses at Syracuse University, especially in two versions of my course titled "Early Modern Melancholy, Madness and Meaning," helped me both to broaden and refine my thinking on the subjects of this book, as did audiences at meetings of the Renaissance Society of America, History of Science Society, and the Pacific Northwest Renaissance Society. I am also indebted to graduate students in my "Introduction to Early Modern Studies" and "Early Modern Minds and Bodies" seminars. Among these, I am particularly grateful to Melissa Welshans, Amy Burnette, and the late Joseph Hughes for their insights and enthusiasm.

Many libraries and librarians are to be thanked for facilitating this book's writing and production. Syracuse University librarian Patrick Williams and staff in our Interlibrary Loan office routinely obtained materials in a pinch. Our preservationists staved off disaster when my office was visited by bookworms. Librarians at Christ Church, Brasenose, and Lincoln colleges, the Bodleian Library, English Faculty Library at Oxford, Wellcome Library, and the Osler Library for the History of Medicine were particularly generous with their time and assistance. Staff at the Bodleian Library, Houghton Library, University of Toronto Library, and Cornell University Library helped to obtain images and permissions for their reproduction here.

Erika Gaffney has been a champion of this project from the start. I am indebted to her and to the series editors, Henry S. Turner and Mary Thomas Crane, for taking a chance on a Burton book and for procuring such thoughtful and incisive reader reports. I pledge a debt of gratitude to my anonymous readers for their encouragement, challenges, and corrections. Joseph Kappes helped with the mammoth task of digitizing my bibliography. Mary Beth Hinton and Stephanie Peake greatly eased the pangs of delivering my first book with their patient and assiduous proofreading and copy-editing.

Research for this book was conducted during a leave granted by the College of Arts and Sciences at Syracuse University and underwritten by funding that also made possible visits to libraries in the UK, Canada, and United States. Parts of this book have appeared in print previously. I wish to thank the editors of *English Studies in Canada* for their permission to reprint parts of my article, "Francis Bacon, Robert Burton, and the Thick Skin of the World," 34.1 (2008): 59–83, in Chapter 2. Chapter 3 is a revised version of "Exhilarating the Spirits: Burtonian Study as a Cure for Scholarly Melancholy," *Studies in Philology* 111 (2014): 486–520. I am grateful to the anonymous readers at this journal for their invaluable suggestions and to the editors for permission to reproduce material from this publication.

I come last to those who come first. My children, Alethea and Eden, whose acuities served as the inspiration for this book, have borne my distraction during its writing—a period that spans the better part of their lives and whose completion has happily coincided with the arrival of their sister, Lyra. Perla and Sheldon, Maureen and Glenn showered their grandchildren with attention in my absence. That we have emerged hale and whole is a testament to the extraordinary caregiving of my husband Ryan and to the unwavering support of my late father and his brothers, Thomas and Miron. Ryan's constant devotion and labor made every effort that went into this book possible and taught me the lesson that is at its heart: that care cures. An engineer by training, my father listened patiently as I worked through each knot and puzzle. Every success herein bears witness to his love, intelligence, and curiosity. This book is dedicated to his memory and to the sustaining, medicinal love of my husband and children.

Introduction

Robert Burton, librarian of Christ Church College, wrote only one book that we know of during his long tenure at Oxford.[1] "Burton's Melancholy," as it was known in the seventeenth century, went to press for the first time in 1621 under the full title *The Anatomy of Melancholy: What it Is. With All the Kindes, Causes, Symptomes, Prognosticks, and Severall Cures of It. In Three Maine Partitions, with their severall Sections, Members, and Subsections. Philosophically, Medicinally, Historically Opened and Cut Up*. None of the editions ever bore the author's name on the title page. Each edition is attributed, rather, to Democritus Junior, whose name is printed directly above the advertisement that the book contains "a Satyricall Preface, conducing to the following Discourse." Beneath this advertisement on the title pages of the first two editions we find a caption, which he credits to Macrobius: "*Omne meum, Nihil meum*"[2] (Figure I.1). Burton thus clues the reader to the satirical character of his book and, through the Macrobian tag, the fact that the book is a *cento*, a pastiche of borrowed texts arranged in a typically subversive manner. By the third edition (1628), along with the addition of a complex emblematic title page that included his portrait in miniature, Burton would replace the Macrobian tag with one taken from Horace: "*Omne tulit punctum, qui miscuit utile dulci*"—he who mingles the practical and the pleasurable wins the prize, or, more literally, "gets the point" (Figure I.2). The caption instructs the reader who hopes to profit from the book to approach it *sympathetically*, that is, with a willingness to be transformed, especially by the pleasures of the experience. The present study is an attempt to demonstrate and elaborate this therapeutic principle by situating it in its rhetorical, physiological, theological contexts. My introduction aims first, however, to contend with the history of critical resistance both to sympathetic readings of the *Anatomy* and to the positively transformative powers of the imagination in Burton's book.

---

[1]   He did, however, write several short poems and at least two Latin academic dramas, *Alba* and *Philosophaster*, neither of which was published during his lifetime and only the latter of which survives.

[2]   "All mine and nothing mine." As the Clarendon editors point out, the Latin phrase captures the spirit of Macrobius' preface to the *Saturnalia*, but does not appear therein. It is, however, used by Lipsius to describe his cento, the *Politica*, discussed in greater detail in Chapter 1. See Robert Burton, *The Anatomy of Melancholy*, ed. Thomas C. Faulkner, Nicolas K. Kiessling, and Rhonda Blair, Introduction and Commentary by J.B. Bamborough and Martin Dodsworth, 6 vols. (Oxford: Clarendon Press, 1989–2000), 4:26. Translations and bibliographic notes, unless otherwise specified, are borrowed from this edition. All quotations from the *Anatomy* refer to this edition as well, unless otherwise indicated, and will hereafter be cited parenthetically in the text.

THE

ANATOMY OF

MELANCHOLY:

WHAT IT IS.

WITH ALL THE KINDES, CAV-
SES, SYMPTOMES, PROGNOSTICKS,
AND SEVERALL CVRES OF IT.

IN THREE MAINE PARTITIONS,
with their feuerall SECTIONS, MEM-
BERS, and SVBSECTIONS.

PHILOSOPHICALLY , MEDICI-
NALLY, HISTORICALLY
opened and cut vp,

BY
DEMOCRITVS *Iunior.*

With a Satyricall PREFACE, conducing to
the following Difcourfe.

The fecond Edition, corrected and aug-
mented by the Author.

MACROB.
Omne meum, Nihil meum.

AT OXFORD,

Printed by JOHN LICHFIELD and JAMES SHORT,
for HENRY CRIPPS. *Ao Dom. 1624.*

Figure I.1   Title page, Robert Burton, *The Anatomy of Melancholy*, 1624. Division of Rare and Manuscript Collections, Cornell University Library.

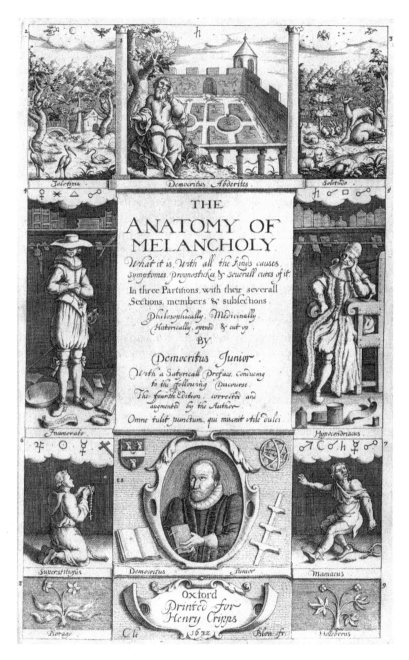

Figure I.2   Christoph Le Blon, engraved title page to Robert Burton,
The Anatomy of Melancholy, 1632 (first printed in the 1628
edition). Division of Rare and Manuscript Collections, Cornell
University Library.

Burton sent the first edition of the *Anatomy* to print with an apology for its unrevised state that he would keep in each of its subsequent revisions:[3] "One or two things yet I would haue amended if I could, That is, first to haue reuised the copie, and amended the stile which now floues *ex tempore*, as it was first written: but my leasure would not permit, *Feci nec quod potui nec quod volui.*"[4] In the second edition (1624) and all editions thereafter, Burton elaborates the excuse of temporal urgency into a defense of his "extemporean stile" and its implicit "plainness":

> as a Beare doth her whelps, to bring forth this confused lumpe, I had not time to licke it into forme, as shee doth her yong ones, but even so to publish it, as it was first written *quicquid in buccam venit*,[5] in an extemporean stile, as I doe commonly all other exercises, *effudi quicquid dictavit Genius meus*,[6] out of a confused company of notes, and writ with as small deliberation as I doe ordinarily speake, without all affectation of big words, fustian phrases, jingling termes, tropes, strong lines, that like *Acesta's* arrowes cought fire as they flew; straines of wit, brave heats, elogies, hyperbolicall exornations, elegancies, &c. which many so much affect. (1:17)[7]

Heaped synonyms for rhetorical flourishes utterly contradict Burton's professed plain speaking. In the very sentence that he tells us he avoids "big words" and "fustian phrases," we have no less than seven collocations, one extended simile, and a big and fustian synonym, "hyperbolicall exornations," for inflated fussiness. Burton plays sound against sense, imitating the ornamented style he claims to eschew in artful remonstration of those who think that plainness and honesty go hand in hand.

The chapters of this study will have much to say about Burton's facetious claim to plainness. I argue, especially in the first chapter, that in his refusal to "reveal himself" Burton rejects contemporary exhortations to confessional transparency, modeling instead (in the petulant but impressible character of Democritus Junior)

---

[3]   Burton continued to revise and republish the *Anatomy* for the remainder of his life, sending it to print in four more editions before his death in 1640. At the time, he was completing a sixth edition, which would be published 10 years later.

[4]   Robert Burton, *The Anatomy of Melancholy* (Oxford, 1621), 10. Edward Bensly, whose notes and working papers (together with those of his predecessor, Aldis Wright) were used to prepare the commentary to the Clarendon edition, suggested that the Latin phrase above (meaning, I have achieved neither what I was capable of nor what I wished) is a reworking of Cicero, *De Oratore* 3.61.228 (4:35–6).

[5]   "Whatever came into my mouth" (4:36).

[6]   "I poured forth whatever my Genius dictated" (4:37).

[7]   The Clarendon version of the passage cited above includes further synonyms and phrases describing the rhetorical excess that Burton claims to be avoiding that were added to the 1628, 1632, and 1651 editions. In preparing their collation, the Clarendon editors followed the 1632 edition, chosen because it is the "first edition to represent the *Anatomy* in near-final form," containing 97.9 percent of the words in the last edition he authorized and because there is convincing evidence that Burton read the proofs and was responsible for its stop-press corrections (1:liii–liv).

a privileged melancholic style that takes aim at popular Puritan and Neostoic ideals of rhetorical temperance and affective restraint. Readers even passingly familiar with the *Anatomy* as it is described in modern scholarship will likely find this argument surprising. It runs against a general view of Burton as the Oxford recluse who obsessively stockpiled information about melancholy for the purposes of protecting himself and others from the very things I claim he defends: namely, a healthy solubility or openness of mind, body, and spirit, made possible by harnessing the salutary powers of the imagination.

The popular portrait of an "anxious" Burton derives from readings of the *Anatomy* that mistake Burton's use of his sources for, at best, neutral appraisal and, at worst, earnest endorsement. Passing references to the *Anatomy* in modern historiographies of gender, subjectivity, and early modern prose routinely overlook the fact that the *Anatomy* baldly declares itself to be a cento—an ancient and ludic form of composition that delights in ventriloquism and juxtaposition, that cuts up and rearranges a master text (or texts) so as to make it speak in ways sometimes wholly contradictory to its original meaning. The art of the cento is not unlike the art of the comic impersonator, whose prosopopoeia works by striking precisely the right balance between imitation and exaggeration. Subtle inflections and infelicities in the comic's impression give the lie to its ironic pantomime. Likewise, witty elisions, circumventions, and juxtapositions reveal the canny subterfuge that Burton wreaks with his sources. However, just as there is danger in directness, there is also danger in too-subtle parody being mistaken for parroting. As we will see in the first chapter, Burton acknowledged and anticipated this risk, although, perhaps, not to the degree that was warranted in his case. The antipathy toward "stylistic" analysis in late twentieth and early twenty-first-century literary scholarship, combined with the increasing availability of searchable electronic archives of early modern texts, has encouraged a kind of consultative style of reading that is ill-equipped to detect such subtleties of tone or context, much less the sophisticated and subversive bibliographical game that Burton plays with the reader.[8] But to explain the fate of the *Anatomy* in terms solely of the present state of the discipline is to occlude the more complex history of its relative neglect.

A Brief History of Burton Studies

While numerous twentieth-century scholars have observed the satirical qualities of the *Anatomy*—one dissertator noting that "only the satirist would take so much time to assert that he is *not* doing precisely what he *is* doing"[9]—the more prevalent approach has been to take Burton's professed plain speaking, his declaration that he "calls a spade a spade" (1:17), far less ironically. This more earnest interpretation

---

[8] For an assessment of the weakness of historicist research with respect to stylistic analysis and a call for a return to "slow" reading in early modern studies, see Marjorie Garber, "Shakespeare in Slow Motion," *Profession* 2010, no. 1 (2010): 151–64.

[9] Robert Wilkerson, "This Playing Labour: The Preface to Burton's *Anatomy of Melancholy* as Satirical Apologia" (PhD diss., Georgia State University, 1975), 128.

of Burton's "plain" style may be traced back at least as far as Morris Croll's early twentieth-century essays on the "Attic" or Senecan style in late Renaissance prose, which he somewhat opaquely classified as a species of the baroque. Croll argues that the objective of the Attic writers was not to persuade "by the sensuous appeal of oratorical rhythm," but by an almost confessional mode of transparent, documentary thought: "by portraying ... exactly those athletic movements of the mind by which it arrives at a sense of reality and the true knowledge of itself and the world."[10] These movements could be witnessed in long series of absolute and participial constructions, appositional members, and relative clauses of the famously intractable prose of Browne, Burton, and Montaigne, as well as in the "curt" rather than "loose" style of Bacon, Lipsius, and Pascal. Croll counted Burton as an Attic writer, named after the so-called practical and unadorned style of the fourth- and fifth-century BC rhetoricians, less for his rejection of ornament (which he admits is inconsistent) than for what he viewed as Burton's desire to document his patterns of thought and discovery: "not a thought, but a mind thinking."[11]

Unlike his colleagues in the early twentieth-century departments of art and music history, Croll and his immediate successors in English literary studies tended not to think about the prose of the late sixteenth and early seventeenth centuries (even that literature they designated by the term "baroque") as mannered or stylized. Rather, Croll regarded the aim of baroque prose as that of manifesting thought from mind to quill with unadulterated directness or immediacy. With a zeal for the virtue of plainness that would find its fullest form in R.F. Jones, Croll writes that the signature of the Attic style was its compulsion to bear witness to the inception of thought, "the moment of expression ... in which the idea first clearly objectifies itself in the mind, in which, therefore, each of its parts still reserves its own peculiar emphasis and an independent vigor all its own."[12] Like George Saintsbury and Barrett Wendell before him, Croll regarded the seemingly unadorned expression of early seventeenth-century English prose as the last gasp of unspoiled genius before self-consciousness turned Renaissance invention into affectation and sarcasm.[13] The moment of aesthetic innocence captured in this

---

[10]   Morris William Croll, "'Attic Prose' in the Seventeenth Century," *Studies in Philology* 18, no. 2 (1921): 95. Expanding upon Croll, Frank Warnke situates the "Attic" style in the rough and uneven aesthetic of a transcontinental literary baroque: "The ideal is not the smooth and persuasive oratorical refashioning of ideas already formed but rather the vital expression of ideas in the process of formation" (*Versions of Baroque: European Literature in the Seventeenth Century* [New Haven, CT: Yale University Press, 1972], 41). Morris William Croll, "The Baroque Style in Prose," in *"Attic" and Baroque Prose Style: The Anti-Ciceronian Movement*, ed. J. Max Patrick and Robert O. Evans (Princeton, NJ: Princeton University Press, 1969), 228.

[11]   Croll, "The Baroque Style in Prose," 210.

[12]   Ibid. The high praise Croll lavishes on these writers for their plainness is coded in the specific terms of late nineteenth-century associations between rhetorical transparency and liberal masculinity.

[13]   See George Saintsbury, *Specimens of English Prose Style from Malory to Macaulay* (London: Kegan Paul, 1885); Barrett Wendell, *Temper of the Seventeenth Century in English Literature* (New York: Scribner, 1904).

prose is, "in brief, the moment in which truth is still *imagined*."[14] The ideological promotion of plainness in Croll's own writing has yet to be properly examined in light of the fraught attitudes toward the value of aesthetic pleasure during the early professionalization of English studies. Meanwhile, despite numerous attempts to reposition the analysis of early modern English prose around the axis of its paradoxical and ironic aspects,[15] Croll's Attic theory has remained the most widely cited account of the so-called "plain style," in which Burton has retained his ill-fitting place.[16]

With the exception of his appearance in Croll's influential essays, the study of Burton in the early twentieth century was predominantly bibliographical and was led by the celebrated physician and bibliophile Sir William Osler (1849–1919), who began the process of reassembling Burton's private library while serving as Professor of Medicine at Oxford.[17] Osler would famously declare the *Anatomy* the greatest of all medical treatises written by a layman.[18] Bibliographical research dominated Burton studies until just before mid-century, at which point psychoanalytic critics had already begun to regard the *Anatomy* as a portrait of the author's psychological instability.[19] A joint study by one literary scholar

---

[14] Croll, "The Baroque Style in Prose," 210. Croll's nostalgia for a perceived rhetorical innocence in these texts may be viewed as an attempt to validate them as objects of study for a modern English professoriate suspicious of what they regarded as the belletristic interests of the previous generation. See my article, "The Forbidden Pleasures of Style," *Prose Studies* 34, no. 2 (2012): 115–28.

[15] See Joan Webber, *The Eloquent "I": Style and Self in Seventeenth-Century Prose* (Madison: University of Wisconsin Press, 1968); Rosalie Colie, *Paradoxia Epidemica: The Renaissance Tradition of Paradox* (Princeton, NJ: Princeton University Press, 1966); Anna K. Nardo, *The Ludic Self in Seventeenth-Century English Literature* (Albany: State University of New York Press, 1991).

[16] See Debora Shuger, "Conceptions of Style," in *The Cambridge History of Literary Criticism*, ed. Glynn Norton, vol. 3 (Cambridge: Cambridge University Press, 1999), 181–6. Shuger notes the almost total scholarly agreement with Croll's theses until Marc Fumaroli's French study of Renaissance rhetoric, *L'âge de l'éloquence* (1980). The predominance of critical work on early modern, "Northern" rhetoric has largely remained the province of French theorists and attests to continued under-attention to the specificity of English baroque, or Attic, prose. On the persistence of Croll's theses (via their resurrection in the 1960s), see Daniela Havenstein, *Democratizing Sir Thomas Browne: Religio Medici and Its Imitations* (Oxford: Clarendon Press, 1999), chap. 5.

[17] See Edith Gittings Reid and Sir William Osler, *The Great Physician: A Short Life of Sir William Osler* (London and New York: Oxford University Press, 1931), 221.

[18] Sir William Osler, *Selected Writings of Sir William Osler, 12 July 1849 to 29 December 1919* (London: Oxford University Press, 1951), 90.

[19] See Richard Leonard Nochimson, "Robert Burton: A Study of the Man, His Work, and His Critics" (PhD diss., Columbia University, 1967). For a critique of this position, see Wilkerson, who reads the book as a thoroughly satiric critique of folly and complains that, despite the influence of Frye's *Anatomy of Criticism*, scholars continue to read the *Anatomy* as "assertive writing" rather than "literary construct" ("This Playing Labour: The Preface to Burton's *Anatomy of Melancholy* as a Satiric Apologia," 10).

and a medical psychiatrist shows another side of the same psychoanalytic turn. Bergen Evans and George Mohr shed light on what they describe as Burton's prescient psychodynamic approach to melancholy, arguing that the author came by this understanding through his own experiences of a disease that originated in childhood neglect.[20] Lawrence Babb, whose *Sanity in Bedlam* reigned as the most cited literary history of early modern madness for almost a half century, also promoted the view of the *Anatomy* as a reflection of its author's illness.

More stylistically sensitive approaches to the *Anatomy* from mid-century through the late 1970s may be found in a series of articles by John Lievsay and David Renaker, as well as in dedicated chapters of Rosalie Colie's *Paradoxia Epidemica: The Renaissance Tradition of Paradox* and Joan Webber's *The Eloquent "I": Style and Self in Seventeenth-Century Prose*, two extraordinarily learned critiques to which the present study is greatly indebted.[21] Jean Simon's *Robert Burton et l'anatomie de mélancolie* (1964) presents one of the most sustained stylistic readings of the *Anatomy* in twentieth-century scholarship, but the fact that his never-translated French monograph was one of only a small handful devoted to Burton in the second half of the last century speaks volumes about the marginalization of the *Anatomy* in Anglophone early modern studies.

In his 1972 *Self-Consuming Artifacts*, Stanley Fish argues that the *Anatomy* offers a desolate view of melancholia as the irremediably self-cannibalizing condition of late humanism and thereby set the tone for the subsequent 30 years of scholarship on seventeenth-century prose style.[22] Fish reads Burton's *copia* as a skeptical reflection of the universality of melancholic disease: "Nothing stands out in Burton's universe, because nothing—no person, place, object, idea—can maintain its integrity in the context of an all-embracing madness." The prefatory Utopia is, according to Fish, "just one more barrel, one more false promise, one more substanceless hope for sanity and order, and, like the others, it surfaces for a few brief moments before the advancing tides of melancholy rise to overwhelm and obliterate it."[23] Stylistic approaches to the *Anatomy* since Fish have by and large supported his diagnosis of Burton's rhetorical excess as an indictment of humanist learning. Some scholars have argued that the *Anatomy*'s erratic style, hyperbolic rhetoric, and misleading synoptic tables lampoon the hubris of late

---

[20]   Bergen Evans and George Joseph Mohr, *The Psychiatry of Robert Burton* (New York: Columbia University Press, 1944).

[21]   John   Lievsay,   "Robert   Burton's   De   Consolatione,"   *South   Atlantic Quarterly* 55 (1956): 329–36; David Renaker, "Robert Burton and Ramist Method," *Renaissance Quarterly* 24, no. 2 (1971): 210–20; David Renaker, "Robert Burton's Tricks of Memory," *PMLA* 87, no. 3 (1972): 391–6.

[22]   For a view of this phenomenon *vis-à-vis* Thomas Browne especially, see Havenstein, *Democratizing Sir Thomas Browne*, 1–5.

[23]   Stanley Eugene Fish, *Self-Consuming Artifacts: The Experience of Seventeenth-Century Literature* (Berkeley: University of California Press, 1972), 329.

Renaissance encyclopedism.[24] Others, taking the view that Burton's rhetorical performance is less deliberate, have viewed the *Anatomy* as a desperate, reactionary "attempt to overwrite an anxiety about the uncontrollable expansiveness of his subject."[25]

Disciplinary aversions to formal and stylistic reading have precipitated nothing short of an epidemic of literalist misreadings of the *Anatomy* in the past several decades. Many such instances may be found in the scholarship that Richard Strier has dubbed the "new humoralism" (denoting the Foucauldian focus on compelled forms of subjectivity that this branch of early modern body-studies shares with new historicism).[26] The new humoralists emphasize the determining power of humoral psychology within early modern views of embodiment. While this scholarship has usefully challenged certain post-Cartesian assumptions about the history of western subjectivity, it has imposed its own anachronistic interpretations of physiological and spiritual solubility as intrinsically anxiety provoking. Mark Breitenberg, following Gail Kern Paster's lead, describes the Burtonian body as a body under siege by a host of unruly passions and regards the copiousness of Burton's prose as an index of its perpetual "danger of overflow and transgression."[27] He refers to Burton's melancholy as internal otherness, "an Other not beyond the pale but more insidiously present within" and equates this alien self with a monstrous femininity, which Burton exorcises in his incontinent prose.[28]

The prevailingly anxious view of the *Anatomy* that one witnesses in the new humoralism (and the wider bodily turn of early modern studies to which it belongs)

---

[24]   See, especially, Robert Grant Williams, "Disfiguring the Body of Knowledge: Anatomical Discourse and Robert Burton's *The Anatomy of Melancholy*," *ELH* 68, no. 3 (2001): 593–613; Renaker, "Robert Burton and Ramist Method."

[25]   See Christopher Tilmouth, "Burton's 'Turning Picture': Argument and Anxiety in *The Anatomy of Melancholy*," *The Review of English Studies* 56, no. 226 (2005): 543. See also Leonard Goldstein, "Science and Literary Style in Robert Burton's 'Cento out of Divers Writers,'" *Journal of the Rutgers University Library* 21 (1958): 55–68. Goldstein suggests that Burton's *Anatomy* documents an anxious response of a very specific kind: i.e., that Burton's *enumeratio* "unconsciously and compulsively expresses the quantitative side of [an emerging] science," and he views Burton's contradictions as "the scientific desire for objectivity in a mind not fully conscious of its method of analysis" (67–8).

[26]   See Introduction, "Back to Burkhardt," Richard Strier, *The Unrepentant Renaissance: From Petrarch to Shakespeare to Milton* (Chicago: University of Chicago Press, 2011).

[27]   Mark Breitenberg, *Anxious Masculinity in Early Modern England* (Cambridge: Cambridge University Press, 1996), 46.

[28]   Ibid., 37–8. Breitenberg's reading follows the "psychological materialist" approach that Gail Kern Paster takes in *The Body Embarrassed* and *Humoring the Body*. In the latter book, Paster turns to philosopher Charles Taylor to restate the literal and phenomenological significance of a humoral system wherein "black bile doesn't just cause melancholy" but "somehow resides in it" (Gail Kern Paster, *Humoring the Body: Emotions and the Shakespearean Stage* [Chicago: University of Chicago Press, 2010], 5).

may be viewed as an extension of late twentieth-century psychoanalytic and poststructuralist criticism, with its symptomatic readings of early modern writing as either the expression of violence against a phantasmic Renaissance ego ideal or the shoring up of its ruins. Representing the former approach (and drawing heavily on Lacan in so doing), Grant Williams characterizes the *Anatomy* as a precocious deconstruction of the encyclopedic impulse, a "disfiguration" of text that "brings out the monstrous condition of textuality" in heaps and lists that ironize and denounce humanist ambition.[29] This reading obscures both the philosophical motives and the therapeutic logic of Burton's rhetorical excess and instability. My book argues for a different vocabulary to describe these features and for an approach that is more sensitive to their felicitous or therapeutic effects. Such an approach yields a very different appreciation of the *Anatomy*—one that heralds its achievement outside of its appeal to postmodern sensibilities and rather of its own organic and philosophical commitment to a poetics of copia, or abundance. That Burton's signature "etcetera" marks incompleteness is clear. What is less clear is why such open-endedness need be understood as renunciatory, even when replete with irony.[30] This begs further questions about the historiography of early modernity that this book hopes to raise and that the remainder of this introduction will take up, namely: How have modern preoccupations with fragmentation distorted our readings of cosmic and rhetorical plenitude? Moreover, how has the professional institutionalization of rhetorical plainness militated against the recognition of Burton's willful inauthenticity and its therapeutic intent?

Transforming and Transformative Melancholy

This book understands Burton's theatricality as a technique for delivering and disguising both social critique and direct physic. Generic theories of satire, Menippean (as Frye suggested) or otherwise, are inadequate to the task of describing these functions in the *Anatomy*.[31] Ritual anthropologist Victor Turner contrasts the normalizing function of satire with the potential subversion of "entertainment." He notes that the word "entertain" derives from the Old French, *entretenir*, which means "to hold apart," or as he glosses it, to create a space in which destabilizing performance may occur. The space of "entertainment" is "liminoid," typically removed from "the mainstream of productive or political events." Turner lists universities and institutes of learning as examples of such theoretically neutral

---

[29]   Williams, "Disfiguring the Body of Knowledge," 593; 597.

[30]   Stanley Fish's essay, "Thou Thyself Art the Subject of My Discourse," in *Self-Consuming Artifacts*, argues that Burton tantalizes the reader with the prospect of escape from a cosmology of despair only to reconfirm that there is no escape, only cold comfort in the universality of human misery.

[31]   Northrop Frye, *Anatomy of Criticism: Four Essays* (Princeton, NJ: Princeton University Press, 1957), 311–12. See also W. Scott Blanchard, *Scholars' Bedlam: Menippean Satire in the Renaissance* (Lewisburg, PA: Bucknell University Press, 1995).

spaces where "all kinds of freewheeling, experimental cognitive behavior as well as forms of symbolic action, might take place."[32] Taking a more skeptical view, Michel Foucault regarded the academic system as a machine for the reproduction of hegemonic power, even if "only the most visible, the most sclerotic and least dangerous form of this phenomenon."[33] Burton, who spent his entire adult life at Oxford, had much to say about institutional hegemony and the corruption of the universities, but his is a critique of the sort that could only be written from within.

Turner offers us another, more helpful, category by which to understand what it is that Burton is doing in the *Anatomy*, and that is play, by which I do not mean the ironic "playing" that poststructuralist readings of Burton have emphasized.[34] I mean, rather, the generative and therapeutic sense of play as a method for the restoration of the spirits as understood by early modern physicians who were informed both by classical and Christian traditions regarding the care for the soul. Turner constructs a lexical ethnography of dictionary entries for the word "play" that locates its postindustrial meaning in the conceptual opposition of light and heavy, free and obligated, joking and serious.[35] As we will see in Chapter 3, these structural oppositions have roots in medieval faculty psychology. Likewise, the account of play as transformative and efficacious, which Turner draws out from Johan Huizinga's cultural history and the developmental psychology of Donald Winnicott and Gregory Bateson, has ancient precedents in the restorative rituals of comedy, sport, and a manner of literary and scientific play that understands itself to be spiritually, politically, and physiologically transformative. I argue in the chapters ahead that Burton's ludic performance aims both to restore or recreate the reader's—and his own—melancholic spirits and, at the same time, to alter the reader's understanding of melancholy altogether.

The central claim of this book is that Burton's cento transforms melancholy from disease, as it is represented in classical and neoteric sources, into a kind of spiritual privilege that draws on the impressionability of the melancholic imagination. The traditional hallmarks of the melancholic personality—suggestibility, vulnerability, and irrationality—become spiritual resources insofar as they may be cultivated to allow for greater compassion and awareness of divine presence. Burton's prolix and seemingly erratic and irrational style imitates and exaggerates the associative or sympathetic reasoning characteristic of the melancholic personality.

---

[32]   Victor W. Turner, *From Ritual to Theatre: The Human Seriousness of Play*, vol. 1, Performance Studies Series (New York: Performing Arts Journal Publications, 1982), 41.

[33]   Michel Foucault, *Power/knowledge: Selected Interviews and Other Writings, 1972–1977*, ed. and trans. Colin Gordon (New York: Pantheon Books, 1980), 52.

[34]   See Nardo, *The Ludic Self in Seventeenth-Century English Literature*, 140–57. Nardo offers the most sustained analysis of the *Anatomy* as "play" that I have been able to find. However, she regards the book as a game whose principal purpose is the author's self-distraction. Any reader benefit that arises from this exercise is coincidental: "Written as play to cure the author's melancholy, *The Anatomy* becomes play to cure the reader's melancholy" (153).

[35]   Turner, *From Ritual to Theatre*, 33–4.

As some scholars have noted, this seems in part to be intended as a means of appealing to a reader who is affected by similarly irrational habits of mind. It has the further effect, however, of underscoring the ethical potential and cosmic power of what I refer to in this study as "mimetic sympathy." By this I mean the capacity of the imagination to facilitate what is referred to in occultist tradition as "actions at a distance," meaning transformations between seemingly distant or disparate things through hidden resemblances.[36] Simply put, I argue that Burton's stylistic irrationality invokes as it imitates the cosmic and ethical force of sympathy, modeling a treatment for melancholy that refines rather than suppresses melancholic unreason.

By speaking of the poetics of sympathy in the *Anatomy* I risk the censure of critics who remain suspicious of any effort to uncover authorial intent in Burton's seemingly uncontrolled verbal feast. Mary Murphy Schmelzer points to Ruth Fox's analysis of the *Anatomy*'s synoptic tables (Fox argues that they are predictably unreliable) as illustration of the "ingenious" but semantic argument that Burton's "abrogation of order and rule constitutes the order of the text."[37] Copia, she says, may have been the prevailing epistemology of the late Renaissance, but the excess to which Burton takes it points to the absence at the center of such abundance.[38] Even as she claims to be motivated by a desire to avoid anachronism, Schmelzer draws conclusions about the sum of Burtonian copia that strike me as distinctly modern. The *Anatomy*, she says, "reveals the precarious underside of a discourse which recognizes that language can never be present to that which it describes."[39] Burton's abundance becomes nought in this reading of Burtonian copia: "The text effects the reductive transformation of everything into nothing by means of an annihilating excess."[40] The translation of everything into nothing and abundance into absence is a conspicuously modern and arguably reductive habit of mind. Early moderns seem to have been better able to sustain wonder and doubt simultaneously and to express these through a playfulness

---

[36]   Marcel Mauss uses the term "mimetic sympathy" ("*sympathie mimétique*") to describe magical transformations by force of similarity rather than continuity, i.e., indirect "resemblance" rather than proxy. See *A General Theory of Magic* (London: Routledge, 2005), chap. 3, "The Elements of Magic." Foucault's account of the four similitudes that make up the correspondence system of the "age of resemblance" is indebted both to Mauss and his sources, especially James George Frazer, *The Golden Bough: A Study in Magic and Religion*, 3rd ed., vol. 3 (London: Macmillan, 1911).

[37]   Mary Murphy Schmelzer, *'Tis All One: "The Anatomy of Melancholy" as Belated Copious Discourse* (New York: Peter Lang, 1999), 25. See Ruth A. Fox, *The Tangled Chain: The Structure of Disorder in "The Anatomy of Melancholy"* (Berkeley: University of California Press, 1976).

[38]   Schmelzer, *'Tis All One*, 55.

[39]   Ibid., 84. Schmelzer equates the failure of linguistic signification (the central loss out of which she believes Burton's prolixity dilates) with the sinful state of lapsed humanity (92–3; 104–5).

[40]   Ibid., 85.

that has been anachronistically misconstrued as trifling or unserious. As we shall see in Chapter 4, much more resides under the dictum "'tis all one" than either assimilative holism or ironic dismissal. The interpretation of Burtonian copia, and of Burton's oft-repeated tag "'tis all one" as "'tis all nought," is a prevailing one in recent studies of the *Anatomy* and one this book hopes to counter.

In his *Book on Games of Chance*, Girolamo Cardano writes that the advantages of play are that we "obtain relaxation from anxiety and a pleasure from which we arise ready and eager for serious business."[41] Burton's therapeutic playing presses against this notion of proscribed play that only restores the body so that it might take up more useful employments. Cardano, however, understood other benefits of play beyond its recuperative value. He suggests that play allows us to better understand the characters of our fellows, "for play is ... a rack on which anger, greed, and honesty or dishonesty are made clear."[42] Burton similarly intimates that the character of his reader will be revealed in the way they play his game, detecting its ironies as well as its encomia. He suggests, moreover, that such subtle reading is crucial to the art of harnessing and refining the transformative powers of melancholy.

In Defense of Melancholy

One of the principal arguments of this book, and the focus of its first chapter, is that Burton casts the amplitude of the melancholic imagination as magnanimity against what he seemed to regard as the pusillanimity of popular Christian Neostoicism. I argue that his exaggerated rhetorical and somatic *uncontrol* rejects the tranquility promoted by Lipsius, Du Vair, and the ubiquitous spiritual hygiene books of the late sixteenth and early seventeenth centuries. He exposes the contradictory counsel offered in such books to be imperturbable without being intractable or "hard-hearted." As Christopher Brooke has recently reminded us, it was a commonplace of anti-Puritan rhetoric in the early seventeenth century to represent the "precisianist" spirit as proudly impervious.[43] This commonplace drew on the deeply rooted Augustinian critique of Stoicism that one finds in the writings of the Church Fathers, who had accorded a special status to a godly sadness, or *tristitia*, that was imitative of Christ's suffering. Such sadness comported with and was seen to be propaedeutic to piety so long as it was properly managed and distinguished from an inward wretchedness (*aegritudo*) that leads either to sloth (*acedia*) or prideful despair.[44]

---

[41]   Girolamo Cardano, *The Book on Games of Chance (Liber de Ludo Aleae)* (New York: Holt, Rinehart and Winston, 1961), 4.

[42]   Ibid.

[43]   Christopher Brooke, *Philosophic Pride: Stoicism and Political Thought from Lipsius to Rousseau* (Princeton, NJ: Princeton University Press, 2012).

[44]   Jeremy Schmidt, *Melancholy and the Care of the Soul: Religion, Moral Philosophy and Madness in Early Modern England* (Aldershot, UK: Ashgate, 2007), 22–4.

The promotion of the melancholic imagination in the Florentine Renaissance had greater debts to the semi-ennobled condition of melancholy in patristic and medieval Christianity than the Burkhardtian narrative has made explicit. Genial representations of the melancholic temperament in the Renaissance drew on complex Christian understandings of the passions and the melancholic complexion as both a powerful aid and an obstacle to spiritual growth. Hugh of St. Victor, for instance, "emphasized with the utmost clarity that it was entirely a matter for men's will-power to turn the conditions even of this complexion to advantage."[45] Ancient and late antique Neoplatonists designated those who showed signs of having been "born under the sign of Saturn" with special powers of divination and prophecy.[46] According to this tradition, melancholics were deemed to have "forward" imaginations that extend outward in a kind of sympathetic reaching that makes them potentially prescient. The Florentine account of melancholic genius elaborated this role of the melancholic imagination that had long been associated with the occult.[47] I argue throughout this book that Burton both inherits and revises this tradition by rendering melancholy genius as a state of exceptional, if potentially excruciating, sympathetic acuity: a capacity to perceive powerful connections between seemingly unlike things that has profound spiritual as well as intellectual and artistic value.

Burton's Spiritual Therapeutics

The appearance of the Clarendon *Anatomy* has helped to revise a number of the misperceptions of the book detailed above. Decades in the making, this first fully annotated critical edition has made the complexity of the *Anatomy* manifest for a new generation of scholars who have increasingly turned their attention to Burton's rhetorical, if not his "stylistic," performance.[48] Angus Gowland has emphasized the *Anatomy*'s debts to classical rhetoric, arguing that the book should be viewed in the tradition of *epideixis*—a branch of oratory wherein arguments

---

[45]   Raymond Klibansky, Erwin Panofsky, and Fritz Saxl, *Saturn and Melancholy: Studies in the History of Natural Philosophy, Religion, and Art* (New York: Basic Books, 1964), 109.

[46]   "What for Plotinus had been essentially a mythical allegory, and for Proclus a cosmological relationship, becomes for Macrobius (or his source) a genuine astrological doctrine of planetary influence" (ibid., 155).

[47]   Lynn Thorndike, *A History of Magic and Experimental Science*, vol. 1 (New York: Macmillan, 1923), 153.

[48]   In addition to articles and monographs by Angus Gowland and Mary Ann Lund detailed below, see Douglas Trevor, *The Poetics of Melancholy in Early Modern England* (Cambridge: Cambridge University Press, 2004), chap. 5; Adam Kitzes, *The Politics of Melancholy from Spenser to Milton* (New York: Routledge, 2006), chap. 5; and Drew Daniel, *The Melancholy Assemblage: Affect and Epistemology in the English Renaissance* (New York: Fordham University Press, 2013), chap. 5.

are sounded less to persuade than to elucidate the rhetor's skill in reciting them.[49] This designation of Burton's rhetorical aim as epideictic rather than deliberative or judicial obscures both the book's explicitly stated therapeutic aim as well as its less explicit philosophical and theological arguments.

Burton's plainness about his motivations for writing the *Anatomy* is uncharacteristically clear and un-ironic. He writes, he says, to ease himself and "helpe others out of a fellow-feeling" (1:8–9). While this therapeutic intent has been observed and commented upon by numerous scholars, my understanding of its logic differs considerably from those who have preceded me. Patricia Vicari, for instance, has argued that the book holds up a pedagogical mirror to recalcitrant sinners, eliciting precisely those penitential impulses that Burton holds responsible for the epidemic of spiritual melancholy.[50] My approach to the *Anatomy* is more complementary to the one taken by Mary Ann Lund in her recent study.[51] Lund refers to the *Anatomy* as "bibliotherapeutic," by which she means that Burton offers direct salve for religious melancholy with a host of rational, nearly Arminian arguments against the doctrine of predestination. I extend Lund's reading of Burton's critique of Puritan theology by situating it in the context of early seventeenth-century anti-Stoic sentiment. Unlike Lund, however, I emphasize the *irrational* qualities of Burton's technique. I draw on representations of the power of the imagination in Renaissance rhetorical theory to account for Burton's bibliotherapy in cognitive, physiological, and performative terms. My contextualization of Burton's use of pathos builds on the work of scholars such as Wayne Rebhorn and Deborah Shuger who have brought the influence of Quintilian, Hermogenes, and other proponents of the *movere* tradition on Renaissance rhetorical theory to light, correcting the misperception that the Renaissance had no other prose models except the so-called plain style, ironically both attributed to Cicero and referred to as "Anticiceronian."[52] I am hardly the first to note that the *Anatomy* offers a kind of literary medicine to Burton's readers.[53] What my book hopes to contribute is a keener appreciation of the ways his bibliotherapy and rhetorical cure would have been understood to work in physiological terms and in accordance with more salutary views of the early modern imagination than have been widely acknowledged.

---

[49] Angus Gowland, "Rhetorical Structure and Function in *The Anatomy of Melancholy*," *Rhetorica: A Journal of the History of Rhetoric* 19, no. 1 (2001): 1–48.

[50] E. Patricia Vicari, *The View from Minerva's Tower: Learning and Imagination in "The Anatomy of Melancholy"* (Toronto, ON: University of Toronto Press, 1989).

[51] Mary Ann Lund, *Melancholy, Medicine and Religion in Early Modern England: Reading "The Anatomy of Melancholy"* (New York: Cambridge University Press, 2010).

[52] Wayne A. Rebhorn, *The Emperor of Men's Minds: Literature and the Renaissance Discourse of Rhetoric* (Ithaca, NY: Cornell University Press, 1995); Debora Shuger, *Sacred Rhetoric: The Christian Grand Style in the English Renaissance* (Princeton, NJ: Princeton University Press, 1988).

[53] In addition to Lund, see Martin Heusser, *The Gilded Pill: A Study of the Reader-Writer Relationship in Robert Burton's "Anatomy of Melancholy"* (Tübingen: Stauffenburg, 1987).

Pneuma: Air, Spirit, and Imagination

One of the principal contexts for Burton's bibliotherapeutics is the pneumatic account of spirit found in Renaissance faculty psychology and the almost completely overlooked history of the imagination that is, as Keith Hutchison and Koen Vermeir have observed, also the history of air.[54] Shigehisa Kuriyama writes that "the imagination of winds is virtually invisible in the historiography of medicine."[55] This invisibility has been equally pervasive in the lamentably discrete historiographies of rhetoric and the imagination.[56] While the pneumatic account of the spirits and *species* (visible, optical, and audible) has been amply discussed by historians of art and music, optics, and acoustics, this has not been true for literature.[57] The ecological model of early modern cognition observed by John Sutton and Koen Vermeir, who have written at length about the "sponginess" of the early modern brain and the vapors of the imagination,[58] has yet to command the attention of literary scholars who have been more interested, of late, in the internal scheme of Galenic humoralism.[59] As a consequence, the discussion of

---

[54]   Keith Hutchison, "What Happened to Occult Qualities in the Scientific Revolution?" *Isis* 73, no. 2 (1982): 233–53; Koen Vermeir, "The 'Physical Prophet' and the Powers of the Imagination. Part I: A Case-Study on Prophecy, Vapours and the Imagination (1685–1710)," *Studies in History and Philosophy of Science Part C: Studies in History and Philosophy of Biological and Biomedical Sciences* 35, no. 4 (2004): 561–91.

[55]   Shigehisa Kuriyama, *The Expressiveness of the Body and the Divergence of Greek and Chinese Medicine* (New York: Zone, 2002), 234. Kuriyama traces the genealogy of an "inward" style of western subjectivity not to the Christian reinterpretation of spirit as soul, or to anatomical empiricism, but rather to Galen's translation of the windy, atmospheric, climactic, environmental pneuma of Hippocratic medicine as an internalized nervous spirit (ibid., 260). For the classic argument that this process rather derives from the Christianization of the pneumatic spirits as *spiritus* or soul, see Gérard Verbeke, *L'évolution de la doctrine du Pneuma: du stoicisme à S. Augustin* (Paris: Desclée de Brouwer, 1945).

[56]   See Gary Tomlinson, *Music in Renaissance Magic: Toward a Historiography of Others* (Chicago: University of Chicago Press, 1993); Penelope Gouk, *Music, Science, and Natural Magic in Seventeenth-Century England* (New Haven, CT: Yale University Press, 1999); D.P. Walker, *Spiritual and Demonic Magic: From Ficino to Campanella* (University Park: Pennsylvania State University Press, 2000).

[57]   See essays in Christine Göttler and Wolfgang Neuber, *Spirits Unseen: The Representation of Subtle Bodies in Early Modern European Culture* (Leiden: Brill, 2008).

[58]   John Sutton, "Spongy Brains and Material Memories," in *Environment and Embodiment in Early Modern England*, ed. Mary Floyd-Wilson and Garrett A. Sullivan Jr. (Houndmills, UK, and New York: Palgrave Macmillan, 2007); John Sutton, *Philosophy and Memory Traces: Descartes to Connectionism* (Cambridge: Cambridge University Press, 1998); Vermeir, "The 'Physical Prophet' and the Powers of the Imagination. Part I."

[59]   On the overinvestment of recent literary scholarship in early modern humoralism at the expense of a richer appreciation of the occult powers of sympathy and antipathy, see the Introduction to Mary Floyd-Wilson, *Occult Knowledge, Science, and Gender on the Shakespearean Stage* (Cambridge: Cambridge University Press, 2013).

the medical and spiritual meanings of air in early modern literature remains a limited one, subsumed within a generally flattened understanding of the Galenic non-naturals (air, diet, evacuation, exercise, rest, and passion) as perilous and peripheral rather than essential to one's spiritual and physical well-being.[60] A chief aim of the present study will be to illuminate the pneumatic dimensions of Burton's sympathetic medicine by identifying the powerful relationships between air, imagination, and spirit that inform it.

Among the relatively few literary scholars who have treated the subject, Gail Kern Paster gives one of the most detailed accounts of the pneumatic conditions of early modern embodiment, but moves rather too quickly from identifying the solubility of the body to declaring its threat. "It is not surprising," she writes, "that the humoral body should be characterized not only by its physical openness but also by its emotional instability and volatility."[61] In her effort to body forth the literal meanings of early modern humoral images, Paster discounts the powers credited to the early modern imagination that were understood to broker interactions between psyche and soma. In so doing, she naturalizes the immanence of an early modern "civilizing process" without considering the specific theological, socioeconomic, and philosophical conditions under which it was codified. Whereas Paster's analysis emphasizes "the forces understood to threaten" the humanist desire for "self-sameness" and "manly constancy,"[62] my study calls attention to the virtues associated with the more labile forms of selfhood that obtained from more positive views of physiological and psychic impressionability in the early modern period.

Timothy Reiss refers to such views of the body's impressionability as "passible" rather than passive, as the former is closer to the Latin and Greek terms of origin, *passibilis* and *pathetikos*, that "named any aspect of the soul to be affected by something."[63] Reiss reminds us that Aristotle understood the condition of human *being* as the possession of a movable soul, literally, a soul capable of motion, or *perturbation*: "Thus was it distinguished from eternal, universal/divine *im*passible soul." "Possibility," says Reiss, "was the fundamental nature of the human being *as* human. Its relation to the endlessly multiple matter, qualities, and events of its surroundings—divine, animate, social, physical—was one of being always and

---

[60]   A notable exception appears to have concentrated around readings of Hamlet and its suggestively foul air. See Carla Mazzio, "The History of Air: Hamlet and the Trouble with Instruments," *South Central Review* 26, no. 1 (2009): 153–96; Carolyn Sale, "Eating Air, Feeling Smells: Hamlet's Theory of Performance," *Renaissance Drama* 35 (2006): 145–68.

[61]   Paster, *Humoring the Body*, 19.

[62]   Ibid., 22.

[63]   Timothy J. Reiss, *Mirages of the Selfe: Patterns of Personhood in Ancient and Early Modern Europe* (Stanford: Stanford University Press, 2003), 96. The categories "active" and "passive" refer, in Aristotelian thought, to categories of actuality and potentiality, *entelechia, energeia*, and *dunamis*, which "did not readily apply to humans in whom active and passive intertwined to compose their *reactive* possible nature—for which Aquinas used the terms *passio* and *passibilis*" (ibid.).

constantly affected by simply being in them," or "more exactly, being *of* them," and not simply as the recipient of such environmental influence. Rather, "the living body affected its physical surroundings as they affected it, for good or ill. [64]

Reiss's account of reactive passibility is reinforced by the pneumatic account of spirit that was the heart of Stoic cosmology, the foundation of Hippocratic medicine, and the oft-overlooked support for the Neoplatonist promotion of the powers of the imagination.[65] The Stoics held that the passible soul is composed of pneuma, a substance made up of fire and air that is the principle of life and the essence of divine reason, or *logos*. Stoicism, as Gérard Verbeke writes, "is a kind of materialistic pantheism, and teaches that even the immanent divine Spirit is corporeal."[66] We see this in Aristotle's explanation that pneuma is both "enclosed in the semen" and "analogous to the element which belongs to the stars."[67] In some early sources, pneuma is represented as emanating from the blood in hot exhalations, or entering the blood via the breath and penetration of the external air in which it is always present. Later Greek sources distinguish vital pneuma from psychic pneuma, localizing the former in the left ventricle of the heart and the latter in the brain. The vital pneuma in the heart was, in fact, thought to circulate through an arterial system that transported pneuma, not blood.[68]

The third-century Neoplatonists did not reject this Stoic doctrine as much as they offered a new interpretation of it, rendering pneuma the spiritual intermediary between body and soul.[69] Porphyry and Plotinus emphasized the role of pneuma as a bridge between the material and immaterial, the corporeal and the divine. Christian Neoplatonists elaborated the Porphyrian distinction between the corporeal and incorporeal spirits but also emphasized the interrelationship

---

[64]   Ibid., 96–7.

[65]   See Ioan P. Culianu, *Eros and Magic in the Renaissance* (Chicago: University of Chicago Press, 1987), chap. 1. The idea of a material spiritual essence animating the body and soul was common to Greek, Arabic, and ancient Jewish philosophy (pneuma, like the Arabic "rouh" and the Hebrew "ruach," refers both to wind or air and the divine principle that animates the body) and was easily assimilated into a Christian metaphysics of incarnation and transubstantiation, but proved somewhat more difficult for medical and theological reformers, who strove anew to distinguish divine from bodily and mundane spirits. As we shall see in Chapter 2, this uneasiness is especially evident in late sixteenth- and early seventeenth-century debates over the causes of melancholy and its distinction from spiritual disease.

[66]   Gérard Verbeke, *The Presence of Stoicism in Medieval Thought* (Washington, DC: Catholic University of America Press, 1983), 4.

[67]   Aristotle, *Generation of Animals*, trans. Arthur Leslie Peck, Loeb Classical Library (Cambridge, MA: Harvard University Press, 1943), 171.

[68]   This medical conception of pneuma seems to predate the philosophical doctrine of pneuma as it is associated with Zeno and Chrysippus. Giorgio Agamben suggests that the philosophical doctrine of pneuma might have developed out of medical practice and observation. See Giorgio Agamben, *Stanzas: Word and Phantasm in Western Culture* (Minneapolis: University of Minnesota Press, 1993), 91–2.

[69]   Verbeke, *The Presence of Stoicism in Medieval Thought*, 41.

between the two as mediated by the power of the imagination, which would be so greatly elaborated by the Florentine Neoplatonists. Synesius of Cyrene regarded the imagination as the most complete and perfect because most direct sense, reversing the terms by which the imagination had traditionally been regarded as suspect.[70] In *On Dreams*, his commentary on the Chaldean Oracles, he argues that the imagination is the mechanism by which the images (*eidoloi*) that one acquires during one's life persist after death. Beyond this ennobling of the imagination as the faculty responsible for the immortalizing of memory (if not the soul itself), what is most notable for our purposes is the principle by which Synesius understood this process to occur. According to Synesius, the *eidolon* retains properties of the pneuma through which the soul passes on its travels before birth and after death. This retention is made possible because image, imagination, and soul share a material resemblance with pneuma that allows for their hylomorphism.[71] Synesius' reasoning relies on the principle of sympathetic attraction—the idea that like seeks out like and that matter transforms or may be transformed by the power of analogy or resemblance.

The chemical revolution of the late sixteenth century foregrounded the curative potential of sympathetic transformations. Paracelsus, the self-proclaimed Luther of medicine, rejected Galenic medicine for what he regarded as its pagan emphasis on the internal causes of disease and its blindness to the determining influence of external forces and spirits.[72] One of the key motivations of early modern pharmacology was, indeed, to provide a material account of grace and its physical properties and effects—a fact still largely underappreciated in the historiography of medicine.[73] Paracelsus drew on the cosmologies of folk medicine and natural magic that understood all of creation to be interwoven in a fabric of sympathetic relation. In folk medical tradition, therapeutic uses of certain plants could be divined by their resemblance to the organs or functions they supported. These structural resemblances were not merely symbolic; that is, they did more than simply point to the hierarchical order of the Christian macrocosm, as earlier Renaissance scholars suggested. Mimetic resemblances could be manipulated, simulated, or exaggerated for efficacious purposes, both salutary and nefarious. The anti-occult sentiment that one finds in early to mid-seventeenth-century writers such as Francis Bacon and Daniel Sennert is not skeptical but cautious,

---

[70] Synesius, *The Essays and Hymns of Synesius of Cyrene*, trans. Augustine Fitzgerald (Oxford: Oxford University Press, 1930), 2:333.

[71] Jay Bregman, *Synesius of Cyrene: Philosopher-Bishop* (Berkeley: University of California Press, 1982), 148–50.

[72] Walter Pagel, *Paracelsus: An Introduction to Philosophical Medicine in the Era of the Renaissance* (Basel: Karger, 1982); Andrew Weeks, *Paracelsus: Speculative Theory and the Crisis of the Early Reformation* (Albany: State University of New York Press, 1997).

[73] Charles Webster, "Paracelsus: Medicine as Popular Protest," in *Medicine and the Reformation*, ed. Ole Peter Grell and Andrew Cunningham (London: Routledge, 1993); Ole Peter Grell, *Paracelsus: The Man and His Reputation, His Ideas and Their Transformation* (Leiden: Brill, 1998).

and it echoes the concerns of Renaissance natural magicians, such as Ficino and Agrippa, who illustrated that one could both transform and be transformed by the subtle powers of evocation and mimetic suggestion.

Burton's spiritual therapy draws on medical, cosmological, and theological accounts of the spirits in which the capacity of the imagination to heal by the power of sympathy is deeply writ. I argue that this power takes on a newly ethical force in the *Anatomy of Melancholy* as Burton assimilates the cosmic powers of sympathy to sympathy as compassionate feeling, which he prescribes as the antidote to a melancholic pandemic caused not by the perturbations of the care-worn spirit (as the Neostoics had argued), but by the absence of care and community. I further suggest that in so doing, Burton offers a potent critique of an emerging model of dispassionate scholarship that helps to illuminate the conditions under which his own promotion of the powers of sympathy and the imagination has been obscured.

Analogy and (the Opposite of) Science

Historians of science and literature have traditionally spoken of the analogical mode of premodern thought as if it were an arrested state of cultural development. While no longer admissible in such reductive terms, the bias against analogical and sympathetic reasoning manifestly persists in the historiography of these subjects.[74] In his influential account of the "occult" and "scientific mentalities" in the Renaissance, Brian Vickers insists that the distinction between the two lay in their divergent approaches to analogy. According to Vickers, analogy muddles the relationships between cause and effect in the natural world that science is supposed to disambiguate:

> Words are treated as if they are equivalent to things and can be substituted for them. Manipulate the one and you manipulate the other. Analogies, instead of being, as they are in the scientific tradition, explanatory devices subordinate to argument and proof, or heuristic tools to make models that can be tested, corrected, and abandoned if necessary, are, instead, modes of conceiving relationships in the universe that reify, rigidify, and ultimately come to dominate thought. One no longer uses analogies: One is used by them.[75]

Analogy not only describes but enacts the magical thinking that is the mark of the primitive, a point Vickers illustrates with ethnographic platitudes about "traditional African thought," "Vedic hymns," Parsi religion, Sumerian cosmology, Buddhist

---

[74]   See Stephen Pumfrey, "The Spagyric Art; Or, The Impossible Work of Separating Pure from Impure Paracelsianism: Historiographical Analysis," in *Paracelsus: The Man and His Reputation, His Ideas and Their Transformation*, ed. Ole Peter Grell (Leiden: Brill, 1998), 21–52.

[75]   Brian Vickers, "Analogy versus Identity: The Rejection of Occult Symbolism, 1580–1660," in *Occult and Scientific Mentalities*, ed. Brian Vickers (Cambridge: Cambridge University Press, 1986), 95.

doctrine, and the Bible.[76] The conviction under which Vickers seems to labor is that the sciences (historiographical as well as literary) ought to be immune to the seductions of the associative reasoning that is, in his description, the chief characteristic of the "occult mentality."[77]

Vickers's account of the promiscuity of analogical reasoning recalls Foucault's account of the danger of sympathy during the epoch he referred to as the "age of resemblance." Foucault suggested that the assimilatory attraction of "like to like" during this period was deemed to be so strong that if unchecked it would "reduce the world to a point, to a homogenous mass, to the featureless form of the Same," because "all its parts would hold together and communicate with one another without a break, with no distance between them."[78] Only antipathy, sympathy's twin impulse, could keep the annihilative powers of cosmic sympathy at bay and prevent the dissolution of all things into one another. The historical accuracy of Foucault's account of Renaissance epistemology has been widely challenged.[79] My intent here is to foreground some of the ways that Foucault's assessments have precipitated a modern critical tradition of reading literary copia (supplied as it is by the rhetorical modes of analogy and associative reasoning) as either intrinsically anxious or necessarily anxiety inducing for early modern readers. Contemporary scholars largely read early modern copia as a kind of transgressive excess, a determination that fails to capture the affective qualities of wonder and delight attached to the patterns of association and accretion that one finds in Burton's prose.

The associative qualities of the *Anatomy* that I am describing may be best situated within the tradition of natural history writing, a genre that William Ashworth evocatively characterizes by invoking Foucault's account of the "emblematic" worldview. In the world of Gesner and Aldrovandi, an object could only be known by the study of its relationships: "You must know its associations—its affinities, similitudes, and sympathies with the rest of the

---

[76] Ibid., 95–6. For critiques of Vickers's assessments, see William Newman, "Brian Vickers on Alchemy and the Occult: A Response," *Perspectives on Science* 17.4 (2009): 485–8; and more recently, Wouter J. Hanegraaff, *Esotericism and the Academy: Rejected Knowledge in Western Culture* (Cambridge: Cambridge University Press, 2012), 183–9.

[77] It is hard to tell whether the object of Vickers's critique is the occultist mentality of the analogist or of the historian: "The problem with such an associative movement is that the writer risks losing contact with his reader as he moves into more personal thought patterns. The associative process and the preference for concrete over abstract turn analogies into substitutes for argument ... . In collapsing the distinctions between signifier and signified, in confusing literal and metaphorical, the occultist ultimately produces a private language that no one can follow. This is the exact reverse of the goals of the new science" (Vickers, "Analogy versus Identity: The Rejection of Occult Symbolism, 1580–1660," 135).

[78] Michel Foucault, *The Order of Things: An Archaeology of the Human Sciences* (New York: Vintage), 23–4.

[79] See, for instance, Ian Maclean, "Foucault's Renaissance Episteme Reassessed: An Aristotelian Counterblast," *Journal of the History of Ideas* 59, no. 1 (1998): 149–66.

created order."[80] In order to understand the seemingly haphazard connections between the entries of a natural history, Ashworth suggests, we must suspend nineteenth-century taxonomical assumptions and look instead for the pleasure of the heteronymous. Pointing to Gesner's peacock entries, which include ancient descriptions, anatomy, medical uses, recipes, behavior (that it is ashamed of its feet, for instance), legends, proverbs, and appearances in mythology, geography, and geology, Ashworth writes:

> If what you seek is a collection of true statements about the peacock ... or the peacock's place in the taxonomic scheme based [purely] on physical characteristics, then you are bound to be disappointed. ... But if you are interested in confronting, in one place, that complex web of associations that link the peacock with history, mythology, etymology, the rest of the animal kingdom, indeed with the entire cosmos, then you are certain to be richly rewarded.[81]

I suggest that this reward is of a similar kind as the reward Burton offers by his own dilation of the causes, kinds, and cures of melancholy. The *Anatomy* borrows from natural history not only its sense of wonder at a world of cosmological resemblances but its fantasy and philosophy of knowledge as an interweaving of seemingly disparate things. The hypochondriac's fantasies, which we shall study in Chapter 2, mirror the natural historian's in seeing likeness between the unlike. This mimetic recognition allows for the weaving of compilations and concordances whose value rests not in their totalities (these are not encyclopedias) but rather in the dense semantic fields suspended *between* entries. By Foucault's clock, Burton may be a late monument to the copious imagination of Renaissance natural history in its prolix splendor, but the desires that animate the copious imagination clearly do not vanish at mid-century.[82]

Over the 30-year period from the time of the first to the sixth publication of the *Anatomy* (1621–1651), Burton's contemporaries mounted increasingly urgent appeals for the stripping of ornament from the language of natural inquiry, calling for a mode of study based in experience rather than received testimony. The *Anatomy* might then have become an (albeit still much-read) historical oddity by the time of its last seventeenth-century printings in 1660 and 1676. These editions straddle Thomas Sprat's declaration in the *History of the Royal Society* of the triumph of English science and the aptly terse and temperate tongue through which it had come into prominence.[83] The near-contemporaneousness of

---

[80]   William B. Ashworth, "Natural History and the Emblematic World View," in *Reappraisals of the Scientific Revolution*, ed. David C. Lindberg and Robert S. Westman (Cambridge: Cambridge University Press, 1990), 306.

[81]   Ibid.

[82]   On Foucault's impact on the historiography of natural history writing, see the Introduction and Epilogue to N. Jardine, J.A. Secord, and E.C. Spary, *Cultures of Natural History* (Cambridge: Cambridge University Press, 1996).

[83]   Thomas Sprat, *History of the Royal Society* (London, 1667).

these publications might instead point to the heterogeneity and heightened self-consciousness of early English scientific writing. As we will see, the distinction between Burton's topoanalysis and the "experimental method" promoted by Bacon and the founders of the Royal Society is not as clear as it might seem. Burton does not simply reproduce inherited positions on the basis of their established authority. His citations are interrogative, not demonstrative. They record of a certain kind of thought experiment, if not quite of the verisimilar variety that Croll detected.

Burton's histrionic performance of the role of the melancholy scholar might be said to depict the passions of the melancholy scientist. Like the naturalist's fascination with the object of scientific inquiry, the melancholic *idée fixe* represents both the narcissistic and mimetic impulses of wonder. Witness, as Paula Findlen does, the profusion of "mirrors" in the cabinet of curiosity.[84] The melancholic hypochondriac, like the natural historian, translates narcissistic identification into mimetic reproduction. The potential threat—and pleasure—of this kind of mimetic investment is that the scientist and melancholic alike stand to lose themselves to the objects of their curiosity. Melancholia's ancient pedigree as the scholar's disease has as much to do with the assimilatory mechanisms of study as it does the romance of the wan and solitary scholarly life. As a figure poised between the vortices of self and the vicissitudes of the outside world, Burton's heroic melancholic is best personified by his usurping and reinventing of the texts and voices that make up his library and laboratory. The *Anatomy* is a cabinet of overheard and appropriated (or, we might say, hypochondriacally "aggravated") reflections on the wonder that is, for Burton, the melancholic, human condition. In this cabinet, the hypochondriac's strange mimetic conceits emblematize the mimetic relation between the author and the other—between the scholar and the knowable object—while extending, as we will see, a kind of Epicurean grace to the all-too-studious subject congested with self.

Structure of the Book

Chapter 1 argues that Burton's professed stylistic carelessness lampoons Stoic *ataraxia* or "care-*less*" tranquility. I begin by showing how his detailed invocation of the pseudo-Hippocratic "Letter to Damagetes" alerts the reader that, like the misunderstood laughing philosopher, the *Anatomy* is not what it appears to be. This chapter challenges the perception that Burton's citations express agreement with his cited authorities by examining the techniques he uses to undermine them. Situating Burton's ludic cento in its classical contexts (and against Lipsius's graver *Politica*), I weigh the value Burton places on unoriginality against the innovations

---

[84] "The abundance of mirrors and other shimmering surfaces ... placed Narcissus in competition with Proteus, the One and the Infinite. Both images flirted with the danger of losing one's identity, either through excessive contemplation or excessive imitation" (Paula Findlen, *Possessing Nature: Museums, Collecting, and Scientific Culture in Early Modern Italy* [Berkeley: University of California Press, 1994], 303).

of his ventriloquistic subterfuge. The chapter closes by considering the baroque and pastoral contexts for the *Anatomy*'s strategic indirectness, suggesting that Burton invites us to consider the greater forms of intimacy and care made possible by his refusal to speak plainly.

Chapter 2 examines an assortment of delusional conceits associated, since antiquity, with hypochondriacal melancholy. Discussions of these conceits appear as merry anecdotes in numerous early modern hygiene manuals. Burton, however, treats these conceits as objects of wonder. He suggests that the excruciation of the mimetic, melancholic imagination reveals empathic impulses that should inspire rather than simply entertain, as they invite the reader to meditate on the fortunate vulnerability of the human condition and our permeability to the curative powers of suggestion. Comparing early modern depictions of melancholic hypochondriacs to those of spiritual melancholics, such as the infamous Francis Spira, I argue that both expose contradictory incitements to empathy and apathy (soft- and hard-heartedness) as well as to faith and despair in the literature of moral and spiritual hygiene in the late sixteenth and early seventeenth centuries.

Chapter 3 examines the therapeutic logic of Burton's recommendation and demonstration of a study cure that works by recreating and exhilarating the spirits. I situate Burton's understanding of imaginative instrumentality in the contexts of Renaissance faculty psychology, rhetorical theories of affect, and pneumatic accounts of spirit, especially as advanced by the Renaissance Neoplatonists. The second part of the chapter examines Burton's opposition of scholarly melancholy and studious delight. The final section illustrates how Burton's catalogues of curiosities and recommended studies sonically induce wonder as sympathetic medicine for scholarly withdrawal and a powerful antidote against despair.

Chapter 4 traces the pneumatic and hydraulic themes that orient the seemingly haphazard survey of natural wonders that makes up the "Digression of the Ayre." I suggest that Burton's meditations on geological ventilation echo his recommendations for social reform, calling for an "airing out" of stale conventions that is imitated by his centonic "airing" of the authorities. I situate Burton's ecstatic meditations on cosmic vicissitude in the contexts of contemporary representations of Ovidian and Pythagorean transformations and identify the Digression's elevated rhetorical mode as belonging to the tradition of the Longinian sublime, with its eroticized fragmentation of the desiring subject. This leads to a final reflection on Burton's representation of humanist citation as a quasi-erotic exchange of spirit across the distances of time and space.

Method and Madness

Reading *The Anatomy of Melancholy* is necessarily an exercise in bibliography. Burton sends us to more than a thousand sources in almost as many pages. The sense we make of his rhetorical performance depends on the complex interplay between source and citation to which I have applied something of a forensic analysis, tracing the development of arguments and motifs across partitions, members, sections, and subsections. It is often in the tension *between* citations, sometimes spanning vast sections of the book, that Burton's mischief with his sources and evidence of what I will call his "melancholic amplitude" may be witnessed. If Burton's bibliotherapy constitutes a game, my hope is to give some sense of just how intricate and deeply thought a game it is. My method, in so doing, has been to take up the exercise to which Burton invites a willing reader.

In the same extended apology with which he commences his book, Burton claims to have "prostituted his muse" by writing in English, something he insists he conceded to only at the printer's insistence (1:16). And yet, Burton offers powerful medicine in what Michael O'Connell calls the rich, sonic quality of his vernacular prose. O'Connell is among the few scholars who considers the *Anatomy*'s therapeutic oral presence, suggesting that Burton offers us the healing company of his voice.[85] Many modern scholars have regarded this same sonic presence as a noise from which the reader must shield him- or herself so as not to fall prey to the temptation to make sense out of nonsense.[86] My intent has been to follow Burton's sound *and* sense and to make historical sense of the structures of meaning that inhere in their resemblance.

Burton's mimetic style makes dissimilar objects similar, sometimes fashioning ecstatic chains of resemblance. At the same time, Burton trains the ear to be wary of conspicuous similarities and dissimilarities. We become suspicious of his egregious contradictions and inconsistencies, and rightly so, as these often reveal subterfuge ingeniously buried under the cover of pretended error. In following Burton's "ranging Spaniel's" quest that "barkes at every bird he sees, leaving his game [and following] all" (1:4), I have fallen into many a pit, far fewer of them recorded than encountered, but I have also been endlessly surprised by the suggestiveness of Burton's seeming erraticism and the fields of meaning his eccentricities and meanderings, elisions, insertions, and apparent "errors" open up to one who so lists to hunt. I'll conclude with an illustration that returns us to the apologia with which Burton's book, and this introduction, began.

In the expanded Preface of the 1624 edition, Burton adds a note to the apologetic description of his "Extemporean stile." Keyed to this term in the margins, he inserts: "*Stans pede in uno*, as he made Verses."[87] "He" ostensibly refers to Horace, who uses this expression in the *Sermones* to describe Aristophanes' compositional style.[88] In Horace's use, the expression means "with ease" or "with haste," a logical

---

[85]   See Michael O'Connell, *Robert Burton* (Boston: Twayne, 1986), chap. 4, "Words against Melancholy."

[86]   See, especially, Robert Grant Williams, "Heterological Rhetoric: Textual Waste in *The Anatomy of Melancholy*" (London, ON: University of Western Ontario, 1995). Williams calls the *Anatomy* an exercise in "degenerate copia," a "meaningless pile of words" (7).

[87]   Robert Burton, *The Anatomy of Melancholy* (Oxford, 1624), 9. The marginal note, along with the expanded *apologia*, is retained in each subsequent edition.

[88]   Horace, *Sermones*, 1.4:10.

collocation for Burton's "extemporean" style.[89] Speculative as it may be, I'm tempted to hear the resonance of Burton's "*stans pede in uno*," or "on one foot," with the rabbinic expression "*al regel achat*," which has the same literal meaning.[90] In perhaps the best-known legend of the *Babylonian Talmud*, a tale is told of Hillel and Shamai, the leaders of opposing rabbinical schools during the late Second Temple period. These two figures, about whom almost nothing biographical is known, are the iconic Janus-faces, the Democritus and Heraclitus, so to speak, of rabbinic literature.[91] Shamai invariably insists upon the most stringent application of the law, and Hillel perennially finds ways to accommodate the law to human frailty. The redactors of the *Babylonian Talmud* were the descendants of Hillel's academy and pay homage to their predecessor in a series of anecdotal portraits that celebrate Hillel's witty generosity. "Tractate Sabbath" tells the story of a gentile who approached Shamai, offering him this challenge: "Make me a proselyte, on condition that you teach me the whole Torah while I stand on one foot." Shamai dismisses the gentile, "[repulsing] him with the builder's cubit [*binyan*, or ruler] which was in his hand." The man goes to Hillel offering the same challenge, to which the rabbi famously replies: "What is hateful to you, do not to your neighbor: that is the whole Torah ... the rest is commentary; go and learn it."[92]

I would like to consider for a moment the possibility that the *Anatomy* supports a reading of the Horatian "*stans pede in uno*" as cognate with the meaning of the expression "*al regel achat*," known in rabbinical tradition as Hillel's answer to the proselyte. Shamai repels the proselyte with the sharp end or "rule" of the law.[93] Hillel, on the other hand, gives the Torah as one principle rule: the golden rule. The Talmud plays on words here, contrasting Shamai's *binyan* (an instrument of measure) with Hillel's *regel*. The two words are synonyms in Hebrew for a single principle, or law. Like Hillel, Burton ultimately gives a simple answer to a seemingly impossible challenge. The way to avoid melancholy, he says, is to "be not solitary, be not idle" (3:445). But unlike Hillel, Burton gives the copious version as well as the kernel. The *Anatomy* is a kind of "Torah"—an open-ended *summa* of the oral and written word to which the writing citer is always expanding.

---

[89]   There is some debate about whether the term was a compliment or an insult. Charles Knapp argues the latter, challenging a dominant interpretation of the term as *facillime*, proposing "carelessly" instead. See Charles Knapp, "Notes on Horace's Sermones," *The American Journal of Philology* 44, no. 1 (1923): 62–6.

[90]   I have only been able to find one mention of the resemblance between these expressions: Moses Hadas, "Horace, Sermones 1.4.10," *The Classical Weekly* 21, no. 15 (1928): 114.

[91]   Godfrey Taubenhaus, *Echoes of Wisdom: Or, Talmudic Sayings with Classic, Especially Latin, Parallelisms* (Brooklyn, NY: Haedrich & Sons, 1900), 70.

[92]   "Tractate Sabbath," in *The Babylonian Talmud: Seder Moed*, ed. Isidore Epstein, trans. H. Freedman, vol. 1 (London: Soncino, 1938), fol. 31a.

[93]   The word the Talmud gives is "*binyan*," which Freedman, drawing on Rashi's commentary, translates as "builder's cubit" or measuring tool (ibid.). However, it also means "principle," and is therefore cognate with the English construction rule/ruler.

Burton's centonic trick is unabashedly brazen, but it is not the performance of seeming ease connoted by the Horatian reference. Rather, Burton suggests that his one-legged labor is a hobbling and imperfect one that he hopes will do more good in the making and reading than would be had by his silence.

As with every interpretive impulse I've had in writing this book, I submitted this one to the usual examination. What grounds do I have to consider the Talmudic resonance of this inconspicuous marginal note? What access did Burton have to this anecdote as it appears in the Talmud and the broader rabbinic literature in which it is commonplace? Why would it have mattered to Burton to add this texture to his Preface? And down the rabbit hole we go, or don't go. This is the game Burton invites and the choice he leaves to the reader of his labyrinthine text. I could cite proof of Talmudic study at Oxford and Cambridge in the early seventeenth century.[94] I could point you to scholarship on Oxford's Hebraists, men who read, cited, and wrote commentaries of their own on Talmudic tractates, including exact contemporaries of Burton's at Christ Church (men such as John Selden, "Renaissance England's Chief Rabbi," whose *de diis syriis* is cited three times in the *Anatomy*).[95] That the Bodleian owned full sets of the Talmud and Talmudic commentaries by many of the major Jewish commentators who used this expression as a kind of shorthand would prove only that Burton had access to the tradition he elsewhere dismisses as needlessly complex in the conventional trope of learned, ecclesiastical anti-Semitism.[96] My case therefore remains conjectural, more so perhaps in this instance than in the many instances of such speculations that follow. It is not based on the evidence of a single demonstrative sentence anywhere in the book but rather in the resonance between Hillel's and Burton's sagacious generosity. If it is suspect to launch a scholarly monograph with one's most tenuous example, I have only your faith to gain. And if I'm wrong, I don't think Burton would have minded.

---

[94]   See James McConica, ed., *The Collegiate University*, vol. 3, *The History of the University of Oxford* (Oxford: Clarendon Press, 1986), 34; 317–18; Mordechai Feingold, "Oriental Studies," in *The History of the University of Oxford*, ed. Nicholas Tyacke, vol. 4 (Oxford: Oxford University Press, 1997); Stefan C. Reif, ed., *Hebrew Manuscripts at Cambridge University Library: A Description and Introduction* (Cambridge: Cambridge University Press, 1997).

[95]   Jason P. Rosenblatt, *Renaissance England's Chief Rabbi: John Selden* (Oxford: Oxford University Press, 2008); Cecil Roth, "Sir Thomas Bodley, Hebraist," *Bodleian Library Record* 7 (1966): 242–51; Allison Coudert and Jeffrey S. Shoulson, eds., *Hebraica Veritas? Christian Hebraists and the Study of Judaism in Early Modern Europe* (Philadelphia: University of Pennsylvania Press, 2004), chap. 12.

[96]   Burton refers to the Talmud by name in three places, mainly as a synonym for the "*Turks Alcoran*" and the "Papist's *Golden Legend*," that is, to suggest a repository of "grosse fictions, fables, vaine traditions, prodigious paradoxes and ceremonies" (3:370). Given Burton's own compilation of anecdotes, legends, fables, and paradoxes, we have some grounds on which to take Burton's censure with a grain of salt.

Chapter 1
Democritus Junior:
Discerning Care

Early in his discussion of the causes of melancholy by "Discontents, Cares, [and] Miseries," Burton relates the myth of Hyginus to explain why human beings are born to worry:

> Dame *Cura* by chance went over a brooke, and taking up some of the durty slyme made an Image of it; *Jupiter* eftsoones comming by put life to it, but *Cura* and *Jupiter* could not agree what name to give him, or who should owne him. The matter was referred to *Saturne* as Judge; he gave this arbitriment. His name shall be *Homo ab humo, Cura eum possideat quamdiu vivat*, Care shall have him whilst he lives, *Jupiter* his soule, and *Tellus* his body when he dies.[1]

Care has possession of human beings while we walk the earth, and we are only freed from her grip once returned to the ground. The deceivingly simple allegory casts Cura as the mother of misery and at the same time the defining characteristic of humanity. What separates us from mud is our capacity to suffer. The use of "care" as a synonym for trouble has become more or less archaic in contemporary English, persisting mainly in expressions that represent care as an appropriative act, an assumption of burden, for example, when to "take care" is to "take pains" or "take the trouble," but the subject from whom these pains and troubles are taken is more or less obscured. What I would describe as the paradoxical grammar implied by this appropriative understanding of care is at the forefront of Burton's interests in *The Anatomy of Melancholy*. Burton, as we shall see, is profoundly concerned with the relationship between care as fear or worry and care as *caritas* or charity. His promotion of melancholy rests precisely on the idea that the excess cares and supposedly groundless fears suffered by the melancholic attest to a generosity of spirit evidenced in his or her sensitivity to the suffering of others.

In his 1622 translation of Guillaume Du Vair's *De La Constance*, Andrew Court urges readers to guard themselves against vexation, by which he chiefly means pity motivated by pride and commandeered by "opinion."[2] Pity "seizeth

---

[1] Robert Burton, *The Anatomy of Melancholy*, ed. Thomas C. Faulkner, Nicolas K. Kiessling, and Rhonda Blair, Introduction and Commentary by J.B. Bamborough and Martin Dodsworth, 6 vols. (Oxford: Clarendon Press, 1989–2000), 1:271. All references to the *Anatomy*, unless otherwise indicated, are to the Clarendon edition, hereafter cited by volume and page parenthetically in the text.

[2] This translation was published under the title, *A Buckler Against Adversitie, or, A Treatise of Constancie* (London, 1622). Court followed this translation of *De La Constance* with another the following year: *The True Way to Vertue and Happinesse*

vpon our Imagination [and] … standeth out in defiance against true Reason."[3] Men who mourn "do not frame their moane to their sorrow, but to the opinion of those they liue withal."[4] Du Vair's *De La Constance* follows Lipsius's Neostoic bestseller, *De Constantia*, both in argument and form. Both are dialogues in which a sage confidant counsels the disconsolate narrator to find inner tranquility amidst war and political upheaval by vigilantly guarding one's passions and ordering one's affairs: "As long as this Order is kept in the managing of mans life … he is in an exceeding happy estate."[5] Burton, by contrast, argues that we suffer not because we are riddled with worldly cares and needless occupations but because we care and feel too little. Discontent is in fact propaedeutic to human compassion in the *Anatomy*'s moral vision. Burton's *homo apatheticus* "sits at a table in a soft chaire at ease, but hee doth not remember in the meane time, that a tired waiter stands behind him." Turning poignantly to the Stoic philosopher (and former slave) Epictetus for authority, Burton reminds the reader that "*he is a thirst that gives him drinke*" (1:277).[6] That being said, the defense of compassionate suffering is couched throughout the *Anatomy* in therapeutic rather than abstractly ethical reasoning. Compassionate feeling is instrumental toward a cure for melancholic withdrawal as it is the foundation of companionship, and company—as Burton so often reminds—is both the best prevention and remedy for melancholy.

Burton stresses that our capacity to suffer is our capacity to move and be moved, to love and be loved. Those who care not "love not, are not beloved againe." He renders Stoic *apatheia* a kind of aristocratic insouciance, a callous indifference. The unfeeling man

> feasts, revells, and profusely spends, hath variety of robes, sweet musick, ease, and all the pleasure the world can afford, whilest many an hunger-starved poore creature pines in the street … . Hee lothes and scornes his inferiour, hates or

---

(London, 1622–1623). Eleven works attributed to Du Vair were printed in English during the seventeenth century. These include *The Holy Loue of Heauenly Wisdom* (London, 1594), *The Moral Philosophie of the Stoicks* (London, 1598), *A Most Heauenly and Plentifull Treasure, or, A Rich Minerall Full of Sweetest Comforts* (1609), *Holy meditations Vpon Seauen Penitentiall and Seauen Consolatory Psalmes of the Kingly Prophet Dauid* (1612), and *Holy Philosophy* (1636). Charles Cotton retranslated *Philosophie morale des Stoiques* in 1664.

[3]   Du Vair, *A Buckler Against Adversitie*, 12.

[4]   Ibid., 14. Du Vair infantilizes and emasculates those unable to resist Opinion's siege upon the "citadel" of reason, suggesting that all weepers are, in essence, weepers for hire: "Did not such people betray their owne Reason … and purposely prostitute their manlinesse?" (ibid.)

[5]   Ibid., 11.

[6]   As Angus Gowland points out, Epictetus was a key source for sixteenth-century Neostoic writers such as Lipsius and Du Vair ("Consolations for Melancholy in Renaissance Humanism," *Societate Şi Politică* 6, no. 11 [2012]: 31). See also Jill Kraye, "Moral Philosophy," in *The Cambridge History of Renaissance Philosophy*, ed. C.B. Schmitt and Quentin Skinner (Cambridge: Cambridge University Press, 1988), 370–72.

emulates his equall, envies his superiour, insults over all such as are under him, as if he were of another *Species*, a demi-god, not subject to any fall, or humane infirmities. (1:277)

This portrait draws on a storehouse of classical and neoteric caricatures of the Stoic as someone who believes himself invulnerable and whose apathy manifests as cruelty rather than merely indifference: "caring for none else [but themselves], *sibi nati*," such men "seeke all meanes to depresse ... those whom they are by the lawes of nature, bound to relieve and helpe" (1:277).[7] Burton underscores the point that malice frequently results from the unnatural policing of empathy. The untrammeled pursuit of tranquility hardens the heart, inuring a person to the signs of his or her fellow's suffering: "they will let them cater-waule, starve, beg, and hang, before they will any wayes (though it be in their power) assist, or ease: so unnaturall are they for the most part, so unregardfull: so hard hearted, so churlish, proud, insolent, so dogged, of so bad a disposition." Whereas empathy refines and elevates the human spirit, cynicism translates man into animal—literally doglike, from the greek κυνικός (kynikos), meaning canine.[8] And "being so brutish, so divelishly bent one towards another," he asks, "how is it possible, but that we should be discontent of all sides, full of cares, woes and miseries" (1:277)?

Burton's rejection of Stoic tranquility draws on a well-established tradition of ecclesiastical skepticism about the compatibility of Stoic and Christian moral philosophy that reaches back to early Patristic writers, chief among them Augustine, who argued that the ennobling of tranquility undermined the power of the passions to induce the humility and compassion necessary for charitable acts, penitence, and salvation. Versions of this critique appear even amidst the early Florentine responses to Senecan humanism[9] and persist in both Catholic and Protestant responses to popular Christian Neostoicism in the sixteenth century.[10] Calvin's indictments of Stoic notions of virtue were widely reproduced by French

---

[7]   See Gilles D. Monsarrat, *Light from the Porch: Stoicism and English Renaissance Literature* (Paris: Didier-Érudition, 1984), chaps. 3 and 4. For a more thorough and recent examination of Christian anti-Stoic traditions and their resurgence in seventeenth-century English political writing in particular, see Christopher Brooke, *Philosophic Pride: Stoicism and Political Thought from Lipsius to Rousseau* (Princeton, NJ: Princeton University Press, 2012).

[8]   *Oxford English Dictionary Online*, s.v. "cynic, adj. and n.," accessed November 12, 2012, http://www.oed.com/view/Entry/46638?redirectedFrom=cynic.

[9]   On the repudiation of Stoic dispassion by Coluccio Salutati, Lorenzo Valla, and Bartolomeo Scala, see Jill Kraye, "Stoicism in the Renaissance from Petrarch to Lipsius," *Grotiana* 22, no. 1 (2001): 21–45.

[10]   Calvin vehemently defends himself from accusations that his understanding of Christian predestination too closely resembles Stoic views of fate. He goes to great lengths to distinguish Christian patience from Stoic perseverance, deploying stock representations of Stoic arrogance and hard-heartedness: "You see how to beare the crosse patiently is not to be altogether astonished and without all feeling of sorrowe. As the Stoickes in old time did foolishly describe a valiant harted man ... yea such a one as like a stone was moued with nothinge ..." (*Institution of Christian Religion*, trans. Thomas Norton [London, 1578], 288r).

and English Protestant writers such as Pierre de La Primaudaye and Philippe Du Plessis-Mornay.[11] These were echoed more broadly across the confessional spectrum by writers who drew on Augustinian traditions of anti-Stoic critique.[12] We see these sentiments profoundly at work in what has been dubbed the Ciceronian or grand style of late Renaissance "sacred rhetoric," and indeed, as scholars such as Deborah Shuger and Wayne Rebhorn have argued, Renaissance rhetoric in general, whose aim, according to Melanchthon, was "to move (*permovere*) and incite souls, and to lead ... to certain emotion."[13] The present study hopes to restore Burton to this positive view of the instrumentality of the passions in the service of both spiritual and physical healing. The aim of this first chapter will be to foreground and contextualize key devices in Burton's rhetorical repertoire that work toward these ends. I focus on his use of genre and persona, arguing that Burton's theatrical insistence upon his own anonymity stages a defense of melancholy that valorizes care (as in worry or fear) as the root of compassionate feeling. This defense takes aim at a particularly fashionable literature of moral hygiene as it appears both in the writings of Christian Neostoics such as Lipsius and Du Vair and in the ostensibly anti-Stoic literature of Puritan practical divinity.[14]

My reading departs from the trend in recent scholarship to view Burton as a proponent of Neostoic attitudes toward mental hygiene. According to Angus Gowland, Burton's consolation is "a basically classical conception of the necessity of psychic self-management to tranquility" whose "efficaciousness ... was premised

[11] See Monsarrat, 75–7.

[12] On the repudiations of Stoic determinism, elitism, asceticism, rationalism, and dispassion by Augustinian writers ranging from Valla and Vives to Calvin and Melanchthon, see William J. Bouwsma, "The Two Faces of Humanism: Stoicism and Augustinianism in Renaissance Thought," in *Itinerarium Italicum: The Profile of the Italian Renaissance in the Mirror of Its European Transformations: Dedicated to Paul Oskar Kristeller on the Occasion of His 70th Birthday*, ed. Thomas Allan Brady and Heiko Augustinus Oberman (Leiden: Brill, 1975). In the first part of this seminal essay, Bouwsma identifies Stoic strains in many of the same writers, illuminating the complex interplay between what he refers to as the two dominant impulses of humanism.

[13] Debora Shuger, "Foundations of Sacred Rhetoric," in *Rhetorical Invention and Religious Inquiry: New Perspectives*, ed. Walter Jost and Wendy Olmsted (New Haven, CT: Yale University Press, 2000), 120; Wayne A. Rebhorn, *The Emperor of Men's Minds: Literature and the Renaissance Discourse of Rhetoric* (Ithaca, NY: Cornell University Press, 1995), 84.

[14] On early English Puritan uses of Stoic sources and traditions, see Margo Todd, *Christian Humanism and the Puritan Social Order* (Cambridge: Cambridge University Press, 2002). Jill Kraye takes an opposing view (and one that helps to establish a contextual basis of support for Burton's anti-Stoicism), arguing that the Stoic ideal of *ataraxia* never fully took root in England and that mental hygienists Thomas Wright, Edward Reynolds, and Francis Bacon were hostile to them and more inclined to emphasize the opportunities for the cultivation of virtue in response to and through the use of the passions. See "Ἀπάθεια and Προπάθειαι in Early Modern Discussions of the Passions: Stoicism, Christianity and Natural History," *Early Science and Medicine* 17 (2012): 230–53.

upon some degree of freedom of the will, enabling the rectification of imaginative errors."[15] Gowland therefore finds the *Anatomy*'s concluding commendation of melancholy puzzling, but accounts for this apparent contradiction by suggesting that Burton's consolations did not "seek to remedy dejection with optimism, but aimed to adjust the outlook of the sufferer so that it came into line with a realistic form of pessimism."[16] He regards Burton's adoption of the Democritean mask as a proclamation that the *Anatomy* will prosecute the moral vision of Democritus' lecture in the *Letter to Damagetes*, which teaches that tranquility of mind is the highest good and that the best remedy for the sick, deluded, irrational world is "harsh reproof effected by condemnation and contemptuous laughter."[17] This chapter instead suggests that Burton's adoption of his Democritean mask sets the stage for a profound critique of Stoic *apatheia*. I argue that Burton's purported stylistic carelessness sets up the problem of care and its absence—real, feigned, and misinterpreted—as the peremptory matter of the *Anatomy*'s investigation. I suggest, moreover, that he does so as a way of training the reader to decipher his *cento* and discover the ethics of care promoted under the guise of stylistic and moral insouciance. The first part of the chapter examines Burton's elaborate alibi as a strategy for undermining Puritan and Neostoic exhortations to tranquility and transparency. The second part examines the pretense of accident in Burton's use of the cento, considering his errant citations as further techniques of both self-concealment and tactical disclosure. Challenging Burton's representation (both by himself and others) as a "plain stylist," the final section illustrates how Burton rejects the rhetorical plainness and transparency recommended to and by spiritual physicians as most proper and beneficial for clerical care, offering the reader an alternative whose curative value rests precisely in its opacity and indirectness.

I. Masks of Indifference and Anonymity

Amid the Latin tags copied in the margins of what we may assume to have been his first Latin dictionary,[18] we find evidence of a young Burton diverting himself

---

[15] "Consolations for Melancholy in Renaissance Humanism," *Societate Şi Politică* 6, no. 11 (2012): 26. Gowland concludes this essay by placing Burton in a "gloomy tradition" that has one foot in Roman Stoicism and the other in Nietzsche (ibid., 27). Mary Ann Lund also remarks on Burton's debts to Stoicism in his program for the rectification of the passions (*Melancholy, Medicine and Religion in Early Modern England: Reading "The Anatomy of Melancholy"* [New York: Cambridge University Press, 2010], 190–91) but notes that he rejects the Stoic doctrine of apathy (169) and uses passionate entreaty to persuade or *move* readers toward the goal of moderating the passions instead (32).

[16] Gowland, "Consolations for Melancholy in Renaissance Humanism," 26.

[17] Angus Gowland, *The Worlds of Renaissance Melancholy: Robert Burton in Context* (Cambridge and New York: Cambridge University Press, 2006), 12. In the final chapter of this book, Gowland tempers this argument by suggesting that Burton is more beholden to the Augustinian tradition than to the Stoics (271).

[18] John Withals, *A Shorte Dictionarie for Yonge Beginners* (London, 1566). Burton's copy with marks here described is held at the Bodleian, shelfmark 4° H 26 Art.

by doodling letters and pictures (including chains of what appear to be Elizabethan paper doll-men, attached at the buckler; see Figures 1.1 and 1.2) and scribbling variations of his initials and name. In one rather conspicuous inscription, Burton declares himself to be the book's true owner: "Robert Burton est verius possessor huius libri."[19] This hardly seems necessary given his older brother's inscribed dedication to his "most lovinge brother Robert" on two separate leaves, one of which suggests that the gift commemorated Burton's arrival at Brasenose in 1593.[20] These marks and inscriptions give us a wonderful picture of the young Burton's early and playful attempts at scholarly self-fashioning. But they are most striking in comparison with the adult Burton's reticence to name himself as the author of his own book. I refer not only to the removal of his signature from the second and all subsequent editions of the *Anatomy*'s conclusion, but his theatrical insistence upon keeping his identity secret and presenting the book as the work of one "Democritus Junior."

The Anatomy of Melancholy begins in burlesque, making great show of the author's reticence to be known: "whence he is, why he doth it, and what he hath to say ... I am a free man borne, and may chuse whether I will tell, who can compell me?" With feigned demurral, Burton admonishes the reader for snooping, like the "curious fellow" in Plutarch's *Moralia* who was rebuked for peeking in a basket that did not belong to him: "*Quum vides velatem, quid inquiris in rem absconditam?*[21] It was therefore covered, because he should not know what was in it." We are beckoned and slapped on the wrist for inquiring after the author's identity in a manner that is at once coquettish and a suggestive indictment of the yoked demands for plainness and confessionalism in Puritan moral and spiritual exercises, intimating that these exercises had more in common with the inquisitorial tactics of the counter-reformation than Puritan apologists such as William Perkins were wont to admit.[22] Burton is necessarily more subtle than to suggest this directly and instead presents the demand for transparency as meddling curiosity. He invokes Paul's admonitory dictum against vain curiosity in Romans 11:20, *noli altum sapere, sed time*: "Seeke not after that which is hid" (1:1), suggesting that the book (like the garden of Eden) has been offered for the reader's pleasure, so long as he or she abides by the author's demand for anonymity: "if the contents please thee, *and be for thy use, suppose* the Man in the Moone, *or whom thou wilt to be the Author*; I would not willingly be knowne" (1:1).

---

[19]   Ibid., 21r.

[20]   Ibid., 41r; 58r. The first inscription reads "To his most loving Brother Robert Burton at Oxon: in Brasenose College" and faces the page where Burton's eldest brother, William, seems to have inscribed a prior donation of the book to George.

[21]   "Since you see that it is covered over, why do you ask about what has been hidden?" Translation from the Clarendon *Anatomy* (4:6). Unless otherwise specified, translations of non-English passages in the *Anatomy* are taken from this edition and will be referred to by volume and page number.

[22]   William Perkins, *M. Perkins, His Exhortation to Repentance ... with Two Treatises of the Duties and Dignitie of the Ministrie* (London, 1605), 15; 17.

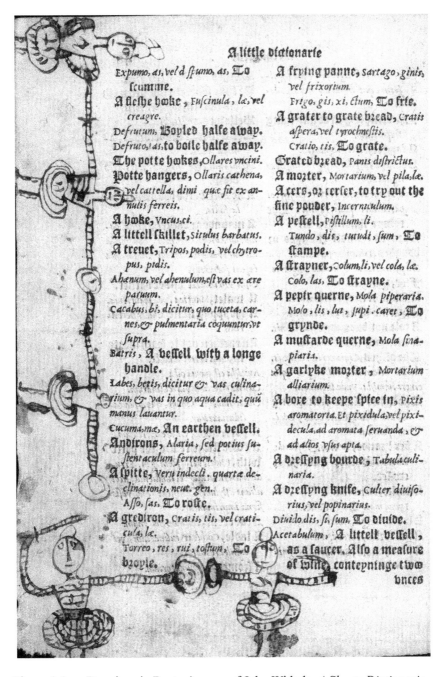

Figure 1.1   Drawings in Burton's copy of John Withals, *A Shorte Dictionarie*, 1566. The Bodleian Libraries, The University of Oxford, 4° H 26 Art, 46v.

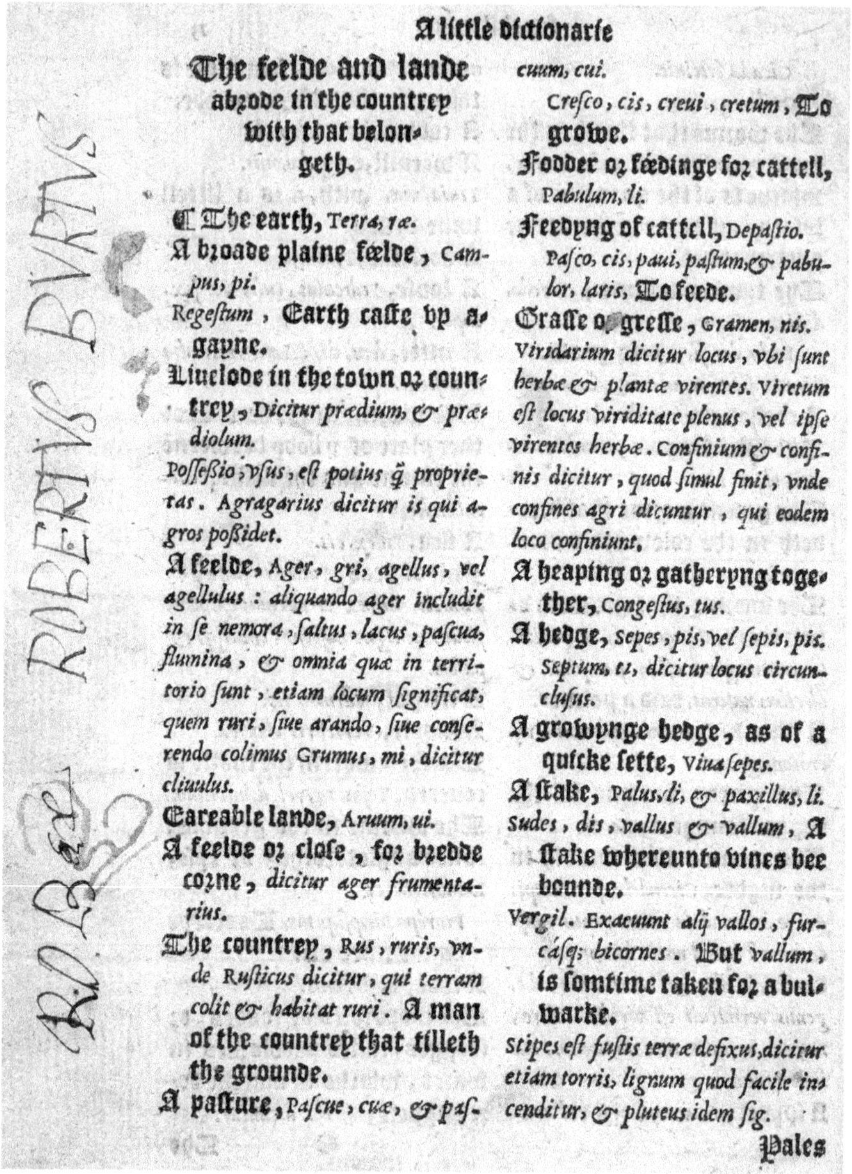

A little dictionarie

The feelde and lande
abrode in the countrey
with that belon-
geth.

¶ The earth, Terra, ræ.
A broade plaine feelde, Cam-
pus, pi.
Regestum, Earth caste vp a-
gayne.
Liuelode in the town or countrey, Dicitur prædium, & præ-
diolum.
Possessio, vsus, est potius q proprie-
tas. Agragarius dicitur is qui a-
gros possidet.
A feelde, Ager, gri, agellus, vel
agellulus: aliquando ager includit
in se nemora, saltus, lacus, pascua,
flumina, & omnia quæ in terri-
torio sunt, etiam locum significat,
quem ruri, siue arando, siue conse-
rendo colimus Grumus, mi, dicitur
cliuulus.
Eareable lande, Aruum, ui.
A feelde or close, for bredde
corne, dicitur ager frumenta-
rius.
The countrey, Rus, ruris, vnde Rusticus dicitur, qui terram
colit & habitat ruri. A man
of the countrey that tilleth
the grounde.
A pasture, Pascue, cuæ, & pas-

cuum, cui.
Cresco, cis, creui, cretum, To
growe.
Fodder or feedinge for cattell,
Pabulum, li.
Feedyng of cattell, Depastio.
Pasco, cis, paui, pastum, & pabu-
lor, laris, To feede.
Grasse or gresse, Gramen, nis.
Viridarium dicitur locus, vbi sunt
herbæ & plantæ virentes. Viretum
est locus viriditate plenus, vel ipse
virentes herbæ. Confinium & confi-
nis dicitur, quod simul finit, vnde
confines agri dicuntur, qui eodem
loco confiniunt.
A heaping or gatheryng together, Congestus, tus.
A hedge, Sepes, pis, vel sepis, pis.
Septum, ti, dicitur locus circun-
clusus.
A growynge hedge, as of a
quicke sette, Viua sepes.
A stake, Palus, li, & paxillus, li.
Sudes, dis, vallus & vallum, A
stake whereunto vines bee
bounde.
Vergil. Exacuunt alij vallos, fur-
cásq; bicornes. But vallum,
is somtime taken for a bul-
warke.
Stipes est fustis terræ defixus, dicitur
etiam torris, lignum quod facile in-
cenditur, & pluteus idem sig.
Pales

ROBERTVS BVRTVS

R D Bx

Figure 1.2   Burton's initials and signature in John Withals, *A Shorte Dictionarie*, 1566. The Bodleian Libraries, The University of Oxford, 4° H 26 Art, 13v.

Despite this thrice-repeated refusal to show himself, Burton agrees, "in some sort," to "satisfy" his reader's curiosity, not by lifting the mask but rather through its onomastic elaboration, giving "a reason, both of this usurped Name, Title, and Subject," or rather, for its denunciation. He will not tell us who he is. Instead, he tells us what this book bearing Democritus' name is not:

> And first of the name of *Democritus*; lest any man by reason of it, should be deceived, expecting a Pasquill, a Satyre, some ridiculous Treatise (as I my selfe should have done) some prodigious Tenent, or Paradox of the Earths motion, of infinite Worlds *in infinito vacuo, ex fortuitâ atomorum collisone*, in an infinit wast, so caused by an accidentall collision of Motes in the Sunne, all which *Democritus* held, *Epicurus* and their Master *Leucippus* of old maintained, and are lately revived by *Copernicus*, *Brunus*, and some others. ... 'Tis not so with me. (1:1)

The assurance that his book will have none of Democritus' philosophical associations is ironized by Burton's claim that this is precisely the sort of book he *would* have written if *he* had written it, which he roguishly insists he hasn't: "*Democritus dixit*," as he'll say at the end of the Preface (1:110).

Burton outwardly dismisses the Epicureanism associated with his alibi, eliding its "prodigious tenents" with the prodigies of ancient mythology: "*Non hic Centauros, non Gorgonas, Harpyasque / Invenies, hominem pagina nostra sapit. / No Centaures here, or Gorgons looke to finde, / My subject is of Man and humane kind*" (1.1). The elegant rendering of Martial, followed by the caption, "Thou thy selfe art the subject of my Discourse," set back from the text as if an aside, should need no glossing (Figure 1.3). Nonetheless, Burton paraphrases and adds further testimony, this time from Juvenal, in an uneven meter that clashes with his iambic translation of Martial. The depreciation from the pure rhyme "kind/find" to the uneven rhyme "sport/report" sonically marks the conspicuousness of Burton's claim that he is merely playing Mercury, indemnified by his own indifference to the message he relays. Burton's vaunted indifference calls attention to the extraordinary contrivance both of the book's design and the author's unflappable facade. His wily denunciation of Epicureanism masks what we might call the argument of the Preface in *anacoluthon*; he is rejecting the mental hygiene approach of the Christian Neostoics with its emphasis on anaesthetic tranquility in order to make room for a more salutary view of the emotions and the vicissitudes of human experience.

Burton's postured indifference allows him to play the *naïf*, to pretend he has no stake in the arguments and opinions he merely recites; but his citations are far from haphazard, as we shall shortly observe, and he is hardly the impartial messenger he claims to be. Burton first tips us off to the artificiality of his flippant pose with his proofs for the commutability of the Democritean and Mercurial masks. "My intent," he says, "is no otherwise to use his name, then *Mercurius Gallobelgicus, Mercurius Britannicus*, use the name of Mercury, *Democritus Christianus, &c.*" The first two titles refer to early newspapers named for the messenger god. The third refers neither to Mercury nor any newspaper but

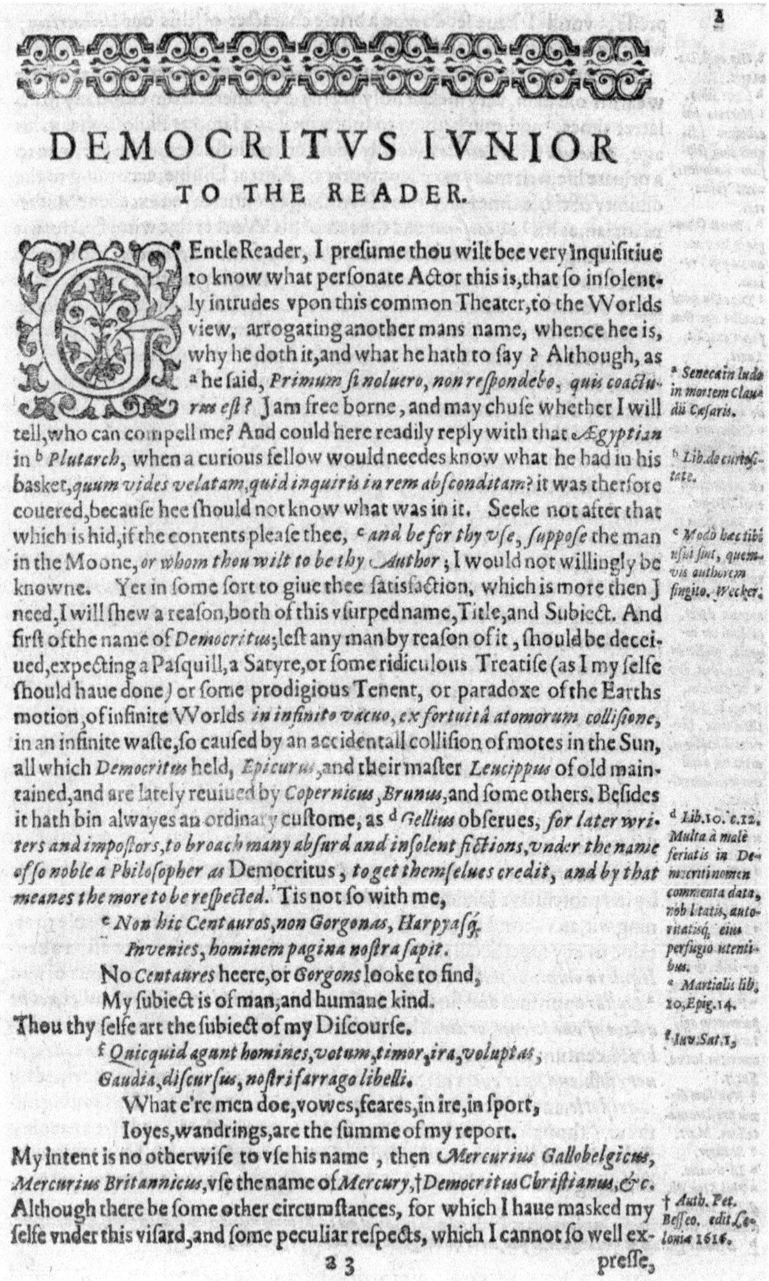

DEMOCRITVS IVNIOR

TO THE READER.

EntleReader, I prefume thou wilt bee very inquifitiue to know what perfonate Actor this is,that fo infolently intrudes vpon this common Theater,to the Worlds view, arrogating another mans name, whence hee is, why he doth it,and what he hath to fay ? Although, as [a] he faid, *Primum fi noluero, non refpondebo, quis coactu-rus eft?* I am free borne, and may chufe whether I will tell,who can compell me? And could here readily reply with that *Ægyptian* in [b] *Plutarch*, when a curious fellow would needes know what he had in his basket,*quum vides velatam,quid inquiris in rem abfconditam?* it was therfore couered,becaufe hee fhould not know what was in it. Seeke not after that which is hid,if the contents pleafe thee, [c] *and be for thy vfe, fuppofe* the man in the Moone, *or whom thou wilt to be thy Author* ; I would not willingly be knowne. Yet in fome fort to giue thee fatisfaction, which is more then I need,I will fhew a reafon,both of this vfurped name,Title,and Subiect. And firft of the name of *Democritus*;left any man by reafon of it, fhould be deceiued,expecting a Pafquill,a Satyre,or fome ridiculous Treatife (as I my felfe fhould haue done) or fome prodigious Tenent, or paradoxe of the Earths motion,of infinite Worlds *in infinito vacuo, ex fortuità atomorum collifione,* in an infinite wafte,fo caufed by an accidentall collifion of motes in the Sun, all which *Democritus* held, *Epicurus*,and their mafter *Leucippus* of old maintained,and are lately reuiued by *Copernicus,Brunus,*and fome others. Befides it hath bin alwayes an ordinary cuftome, as [d] *Gellius* obferues, *for later writers and impoftors,to broach many abfurd and infolent fictions,vnder the name of fo noble a Philofopher as* Democritus *, to get themfelues credit, and by that meanes the more to be refpected.* 'Tis not fo with me,

[e] *Non hic Centauros,non Gorgonas, Harpyafq̃.*
    Invenies, hominem pagina noftra fapit.
No *Centaures* heere,or *Gorgons* looke to find,
My fubiect is of man,and humane kind.
Thou thy felfe art the fubiect of my Difcourfe.
    [f] *Quicquid agant homines,votum,timor,ira,voluptas,*
    Gaudia,difcurfus,noftri farrago libelli.
    What e're men doe,vowes,feares,in ire,in fport,
    Ioyes,wandrings,are the fumme of my report.
My intent is no otherwife to vfe his name , then *Mercurius Gallobelgicus, Mercurius Britannicus,*vfe the name of *Mercury,†Democritus Chriftianus,&c.* Although there be fome other circumftances, for which I haue masked my felfe vnder this vifard,and fome peculiar refpects, which I cannot fo well ex-

a 3   preffe,

[a] *Senecain ludo in mortem Clau dii Cæfaris.*

[b] *Lib.de curiofi tate.*

[c] *Modò hec tibi nfui fint, quem vis authorem fingito. Wecker.*

[d] *Lib.10.c.12. Multa à malè feriatis in De mocriti nomen commenta data, nob litatis, auto ritatisq̃, eius perfugio vtenti bus.*

[e] *Martialis lib, 10,Epig.14.*

[f] *Iuv.Sat.1,*

[†] *Auth. Pet. Beffeo. edit.Co lonia 1616.*

Figure 1.3   "Thou thy selfe art the subiect of my Discourse." Detail from
                Robert Burton, *The Anatomy of Melancholy* (1624), a3. Division of
                Rare and Manuscript Collections, Cornell University Library.

rather to *Le Démocrite Chrétien*, Pierre de Besse's 1615 supplement to the 1612 penitential textbook, *L'Héraclite Chrétien*.[23] In *Le Démocrite Chrétien*, Besse says that contrary to medieval typology, a *Democritus Ridens* who transforms tears into laughter is more Christ-like than the weeping philosopher.[24] The reference to Besse's Christian Democritus announces that among his many roles and masks, the mercurial Democritus Junior is a Christian Democritus whose pastoral task in the *Anatomy* will be to cheer the melancholic reader. By presenting himself as a Christian Democritus, Burton signals his promise to substitute sociable laughter for solemn introspection.[25] In the third partition of the *Anatomy*, Burton will advise strongly against the tactics recommended by contemporary Puritan divines for daily inventories of conscience and ruminating accounts of past sin, but already in the Preface he insinuates that the *Anatomy*'s medicine will not be the "corrosive Chiurgerie" that Richard Greenham recommends to "pricke and pierce our Consciences with the burning yron of the law; and to cleane the wound of the Soule by sharpe threatenings."[26] At the same time, however, the Preface makes clear that Democritus Junior will not offer merely comfortable words but rather a laughter that is at once corrective and communal.

Winfried Schleiner writes that Burton's pseudonym draws on a long tradition in which Democritus' laughter stood for what we might call the "manic" expression

---

[23]   These three names point in very different directions. *Mercurius Gallobelgicus*, the first known printed periodical in Europe, was widely read in England before the lifting of the domestic news ban (Donne infamously accused the publication of libel in his caustic epigram by the same title). After the removal of this ban and the subsequent imposition of a ban on foreign newspapers, England's domestic news market exploded and dozens of circulars that sported Mercury's name appeared, including Marchmont Nedham's *Mercurius Britannicus*, which notoriously attacked King Charles and notable Royalists during the Civil Wars. At the time of the first printing of the *Anatomy*, the reference to *Mercurius Britannicus* must have been to the narrator of Joseph Hall's satirical travel fantasy, *Mundus Alter et Idem*. There are numerous parallels between Hall and Burton that extend beyond their shared experimentation with dystopian writing, but the key one here is that both published their books under the pseudonym of their mercurial narrators.

[24]   Despite the logic of association between Heraclitean sorrow and Christian mercy, there was a prominent tradition of the Christian Democritus in early seventeenth-century art and letters. Pierre de Besse's *L'Héraclite Chrétien* illustrates the same preferences for the Democritean response to suffering as his contemporaries Landino, Erasmus, and Montaigne, the last of whom wrote: "*J'ay bien estimé les larmes de ce dolent, mais je fais encore plus d'estat des mocqueries de ce folastre.*" See Edgar Wind, "The Christian Democritus," *Journal of the Warburg Institute* 1, no. 2 (1937): 180–82.

[25]   For an overview of Puritan introspective exercises and self-discipline placed in the context of the turns to and away from "Pietism" in late sixteenth- and early seventeenth-century England (and, in the latter part of the book, New England), see Theodore Dwight Bozeman, *The Precisianist Strain: Disciplinary Religion and Antinomian Backlash in Puritanism to 1638* (Chapel Hill: University of North Carolina Press, 2004), especially chaps. 6 and 7.

[26]   Richard Greenham, *A Most Sweete and Assured Comfort for all those that are Afflicted in Consciscience* [sic], *or Troubled in Minde* (London, 1595), Diij v–r.

of melancholy. This tradition provided the intellectual patrimony for a specifically utopian variety of Renaissance satire (of which Burton is one example) in which Democritus "expressed his dissent in delirious laughter, which ... could be taken as a sign of being out of tune with the world."[27] As Christoph Lüthy reminds, the figure of Democritus *ridens* makes his earliest appearance in Latin literature alongside Heraclitus, "the weeping philosopher." Lüthy traces this pairing through medieval and Renaissance iconographies, noting the rise, fall, and return of a Senecan preference for Democritean laughter over Heraclitean weeping, the latter preferred for its better resemblance of Christ's tears.[28] Lüthy marks a return in popularity of Democritus in the later fifteenth century, hallmarked by Ficino's evaluation of a double portrait of the two philosophers. Ficino writes: "Why is Democritus laughing? Why does Heraclitus weep? Because the mass of mankind is a monstrous, mad and miserable animal."[29] Ficino's comment is less a contrast of opposing attitudes than an expression of their equal insufficiency to the task of representing human suffering. The iconic pairing underscores the problem of how one literally countenances, that is, puts on or up a face between the self and the suffering of others. Democritus' laughter recognizes the failure of the tragic mode (or mask) to *co-miserate*. His is not laughter at the sufferer but rather at the absurdity of a world in which we are both outside and inside suffering—both agents and acted upon by the indiscriminate swerve of the atom. Democritus never laughs at the singular but rather at the paradigmatic. His comic vision is predicated upon the contiguity of individual experience and therefore foregrounds community where tragedy, however universalizing, foregrounds alienation. However, unlike the Democritus of the pseudepigraphic Hippocratean *Letters*, who denies the uniqueness of suffering, Democritus Junior catalogues each symptom, articulating a universe of melancholy more wondrous for its diversity than tragic in its ubiquity.[30] Still, different as they are, each symptom in the *Anatomy* is a symptom of a kind. Burton's exfoliation of the myriad kinds and cures for melancholy articulates a logic that makes individual sufferers part of a whole.[31]

---

[27]   Winfried Schleiner, *Melancholy, Genius, and Utopia in the Renaissance* (Wiesbaden: Otto Harrassowitz, 1991), 209.

[28]   Christoph Lüthy, "The Fourfold Democritus on the Stage of Early Modern Science," *Isis* 91, no. 3 (2000): 443–79.

[29]   Marsilio Ficino, *The Letters of Marsilio Ficino*, trans. Members of the Language Dept., School of Economic Science, vol. 1 (London: Shepheard-Walwyn, 1975), 104.

[30]   Burton writes that the "*four and twenty letters* ... make no more variety of words in divers languages, than *melancholy* conceits produce diversity of *symptoms* in several persons," using a conspicuously Lucretian figure for *copia* whose circulation as a trope for atomism is traced by Gerard Paul Passannante, *The Lucretian Renaissance: Philology and the Afterlife of Tradition* (Chicago: University of Chicago Press, 2011). Burton uses the same figure again in "Exercise Rectified of Body and Mind" (discussed at length in Chapter 3) to describe the therapeutic sense of infinite variety that obtains from the study of algebra.

[31]   For a view of the reactionary politics associated with this argument and nostalgic invocation of a feudal/agrarian world of merry commoners and community, see

Montaigne helps us to better understand the moral vision and communal sensibility of Burton's Democritean laughter. Of the two alternatives, Heraclitean weeping and Democritean laughter, he prefers the latter: "not because it is more pleasing to laugh than to weepe; but for it is more disdainefull, and doth more condemne us then the other. And me thinkes we can never bee sufficiently despised, according to our merit."[32] Like Montaigne, Burton chooses rather to laugh with Democritus than weep with Heraclitus, because it is more fitting to laugh than cry at the stupidity of men. He declares: "I am of *Democritus* opinion for my part, I hold them worthy to be laughed at, a company of brainsicke dizards, as mad as *Orestes* and *Athamas*, that they may goe *ride the asse*, and all saile along to the *Anticyrae*, in the *ship of fooles* for company together" (1:59). But as soon as he says this, Burton, like Montaigne, turns this dismissal upon itself: "are they fooles? I referre it to you, though you be likewise fooles and Madmen your selves, and I as mad to ask the question" (1:59–60). The pleasure of the Democritean mode for both writers is its comic embrace of human weakness. The Christian Democritus does not stand apart in judgment; he casts his allegiance with the human ship of fools.

Writing from "Experience": Experto Crede Roberto

While he shares an obvious family resemblance with the stock ingénues of humanist satire, Democritus Junior is more complex because he is quite literally a composite of voices. Burton recites the borrowed passages of his cento in a wide cast of narrative personae that features the melancholic scholar and digressive natural philosopher but, also, and indeed more frequently, the religious and moral authorities whose counsel he relays with just enough exaggeration for us to recognize their caricature. Burton channels still more familiar dispensers of therapeutic advice. We are privy to the chattering of the midwife and fishwife along with the learned physician. We hear the ubiquitous counsel of the well-meaning friend and the voices of those afflicted by the many varieties of melancholy under examination: pining lovers, jealous husbands, and desperate penitents alike. These impersonations bring the pains as well as the pleasures of melancholy to life in ways that we shall have occasion to examine in detail in later chapters. My intent here is to note how the elasticity of Burton's narrative persona offers an antidote to the overwrought interiority promoted by English Puritans, known for their "preciseness" in regimens of self-examination and spiritual hygiene.[33]

For John Abernethy, the labor to know the self in all its iniquity is "a great worke, & has neede of a thousand eyes." While this would seem to privilege the

---

Leah S. Marcus, *The Politics of Mirth: Jonson, Herrick, Milton, Marvell, and the Defense of Old Holiday Pastimes* (Chicago: University of Chicago Press, 1989).

[32] Michel de Montaigne, "Democritus and Heraclitus," *Essayes, or Morall, Politicke and Millitarie Discourses*, trans. John Florio (London, 1603), 165.

[33] Bozeman, *The Precisianist Strain*, 89–90. Bozeman's book is in part an attempt to offer a corrective to a traditional historiographical focus on German pietism.

external scrutiny of a public gaze, the emphasis in Abernethy's "nosce te ipsum" is on the inward-looking examination of self: "Begin, and acquaint thy selfe, with thy selfe. By vse and custome learne to take a view of they selfe, that at length thou mayest attaine to some perfect habit in seeing, and knowing thy selfe thorowly."[34] Such knowledge is won by searching "narrowly, euen thy least errours, secret sinnes, priuie corruptions ... *substantially*, searching euery corner; iudging great sins infinite: little sinnes, great ones; and no sinne small." Abernethy's script for the examination of conscience is necessarily incomplete, even as it attempts to be comprehensive: "Spying all sinnes, sparing no sinnes, spending all times herein, neuer ending; the more ye find, suspect the more, that there is some more behind."[35] Whereas such exercises emphasize a view of the self as continuous through time, the *Anatomy* invites the reader to meditate on the plasticity and contingency of the self. Burton's catalogues of diverse kinds, causes, and cures for melancholy replace the inventory taking of personal sin recommended by Abernethy. Moreover, his exaggerated authorial instability undermines the logic of selfhood assumed by the keeping of daily spiritual records or ledgers of conscience.[36] Burton's elaborate burlesque of authorial *personality* rejects not only the Puritan exhortation to "know" and "examine" oneself but the very notion of discrete, autonomous, and *self-same* personhood that this exhortation implies.

My characterization of Burton's resistance to proprietary notions of selfhood might seem to be contradicted by his few but suggestive remarks regarding his motivation for writing about melancholy. Burton famously tells the reader that he writes of Melancholy "by being busie to avoid Melancholy" (1:6), a disease he calls "Mistris *Melancholy*, my *Aegeria*" (1:7) and the "Rocke" upon which he was so fatally driven that this and not a subject more fitting to a learned divine was what he chose to devote his writing to (1:20). However, these statements seem less to be a bid for authority based on personal experience than a statement of intent to render personal suffering into a part of the general cure. Burton announces his therapeutic strategy as one of homeopathic substitution: "I would expell *clavum clavo*, comfort one sorrow with another, idleness with idleness, *ut ex viperâ Theriacum*, make an Antidote out of that which was the prime cause of my disease" (1:7). Writing about

---

[34]   John Abernethy, *A Christian and Heauenly Treatise* (London, 1622), 27.

[35]   Ibid., 28.

[36]   Such as is recommended by example in Richard Rogers, *Seven Treatises* (London, 1603) and by prescription in William Perkins et al., *A Garden of Spirituall Flowers* (London, 1610). Examples of this genre, which goes by many names in the scholarly literature (including Protestant/Puritan spiritual autobiography), are too many to enumerate here but useful surveys may be found in Tom Webster, "Writing to Redundancy: Approaches to Spiritual Journals and Early Modern Spirituality," *The Historical Journal* 39, no. 1 (1996): 33–56; and Ann Thompson, *The Art of Suffering and the Impact of Seventeenth-Century Anti-Providential Thought* (Aldershot, UK: Ashgate, 2003), chap. 1. Webster gives an illuminating overview of the historiography of this genre in the context of ongoing debates (between Peter Lake and Peter White) concerning the orthodoxy/marginality of Calvinism and Puritanism in early modern England.

melancholy translates the "imposthume" of "a heavy heart" by making an antidote from the viper. As he will do throughout the book, Burton emphasizes the greater utility of the cure that transforms melancholy as compared with one that seeks merely to diminish it by dissuasion or distraction. Such wholesale translation calls for an immersion of reader and writer in contemplation of the disease that brings about its own relief.

Burton compares himself to the man who "thought he had some of *Aristophanes* Frogs in his belly, still crying *Brecec'ekex, coax, coax, oop, oop, oop*, and for that cause studied Physicke seven yeares, and traveled over most part of *Europe* to ease himself." He tells us that like the croaking patient-cum-scholar, he "turned over such Physitians as our Libraries would afford" in order to seek comfort, like Cardan and Tully after the loss of their children, by writing a *consolatio* and substituting the intelligibility of written words for the unintelligibility of private pain (1:7).[37] Writing, he says, transforms private grief into a method of public succor: "*Haud ignara mali miseris succurrere disco*,[38] I would help others out of a fellow-feeling, and, as that virtuous Lady did of old, *being a Leaper her selfe, bestow all her portion to build an Hospitall for Leapers*, I will spend my time and knowledge, which are my greatest fortunes, for the common good of all" (1:8). Writing relieves the writer of privacy itself, reconstituting the subject's individual experience as both social and contingent.

From the firsthand experience of suffering comes the authority immortalized in Burton's aphoristic "Experto crede R O B E R T O," trust the expert Robert (1:8).[39] This is the only place in the *Anatomy* (from the second edition on) where Burton names himself, but the claim to authority based on personal experience is ironized by the coincidence of Burton's name and the "Robert" named by the medieval proverb. Burton turns his "real" name into a red herring—an *author effect*—and a particularly ghostly one at that. Who exactly is speaking here? Who summons the name of the author as authority for the author's experience? Burton's hyperbolic

---

[37] The death of the child is the litmus test for Cicero of Stoic reserve. See *Tusculan Disputations* and Richard Strier's discussion of Coluccio Salutati's argument with this in his essay, "Against the Rule of Reason: Praise of Passion from Petrarch to Luther to Shakespeare to Herbert," in *Reading the Early Modern Passions: Essays in the Cultural History of Emotion*, ed. Gail Kern Paster, Katherine Rowe, and Mary Floyd-Wilson (Philadelphia: University of Pennsylvania Press, 2004), 25.

[38] "I learn from my own experience of misfortune to help the unhappy," echoing Virgil, "Non ignara mali, miseris succurrere disco" (*Aeneid*, 1.630).

[39] Literally, "Trust Robert, who has learnt from experience" (4:20). The Clarendon editors hear this as an echo of "experto credite quantus" (*Aeneid*, 11.283) and Ovid, "Odimus inmodicos (experto credite) fastus" (*Ars Amatoria*, 3.511), but the specificity of the name Robert appears to have been established by sixteenth-century uses of this proverb (Ed. Marshall, "Experto Crede Roberto," *Notes and Queries* 7, no. 107 [1877]: 408). It may have had more local currency at Oxford as an expression of melancholy, as one scholar surmises based on its appearance in the epitaph to a 1627 grave for the second of three lost sons of the rector of Exeter College. See J.H.M., "Experto Crede Roberto," *Notes and Queries* 6, no. 144 (1852): 107.

self-naming divides experience and identity, making his "own" name no more secure a *point d'appui* for grasping the author's interiority than the alias by which he signs his book.

Democritus Junior to the Hippocratic Reader

The story of Democritus of Abdera's meeting with Hippocrates was too well known from the multiple Latin translations and publications of the letters attributed to Hippocrates to warrant its exceptionally long and, for Burton, unusually faithful reproduction.[40] This epistolary "novel" tells the story of Hippocrates' summons by the distressed citizens of Abdera to cure their beloved philosopher of his apparent madness. The symptom that chiefly concerns the Abderites is that Democritus seems incapable of empathy, which they diagnose on the basis of his indiscriminate laughter:

> That man of all our citizens who we always expected would be the fame of our city in the present and future ... that man has been made ill by the great learning that weighs him down ... . For, previously inattentive to everything, including himself, he is now constantly wakeful night and day, laughs at everything large and small, and thinks life in general is worth nothing. Someone marries, a man engages in trade, a man goes into politics, another takes an office, goes on an embassy, votes, falls ill, is wounded, dies. He laughs at every one of them ... .

His response to the news of one person's good fortune or another's calamity is, to the Abderites, distressingly unmodulated. Still, even in their simplistic characterization, the philosopher's indifference is not quite callous but somehow charmed:

> The man is investigating things in Hades, and he writes about them, and he says that the air is full of images. He listens to birds' voices. Arising often alone at night he seems to be singing softly. He claims that he goes off sometimes into the boundless and that there are numberless Democrituses like himself. [41]

By averting ear and eye from the cacophony of the Abderites' complaints, Democritus enters into sympathetic commerce with another order, of which we are reminded by the poetic descriptions of melancholy that appear throughout

---

[40]   The sequence of 24 letters, written sometime in the third century, was first translated from Greek into Latin by Rinuccio Aretino between 1434 and 1450. A Latin translation of works assumed to have been authored by Hippocrates, including the epistles, was edited by Fabius Calvus and published in 1525. A complete series of the letters was published in Latin, edited by F. Asulanus in 1526. There were at least three more Latin translations published before Eihard Lubin's popular publication of the letter sequence in 1601. See Hippocrates, *Pseudepigraphic Writings*, ed. and trans. Wesley D. Smith, *Studies in Ancient Medicine*, vol. 2 (Leiden: E.J. Brill, 1990), 45.

[41]   Ibid., 57.

the *Anatomy*. Like the melancholic scholar who features so prominently in the first and second partitions, and like Burton himself in his role as "Democritus Junior," Democritus of Abdera has reputedly been "made ill" by study. Like the melancholic birdmen who appear in Burton's discussion of delusional melancholy (which we will examine in detail in the next chapter), Democritus imitates the nightingale, "singing softly" in the dark. Like Burton digressing upon air, Democritus "goes off into the boundless." Above all, the Abderite philosopher echoes Democritus Junior in his reports that he is multiple: there are "numberless Democrituses like himself."[42] Despite these resemblances, Burton's use of the *Letters* draws greater attention to the relationship between the reader of the *Anatomy* and Hippocrates, the father of diagnostic medicine, than the one between his alias and namesake.

Burton's insistence that he has "inserted" the Hippocratic narrative *"verbatim almost"* is conspicuously accurate, but it only tells half the story. His summary commences with the iconic meeting of Hippocrates and Democritus in the garden, in that famous scene depicted in Letter 17 wherein the philosopher delivers his well-known lecture on folly and vanity. Burton, however, leaves out the details of the exchanges leading up to this moment and the ironic depiction in the preceding letters of Hippocrates as vain, petty, and overly hasty in his medical judgments. Read outside of this sequential context, the lecture in Letter 17 sounds all the conventional notes of Stoic didacticism and loses its ironic force as targeted and deserved reproach. Hippocrates' narrative credibility is in fact undermined and ironized from quite an early point in the letters, if not quite from the start. At first the doctor suspects that the Abderites have misjudged Democritus. He rejects their assessment that the philosopher has gone mad from too much learning, sagely reflecting that such accusations of excess proceed from deficiency in the accuser.[43] He nonetheless accepts the Abderites' invitation to visit the philosopher with great show of the purity of his motives for doing so, but this is cast into some doubt by his boasting that the "Abderites want it proved, and will pay for it, that they don't understand Democritus." We continue to form doubts about the doctor when, in the same letter, Hippocrates asks Dionysius to chaperone his wife while he travels to take this commission. He notes that the request is superfluous and that he has no reason to fear for her honor or safety as she is good and honest and will be guarded by her parents in his absence. But he insists that a friend makes a better chaperone for a wife than a parent, whose judgment is impaired by what he calls an "indwelling desire for amity." Hippocrates is blinded to the possibility of his

---

[42] Ibid., 57. In the decades following the publication of the first edition of the *Anatomy*, there was a small outcropping of treatises and pamphlets attributed to or signed "Democritus Jr." (i.e., *Hell's Intelligencer* and *Wit's Progresse*) and even "Heraclitus Jr." (*England's Ichabod*). One self-styled Democritus Junior explains how he has taken his place in a tradition of social critique that runs from the Abderite Democritus through Burton. Like his Democritean forebears, this Democritus Junior would play the "Countries Physitian" and "be for his labour esteemed a mad man" (Anon., *Democritus Natu Minimus*, 1647, A2).

[43] Hippocrates, *Pseudepigraphic Writings*, 65.

own cuckolding by this arrangement, an irony that undermines the wisdom of his parting remark that a "lack of emotion is wisest in all things."[44]

Hippocrates' pedantry is further underscored in the next letter of the sequence. He has not yet departed for Abdera but is convinced (by nothing more than rumor) that Democritus is either mad or deserves to be reprimanded for seeming so and therefore begins to rehearse his reproach. His earlier suspicion about those who accuse others of excess is replaced with officious certainty that "if excess is wicked, then unremitting excess is more so."[45] Even after a prophetic dream (wherein Truth chides Hippocrates for being deceived by Opinion) the doctor still proves an inadequate auditor for Democritus' lecture. The final strains of Democritus' moralizing speech in Letter 17 provoke Hippocrates' personal indignation at the ingratitude of his patients, and it is this appeal to the doctor's pride rather than his conscience that precipitates his sudden conversion.[46] Given Burton's unusually faithful reproduction of his source narrative, the omission of this final detail seems noteworthy indeed. As he so often does, Burton draws our attention to the elided text. Along with this plot detail, Burton leaves out the doctor's comic interruption of the philosopher's lecture with the complaint that while Democritus has been speaking, he has grown faint with hunger. Hippocrates begs Democritus to let him eat and rest, promising to return the next day for more instruction. In the subsequent letter, also left out of Burton's retelling, Democritus makes clear that the well-fed doctor has failed to show up for his lesson.[47] Democritus chastises Hippocrates for being gulled by appearances, admonishing him to be a more careful diagnostician, and to make "close observation" of "the totality of the structure" before pronouncing disease. He warns the father of clinical medicine of the dangers of partial diagnosis. This irony is not lost on Burton, who seems, in sum, to have related this story as a means of cautioning the reader against such hasty, decontextualized, diagnostic interpretations. The lengthy homage to the Hippocratean epistles insinuates that, like Hippocrates, the reader's character will be revealed in accordance with his or her ability to discern wisdom from pedantry and truth from opinion. We are invoked as the Hippocratic reader of the *Anatomy*, tasked with sorting more from less credible testimony and arguments in Burton's cannily crafted cento.

---

[44]   Ibid.

[45]   Ibid., 67.

[46]   "Really, I expect that your medical science is not even pleasing to them. They are disaffected from everything by their wantonness, and they consider wisdom madness. Yes, I suspect that they have slandered most of your learning through jealousy or ingratitude" (ibid., 91).

[47]   "Greetings. You came to administer hellebore, on the assumption I was mad, persuaded by mindless men in whose judgment my labor was madness … . Consider, if you had found me not writing, but reclining, or walking around slowly, communing with myself, sometimes exasperated, sometimes smiling at my inner thoughts, not attending to conversation of acquaints, but with my mind entirely engaged in intense investigation, you would have thought that Democritus … was the image of madness" (ibid., 93–4).

II. Cento: The Patchwork Cloth

While numerous scholars have noted the formal qualities of the *Anatomy* as a cento, few have endeavored to trace the subversive miscitation and ventriloquism characteristic of this genre in the book.[48] Theodor Verweyen and Gunther Wittig suggest that the cento be understood "not as a generic term but an *écriture*," a writing practice that transposes a set of sentences or syntagms from one context to another, with effects "such as parody, travesty, contrafacture, and pastiche."[49] The "perverse" origins of the cento are, as Mikhail Bakhtin observed, ancient ones indeed. Bakhtin situated the cento in the tradition of Hellenistic writing wherein "forms of direct, half-hidden and completely hidden quoting were endlessly varied," sometimes with reverence, sometimes with irony, and frequently with ambiguous intent.[50] The point of the cento in classical literature was to make something new from the authoritative master-text, typically Virgil.[51] More serious centos were composed from the *Aeneid* exclusively. Ausonius' pornographic *Cento Nuptialis* (c. 374) draws from the *Eclogues* and *Georgics* as well. Classical centos were prized for their successful redeployment of the poet's words in wholly different contexts than those found in the original. Early Christian writers utilized the cento to transform Virgilian verse into prophetic Christian gospel.[52] Ausonius' *Cento* transforms Virgil's martial verses into a pornographic wedding song. He narrates the procession of the bridal couple, from feast to the offerings of gifts and song. Then, with the entry into the bedchamber, Ausonius rips from the *Aeneid*, transforming fragments of text depicting military virtue into a brutal depiction of the bride's deflowering. The blood of the battlefield and the fluidity of the epic landscape are translated into hymenal blood and semen.

With theatrical self-diminishment of the sort Burton will imitate, Ausonius goads his reader to read his "trifling and worthless little book, which no pains has shaped nor care polished, without a spark of wit and that ripeness which deliberation gives." He facetiously dismisses the value of the cento as a "task for the memory only, which has to gather up scattered tags and fit these mangled

---

[48] For exceptions, see Hugo Tucker, "Justus Lipsius and the *Cento* Form," in *(Un)masking the Realities of Power: Justus Lipsius and the Dynamics of Political Writing in Early Modern Europe* (Leiden: Brill, 2010), 163–92; Robert Grant Williams, "Heterological Rhetoric: Textual Waste in *The Anatomy of Melancholy*" (London, ON: University of Western Ontario, 1995).

[49] Theodor Verweyen and Gunther Wittig, "The Cento: A Form of Intertextuality from Montage to Parody," in *Intertextuality*, ed. Heinrich F. Plett (Berlin: Walter de Gruyter, 1991), 172.

[50] Mikhail Mikhaïlovich Bakhtin and Michael Holquist, *The Dialogic Imagination: Four Essays* (Austin: University of Texas Press, 1981), 68.

[51] Conventionally, the cento staged this event as a performance tied to a specific occasion, as with Ausonius' *Cento Nuptialis*, written for the occasion of the wedding of Constantia to Gratian.

[52] See Scott McGill, *Virgil Recomposed: The Mythological and Secular Centos in Antiquity* (Oxford: Oxford University Press, 2005).

scraps together into a whole, and is more likely to provoke your laughter than your praise." Ausonius compares this task to a sort of game of which there are two sorts of players: one fashions wonders, the other, grotesques.[53] Like Burton, he declares that he is of the latter kind:

> You may say it is like the puzzle, which the Greeks have called *ostomachia*. There you have little pieces of bone, fourteen in number and representing geometrical figures ... . By fitting these pieces together in various ways, pictures of countless objects are produced: a monstrous elephant, a brutal boar, a goose in flight ... . But while the harmonious arrangement of the skillful is marvelous, the jumble made by the unskilled is grotesque. This prefaced, you will know that I am like the second kind of player.[54]

The game to which Ausonius refers appears to have been a kind of geometric puzzle that involves 14 pieces or figures arranged from the bisected lines of a parallelogram into various shapes.[55] Out of a fixed number of elements (or syntagms) an infinite number of forms and arrangements are possible. The *ostomachia* is, literally, a contest for the arranging of bones, which is an apt figure indeed for the art of rearranging ancient literary artifacts. The centonist makes something new—sometimes sacred, sometimes profane—out of the "bones" of the venerable fathers.

Insofar as it is a game played with the remnants of the dead, the cento always verges on violation. It disinters even as it preserves the dead in fragments. The centonist's art is rooted in the power of displacement: the power to recast the ways that texts are re-membered. Mary and Richard Rouse have noted the ways in which medieval florilegia, such as the *Florilegium anglicorum*, *Florilegium gallicorum*, and the widely circulated *Manipulus florum* of Thomas of Ireland, determined the choices of literary examples used by contemporary and later writers of treatises and sermons.[56] The authors of classical and medieval compilations were more than merely redactors of quotable libraries. They preserved and in many cases provided the only evidence of the existence of these earlier texts.[57] However, as the Rouses note, the preservation of tradition through the compilation of excerpts disseminates a perpetually fragmented origin. The manuscript and oral traditions of classical and medieval cultures lent themselves to a fragmented preservation of text and tradition that was fundamentally altered but in no way resolved by the rise of

---

[53] Ausonius, *Ausonius*, trans. Hugh G. Evelyn White, vol. 1 (London: Heinemann, 1919), 371.

[54] Ibid., 1:373–5.

[55] Ibid., 1:395–7. White includes a diagram of the figure and an approximation of how one might reconstruct the "helephantus belua" or monstrous elephant that Ausonius mentions.

[56] Mary A. Rouse and Richard H. Rouse, *Authentic Witnesses: Approaches to Medieval Texts and Manuscripts* (Notre Dame: University of Notre Dame Press, 1991).

[57] Ibid., 6.

print technology. The late Renaissance anthologist frequently represented himself as performing the onerous task of sorting the most useful or valuable material from a disorienting sea of print. That being said, the labor of the anthology and cento differ in a significant way: whereas the anthologist culls and collects, the centonist weaves, allying himself more closely with the textilic or tapestry tradition of storytelling than narrative tally or "account." Justus Lipsius complains of the difficulty of this art in the Preface to his own cento, the *Politica*, where he invokes a double analogy for the figure of the centonist that subtly indicates his departure from earlier traditions of the genre. On the one hand he says, "I have here and there joined them together with the cement, so to speak, of my own words," and then likens his craft to the more subtle art of Phrygian tapestry: "In short, just as the Phrygians make one single tapestry out of a variety of colored threads, so I make this uniform and coherent work out of a myriad of parts."[58]

Lipsius's representation of the cento as both a solid thing and a supple art is consonant with his philosophy of the art of government. The *Politica* is a manual for monarchs on how to maintain autocratic rule without recourse to tyranny. Lipsius argues that political order depends upon the cultivation of virtue, temperance, and the submission of political subjects to a single ruler. The subjugation of individual liberty to the prince for the good of all is mirrored in Lipsius's use of the cento format. His book is made up almost entirely of adages and commonplaces, which he "submits" to his purposes and governance. He gives detailed instructions for the reading of his cento, advising the reader to "carefully observe the distinctions between my words and those of others," handily distinguished by font. Lipsius furthermore cautions the reader to "observe the partitions within the text," noting especially the placement of "commas, semicolons, full stops or colons" because, as he warns, "the end of a sentence does not always coincide with the end of a period: but often continues and is connected to the next item." We get no such help or admonition from Burton's cento. Lipsius's reader is instructed to read notes, margins, headings, and subheadings and commanded not to "show yourself in any way difficult or obstinate."[59] This insistence on the manner in which Lipsius's cento ought to be read is in acknowledged tension with the license he takes in making it. Lipsius resolves the problematic openness of his form by declaring dominance over it: "Am I not weaving a Cento (for that is what this work is), in which these departures from the original meaning are always allowed and even praised?"[60] He chooses which voices to include, which to omit, and which to adjust according to his needs. He is the centonist-redactor as *principus*, modeling the art of censure to the autocrat he aims to instruct.

Burton's cento seems both to be aping Lipsius's heavy-handed manipulation of his sources as well as delighting in the audacity of the centonic form *qua*

---

[58]   Justus Lipsius, *Politica: Six Books of Politics or Political Instruction*, ed. and trans. Jan Waszink (Assen, Netherlands: Koninklijke Van Gorcum, 2004), 231–3.

[59]   Ibid., 237.

[60]   Ibid.

insolence and invention. Even as he protests his carelessness, Burton emphasizes the deliberateness and inventiveness of his method. Like Virgil did with Ennius, he says, he has mined the dunghills of the *auctoritas* for the rags out of which he weaves a "rhapsody":

> And for those other faults of Barbarisme, *Doricke* dialect, Extemporanean stile, Tautologies, Apish imitation, a Rhapsody of Rags gathered together from severall Dung-hills, excrements of Authors, toies and fopperies, confusedly tumbled out, without Art, Invention, Judgement, Wit, Learning, harsh, raw, rude, phantasticall, absurd, insolent, indiscreet, ill-composed, indigested, vaine, scurrile, idle, dull and dry; I confesse all ('tis partly affected). (1:12)

The apology for his rude, tumbled, confused, witless insolence is, of course, more than just "partly affected." As Robert Hallwachs and others have observed, the vast majority of Burton's revisions to the 1624 edition consisted of stylistic adjustments found precisely in the "dovetailing" or "stitching" of citations and sentences.[61] These seemingly inconsequential changes give the lie to Burton's claim of artlessness and disclose a much more carefully woven tapestry than the rhapsodic rag heap he claims to have left us. Scholars who have noted inconsistencies and infelicities in the weave, so to speak, of Burton's cento, have mainly concerned themselves with correcting miscitations and properly identifying misattributed sources as opposed to considering the suggestiveness of these errors. A notable exception is David Renaker, who argues that Burton's inaccuracies are often so egregious they call attention to themselves as the flourishes of a deliberately "plastic memory" exercising itself in hyperbole.[62] As Renaker observes, Burton inflates the number of battles attributed to Edward IV, the legions attributed to the Roman republic, and the years attributed to the longest living men. He makes planets larger, plagues more frequent, gods more plentiful.[63] He cultivates elaborate mythologies from the barest kernels of narrative. Renaker notes, for example, a pattern of intensifying exaggeration in the liberties Burton takes with the story of *Cleombrotus*. Burton first refers to this figure as Theombrotus, of *"Theombrotus Ambrociato's* 400," in a list of melancholic persons who renounce the world and "cast all" (their possessions) "into the Sea" (1:279). Later on in the first partition, Burton gives a more prolix account of the tale as a case of inspired mass suicide: "I know not how many hundredths of his auditors, by a luculent oration he made of the miseries of this, and happinesse of that other life, to precipitate themselves. And having read *Platoes* divine tract *de anima*, for examples sake led the way first" (1:437). The story makes a third appearance in Burton's diatribe against the "madnesse" of "superstitious Priests (that tell such vaine stories of immortality, and the joyes of heaven in that other life) that many thousands voluntarily breake

---

[61]   Robert G. Hallwachs, "Additions and Revisions in the Second Edition of Burton's *Anatomy of Melancholy*: A Study of Burton's Chief Interests and of his Style as Shown in his Revisions" (PhD diss., Princeton University, 1942), 11.

[62]   David Renaker, "Robert Burton's Tricks of Memory," *PMLA* 87, no. 3 (1972): 391–6.

[63]   Ibid., 392.

their owne necks, as *Cleombrotus Ambraciotes* Auditors of old ..." (3:378). In the first instance, the figure of Cleombrotus is merely an ascetic. In the second version, he encourages 400 listeners to follow his example of leaping into the sea. In the final instance, Cleombrotus serves as the *locus classicus* of morbid religious extremism that Burton denounces in his own age.

Renaker suggests that Burton combined several versions of the story for hyperbolic effect, but surmises that he did so because he "did not consider accuracy essential and ... may have sensed a positive value in the transformations wrought by his memory."[64] He considers Burton's inconsistencies with the story to be deliberate but vague in purpose. We might however consider how this particular story serves Burton's rhetorical purposes. How, for instance, does it enable the anatomist to comment on the temptation and danger of apocalyptic eschatology (and thereby anticipate Burton's critique of Calvinist theology in the third partition)? How does it represent the susceptibility of the auditor or reader to the sway of authority?[65] What, moreover, does the story suggest about the power of voice and the way in which it can be manipulated and exaggerated, as illustrated even by Burton's own retelling of it?

Tentative as it is, Renaker's reading of Burton's "mistakes" provoked an illuminating response from Frederick Rener, who argued that Renaker had overlooked Burton's place within a classical tradition of *imitatio*, in which the author "was to gather his material (res) from the best sources ... make it his own ... and produce something entirely new and better (Petrarch's 'aliud et melius')."[66] As Rener reminds, the figure most frequently used to illustrate this formula was the bee analogy, as it appears in Seneca's "Ad Lucilium." Burton's own professed use of sources, and of the bee motif as a means of describing this use, indeed locates him in a tradition wherein "the subject matter was taken over from the sources, while the order (*dispositio*) and the formulation (*elocutio*) were the author's own."[67] However, Burton presents the art of centonic arrangement as a subjugation of the source-text to the tastes and desires of the writer, lending a somewhat more capricious and antagonistic twist to the bee analogy.[68] He hints that the artful repurposing of his sources will be "apparent" to the careful reader:

---

[64]   Ibid., 395.

[65]   Burton's inconsistent representation of Cleombrotus may also draw on the vexed interpretive tradition that has tried to reconcile the Cleombrotus in the *Phaedo* (who was absent at Socrates' death) with the depiction in Callimachus' *Epigrams* of a Cleombrotus who flung himself into the sea upon reading the *Phaedo*. See G.D. Williams, "Cleombrotus of Ambracia: Interpretations of a Suicide from Callimachus to Agathias," *The Classical Quarterly* 45, no. 1 (1995): 154–69.

[66]   Frederick M. Rener, "Robert Burton's Tricks of Memory," *PMLA* 88, no. 1 (1973), 143.

[67]   Ibid.

[68]   Timothy Reiss includes Burton's invocation of the bee in his study of anti-autonomous writing in the West, but regards Burton's use of Seneca's analogy as evidence of an approach to writing that makes "something new, yet all somehow coexisting in mutual

apparet unde sumptum sit (which *Seneca* approves) *aliud tamen quàm unde sumptum sit apparet*,[69] which nature doth with the aliment of our bodies, incorporate, digest, assimulate, I doe *concoquere quod hausi*, dispose of what I take. I make them pay tribute, to set out this *Maceronicon*, this method onely is myne owne. (1:11)[70]

Burton's patchwork might be drawn from every resource, but he does not consume these indiscriminately or passively. In keeping with the long and detailed dietary study of the second partition, Burton's digestive metaphor implies that diet not only provides nourishment, it shapes temperament. The centonist's reading is not simply a matter of ingestion for the purposes of regurgitation, it is a practice out of which the writer cultivates the capacity to think and speak, to make one's own words and thoughts known to others. We might note here that Burton does not hold the impressionability of the mind and body as reason to rigidly censor one's reading (or, for that matter, to rigidly police one's eating).[71] His lengthy surveys of dietary advice underscore the diversity of opinion and contingency of each recommendation, suggesting an understanding of diet and physical regimen that assumes extraordinary physiological plasticity. A body may be shaped by custom, climate, diet, dress, entertainment, reading, or changes to any of the above. But the same principle that explains the body's capacity for alteration holds that such changes may be reversed if previous conditions are restored or altered in wholly new ways as subsequently exposed.

Burton repeatedly uses domestic metaphors and analogies to translate reading in particular and academic labor in general into the intimate arts, crafts, and

---

relation" (*Against Autonomy: Global Dialectics of Cultural Exchange* [Stanford: Stanford University Press, 2002], 167). Grant Williams understands Burton's remark that he makes something "of his own" out of the waste of humanism to be a coprophilic statement. He situates the *Anatomy* in the context of late Elizabethan and early Stuart preoccupations with waste and its domestic refinement, suggesting that Burton might have called his book the *Anatomy* after John Harington's *An Anatomie of the Metamorpho-sed Aiax* (1596), the first "toilet book," frequently sold chained to the water closet he invented ("Heterological Rhetoric," Introduction).

[69]   Cf. Seneca, *Epist.* 84.5, "*apparuerit unde sumptum sit, aliud tamen esse quam unde sumptum est appareat*" ("It is apparent where it came from, yet it is apparent that it is something other than from where it came"). Macrobius repeats this tag in the Preface to his *Saturnalia*.

[70]   Compare with Montaigne's language in "Of Practice": "What serves my turne, may happily serve another mans; otherwise I marre nothing, what I make use of, is mine owne" (II.6.220). Hugo Tucker notes the "innutrative" quality of Burton's centonic digestion: "Burton's vision is thus based on the positive metaphors of successful assimilation and imitation, innutrition and digestion" ("Justus Lipsius and the *Cento* Form," 171).

[71]   For a discussion of more anxious views of the physiology of reading, see Michael Schoenfeldt, "Reading Bodies," in *Reading, Society and Politics in Early Modern England*, ed. Kevin Sharpe and Steven N. Zwicker (Cambridge: Cambridge University Press, 2003), 215–43. Schoenfeldt does, however, include Burton in his survey, referring to his use of the digestion metaphor to describe a "deliberate process of vigilant assimilation" (220).

labors of the housekeeper, lover, and parent—odd choices, some have noted, for an unmarried Oxford librarian. Not so odd, however, in the context of the long tradition of treating reading as an integral part of the repertoire of self-cultivation and care. Burton depicts the cento as the expression of an economical or domestic cultivation of the soul that requires industry and resourcefulness. He compares the centonist to the "good hous-wife" who "out of diver fleeces weaves one peece of Cloath," as well as the bee "that gathers Wax and Hony out of many Flowers [to] make a new bundle of all" (1:11). The cento is a tapestry skillfully woven from available threads. Like a good housewife outfitting her home with what she has at her disposal, Burton prides himself on his editorial thrift and care. How do we reconcile these representations of the loving labor of his reading and arrangement with his claims that he chose and cited his material *per accidens* (1:19)? The apparent contradiction is usefully considered in the light of Burton's comments on the accidental manner of the book's composition and wandering nature of his sentences. From these comments we glean a sense of the complex ways in which accident is associated in the *Anatomy* with riddles and revelation, with fortunate error, or an allowance for the possibility of redemption through pleasurable, if potentially transgressive, dilation.

Speaking "Per Ambages"

Burton uses the expression "*per ambages*" to describe the shape, or what George Williamson described as the "amble," of his sentence.[72] In the well-worn argument of Morris Croll, the Senecan or "Attic" sentence (which describes the work of such heterogeneous authors as Browne and Bacon) maps out the lived experience of thought, revealing the immanent genius of the author.[73] Later twentieth-century Burtonists have argued, to the contrary, that the circuitous Burtonian sentence stages the asignifying power of language.[74] Neither interpretation fully recognizes the way in which speaking *per ambages* means to make a riddle or puzzle of oneself or one's meaning. Both Virgil and Ovid use the expression to signify labyrinthine or oracular convolution. In the sixth book of the *Aeneid*, Virgil describes the "winding ways" of Daedalus' temple sanctuary at Cuma and the "riddling visions" of the Cumaean Sybil herself.[75] Ovid repeats the tag associating Daedalus with the arts of technical deception, using the term to describe his design of the Cretan labyrinth.[76] Like Daedalus' labyrinth, Burton's *ambages* are intricate mazes. Like the Sybil's puzzles, his winding, riddling sentences are laden with

---

[72] George Williamson, *The Senecan Amble* (Chicago: University of Chicago Press, 1951).

[73] See Introduction.

[74] For instance, Robert Grant Williams, "Disarticulating Fantasies: Figures of Speech, Vices, and the Blazon in Renaissance English Rhetoric," *RSQ* 29, no. 1 (1999): 50.

[75] "*ipse dolos tecti ambagesque resoluit*" (*Aeneid*, 6.29); "*horrendas canit ambages, antroque remugit*" (*Aeneid*, 6.99).

[76] "*in errorem variarum ambage viarum*" (*Metamorphoses*, 8.160).

meaning that is mirrored by the form in which they are delivered. The Daedalian qualities of Burton's *ambages* are more easily discerned from a wider, forensic perspective. Whereas up close they appear impenetrable, as in the sibylline tradition, broader examination grants a keener view both of their architectonics and their implications.

As Joan Webber observed, Burton associates the *ambage* with the figure of the river, invoking Heraclitus while signaling Democritean sympathies.[77] Democritus Junior's sentences mimic the enigmatic inconstancy of the melancholic subject whose humor most closely resembles the world in flux. Webber calls the *Anatomy* "ever different, yet ever the same, in constant movement and yet keeping the same name and place. It is never finished, and yet always complete, infinitely open and yet bounded."[78] Webber likens this stylistic quality to what she calls the nonstatic persona of the literary baroque, best witnessed in Montaigne's pithy expression of the discontinuity of the self: "My selfe now, and my selfe anon, are indeede two."[79] Burton appears to be invoking the same conceit when he claims to have taken up tone and mask, "now Comical, then Satyricall," as the moment or his mood occasioned:

> 'tis not my study or intent to compose neatly, which an Orator requires, but to expresse my selfe readily & plainely as it happens. So that as a River runnes sometimes precipitate and swift, then dull and slow; now direct, then *per ambages*; now deepe, then shallow; now muddy, then cleare; now broad, then narrow; doth my stile flow: now serious, then light; now Comical, then Satyricall; now more elaborate, then remisse, as the present subject required, or as at that time I was affected. (1:18)

Burton's stylistic inconsistency is a result of his capacity to be "affected." It sharply contrasts with the constancy of both style and self demanded by the Neostoic rhetoricians, privileging instead the freedom to be moved that is, as we will see in chapters ahead, the very sign of and hope for our redemption.

Burton's characterization of his style as both subordinate to the demands of the moment and faithful to the author's experience would seem to support Croll's reading of his sincerity.[80] But, as we were when asked to trust Robert "who

---

[77] Joan Webber, *The Eloquent "I": Style and Self in Seventeenth-Century Prose* (Madison: University of Wisconsin Press, 1968), 113. See also Ellen Louise Hurt, "The Prose Style of Robert Burton: The Fruits of Knowledge" (PhD diss., University of Oregon, 1966), 169.

[78] Webber, *The Eloquent "I,"* 113.

[79] Montaigne, *Essayes, or Morall, Politicke and Millitarie Discourses*, 577. On the poetics of mutability and transformation in baroque art and literature, see Giancarlo Maiorino, *The Cornucopian Mind and the Baroque Unity of the Arts* (University Park: Pennsylvania State University Press, 1990).

[80] Indeed, Burton seems to be drawing on a rhetorical commonplace for the depiction of an improvisatory style associated with music. Poliziano described the recitations of the "improvvisatori sulla lira" musicians in a letter to Pico della Mirandola in a strikingly

knows," we are pressed to consider what it means to speak of the genuineness of a literary persona so clearly predicated on the inconsistency of the self. What kind of authorial experience can we seek to verify when the speaking body pronounces itself as a mask and exaggerates its non-selfsameness? Modern scholars have mainly followed in the Crollian tradition of reading Burton's description of his extemporaneous style earnestly. Williamson and Webber both regard the Burtonian sentence, Burton's *ambage*, as a circuitous progression toward self-discovery. Grant Williams, on the other hand, reads Burton's use of the term out of Puttenham, who designates it as a synonym for *periphrasis*:

> Then haue ye the figure *Periphrasis*, holding somewhat of the dissembler, by reason of a secret intent not appearing by the words, as when we go about the bush, and will not in one or a few words expresse that thing which we desire to haue knowen, but do chose rather to do it by many words.[81]

Williams suggests that Burton's *ambage* is symptomatic of a "degenerate copia" that "obscures a topic with circuitous postponement and multi-directional dispersal." He says that unlike Erasmian copia, Burton's *ambage* "complicat[es] the one with the many," making repetition plural and undifferentiated, usefully recalling the transgressive dilation Patricia Parker described in *Literary Fat Ladies*.[82]

Parker shows how Dudley Fenner and other English Renaissance rhetoricians ally rhetorical discipline to domestic patriarchy, figuring devices such as "disposition" and "partition" in terms of property and treating the proper arrangement of words as analogous exercises for the maintenance of social order.[83] She notes how a similar language of "joincture" and "ends" is invoked to describe properly married words and persons. For instance, she sees a close kinship between Thomas Wilson's cautioning against "the iognyng of woordes that should be parted" and "the Partyng of woordes that should be ioigned" and the marriage vows in the Book of Common Prayer.[84] If legitimate progeny are the proper ends of marriage, what are the ends of properly married words? If Burton rejects the rules of permissible copia, producing reams of dilatory sentences instead, what teleological project might he be understood to be subverting? Moreover, if disciplined language is so closely linked to social discipline, how

---

similar manner: "It was varied, however, as the words demanded, either even or modulated, now punctuated, now flowing, now exalted, now subdued, now relaxed, now tense, now slow, now hastening ..." (quoted in D.P. Walker, *Spiritual and Demonic Magic: From Ficino to Campanella* [University Park: Pennsylvania State University Press, 2000], 20).

[81]   George Puttenham, *The Arte of English Poesie* (London, 1589), 161.

[82]   Williams, "Heterological Rhetoric," 94.

[83]   Puttenham's *Arte of English Poesie*, for instance, conspicuously ties textual ambiguity to the threat of state insurrection. See Patricia A. Parker, *Literary Fat Ladies: Rhetoric, Gender, Property* (London and New York: Methuen, 1987), 99.

[84]   Thomas Wilson, *The Rule of Reason, Conteinying the Arte of Logique*, ed. Richard Sprague (Northridge, CA: San Fernando Valley State College, 1972), 169, quoted in Parker, *Literary Fat Ladies*, 118–19.

are we to interpret the recklessness of Burtonian copia even as it paraphrases and seems to reproduce authoritative positions on marriage, social order, inheritance, "constancy," and "knowing one's place"? We might find some help in the range of meanings that Parker identifies for the term "dilation" in Renaissance English. Parker observes a connection between rhetorical and erotic forms of "dilation" that pervert by extending the gap between the initiation and completion of an act.[85] If sexual and linguistic "perversions" disrupt a shared telos of reproduction, Burton's dilations may be said to be "perverse" even outside of their citational subterfuge because they militate against an ending and refuse rhetorical consummation. We might even say that they undermine a specifically patriarchal *logos* of transmission, making lateral as opposed to hierarchical relations between textual "source" and "successor."

III. The "Plain" Stylist

Burton's own statements about style would appear to accord with the sentiments about rhetorical perversion shared by Fenner and Wilson. He represents his rhetorical approach in a manner that has earned him a rather fixed place in the canon of so-called "plain," Attic or anti-Ciceronian seventeenth-century writers, who have been said to share a commitment to rhetorical transparency as a way of communicating moral sincerity.[86] But Burton is in fact nowhere more egregiously self-contradicting than in the way he presents himself as a plain stylist. This is particularly well illustrated in his critique of rhetorical ornament. He quotes Letter 115 of Seneca's *Moral Epistles*, "On the Superficial Blessings," which ends with the pronouncement that elegance is not a manly garb, "*non est ornamentum virile concinnitas*," but then appends the following ironic caption: "*vox es praeterea nihil, &c*, you are nothing but a voice." The latter hangs off the former, as if the saying attributed to Seneca were merely a gloss:

> *Non est ornamentum virile concinnitas*, as of a nightingale,
> — *vox es praeterea nihil, &c.* (1:18)

The tag is not, however, from Seneca but rather from the *Apophthegmata Laconica* or "Sayings of the *Spartans*" collected in Plutarch's *Moralia*, where it pithily relates the following anecdote: A man plucked the feathers from a nightingale

---

85   According to Parker, the word "dilation" has seven principal meanings in Renaissance English: Neoplatonic generation; time; pride; natural increase; biblical exegesis; strategic delay ("dilatory pleas" such as Hamlet's); and finally, an erotics of prolongation, such as Eve's "sweet reluctant amorous delay" in *Paradise Lost* (*Literary Fat Ladies*, 15–16).

86   See Kenneth John Emerson Graham, *The Performance of Conviction: Plainness and Rhetoric in the Early English Renaissance* (Ithaca, NY: Cornell University Press, 1994); Peter Auski, *Christian Plain Style: The Evolution of a Spiritual Ideal* (Montreal: McGill-Queen's Press, 1995).

and, surprised to see how little meat there was, exclaimed: "You are nothing but a voice." If Burton is here claiming that to write "for the ears" is to be "nothing but a voice," he is contradicted in form and principle by the ventriloquism and vagrancy of his own centonic practice. Democritus Junior is nothing if not a voice, or rather, nothing but a voice made up of voices. The *Anatomy* not only deflects the reader's supposed desire to know the author's biographical identity, it rejects the very idea of a subject beneath the voice. The punch line of the apophthegm contrasts the gorgeous voice of the nightingale to its paltry body. Plucking a nightingale is an exercise sure to disappoint, as the bird's scant meat makes a very poor supper. But the anecdote also warns about the impulse to discern essence by excoriating surface. Burton's suggestion here is not that the remarkable voice dwells in the plumage. Rather, he is heralding the insufficiency (and violence) of the anatomical mode as a means of understanding living things; dead birds don't sing.

Burton's critique of ornament is not wholly ironic, however. Seneca's cited repudiation of oratorical fastidiousness accords with many features of Burton's style. On the whole, his writing is more abrasive than neat, more hyperbolic than ornate, more direct than indirect, but this directness is itself a mannerism, a theatrical device rather than a mode of authorial or pastoral transparency.[87] David Burchell suggests that the more abrasive "Senecan" or "Attic" style was better suited to the task of raising outrage than Ciceronian *concinnitas*, with its more predictable word order and emphasis on lexical and clausal connections. Burton's prose is indeed closer in kind to the inverted word order and the deliberate elisions of connecting particles and prepositions that one finds in Tacitus.[88] If these Tacitean markers may be witnessed in the shape of Burton's sentences, Seneca's influence is even more evident in his preferred rhetorical figures and the abrasiveness of his direct address. E.J. Kenney explains that this quality in Senecan prose "depends for its effect on a series of discrete shocks: paradox, antithesis, graphic physical detail," and the marked absence of the third person (all, except the last, characteristic of Burton's style).[89] Kenney is careful, however, to point out that the roughness of Senecan prose in no way suggests that it is any less contrived than Ciceronian prose; neither, I would add, is its directness any gauge of the author's sincerity.

The modern association of the direct, second-person address (especially when coupled with the first-person pronoun) with greater psychological transparency or intimacy may be traced to conceptions of privacy and publicity that did not obtain in early seventeenth-century England. The congeniality of direct address in modern English contrasts significantly with the thou/you distinction in early modern use. The modern second-person pronoun, "you," effaces the

---

[87]   Mary Ann Lund understands Burton's direct address somewhat less theatrically, as a more intimate pastoral technique intended at reaching the individual reader. See *Melancholy, Medicine and Religion in Early Modern England*.

[88]   David Burchell, "Hobbes, Science and Rhetoric Revisited," in *Science, Literature and Rhetoric in Early Modern England*, ed. Juliet Cummins and David Burchell (Aldershot, UK: Ashgate, 2007), 60–61.

[89]   E.J. Kenney, *Latin Literature* (Cambridge: Cambridge University Press, 1982), 515.

potential affront of such directness, which was typically the manner by which one addressed one's subordinates or extreme familiars in early modern English.[90] The use of the second person in exchanges between persons of equal rank could easily be interpreted as hostile. This same forwardness was, however, well suited to sermons, satires, and other moralistic writings that aimed to attack pride and induce humility, and it is in this way that we might better understand the pastoral purpose of Burton's rhetorical abrasiveness. Burton is both drawing strength from this tradition and undermining its pedantry by imitation. The forwardness of his direct address is continually belied by the fact that we never can be sure where and when Burton is speaking in his own person and where he is parroting, for the purposes of undermining, someone else's direct reproach. At the same time that this uncertainty destabilizes the author-reader relation, it cultivates its own kind of intimacy. Burton's use of the second-person pronoun belongs to what Anne Drury Hall calls the "dense and witty style" of the early seventeenth-century familiar letter that "looks in two directions" by "explicitly speaking to the understandings shared by the writer and his friend" while being "implicitly aware of the large, faceless crowds of those deliberately excluded from this conversation."[91] We are hailed as Burton's intimates to the degree that we recognize ourselves as a kind of private audience, as the familiars to whom he is whispering as if from behind his hand while bellowing for public auditors.

The effectiveness of this double address relies on the impression/illusion of immediacy. E.J. Kenney says of Seneca's style that its effect is that of "an impromptu speaker, developing various aspects of his topic as they occur to him, often at inordinate length and with much repetition." His deficiency is his lack of proportion, "his inability to stop," which is "essentially the attribute of the speaker rather than the writer."[92] Burton embellishes this illusion of spontaneity and incontinence in order to sustain the fiction of the *Anatomy*'s "vacunal pretense." His chatty performance enables him to ventriloquize and retranslate, parrot and invert his authorities under the guise of innocuous repetition. Burton makes precisely this kind of mischief in his whimsical comment on the role of the parrot both as a speaker of truth and a corrupter of speech—a bird who gets it wrong and right in the telling. He calls himself "Swine Minerva," whose truthful speech is met with disdain. He quotes and comically mistranslates the complaint that "sometimes *veritas odium parit*" phonetically into English:[93] "as he said,

---

[90]   For a recent overview of the scholarly debate concerning second-person pronouns in early modern English, see Teresa Fanego, "English in transition 1500–1700: On Variation in Second Person Singular Pronoun Usage," in *Sederi vii: Articles and Essays Presented in the 7th Conference of the Society Held at the University of Coruña, Spain, in March 1996*, ed. S.G. Fernández Corugedo (La Coruna: Universidad de Coruña, 1996), 5–15.

[91]   Anne Drury Hall, "Epistle, Meditation, and *Sir Thomas Browne's Religio Medici*," *PMLA* 94, no. 2 (1979): 235.

[92]   Kenney, 516.

[93]   From Terence's comedy, *Andria*: "*Obsequium amicos, veritas odium parit*" ("Flattery begets friendship, truth enemies"), set in capitals (and rendered into *sententia*) in the 1541 Aldine octavo edition of the *Comoediae* and popularized by Erasmus in

verjuice and oatmeale is good for a Parret" (1:84). The exaggerated deixis of the attribution "he said" comically defers responsibility for the joke, placing the source of the mistranslation elsewhere and allowing the speaker to claim that he is merely reproducing empty sounds. His botched translation moreover coyly mimics the dietary prescriptions of the ubiquitous hygiene books of his day: "*veritas odium parit*"—verjuice and oatmeal are good for a parrot. This is Burton as ingénue *par excellence*.

Apologia and Retraction: Aping Indifference

Burton's Democritean persona stages its own hysterical instability, giving and retracting apology at the end of the Preface in a performance that has accounted, more than any other feature of the *Anatomy*, for the impression that the author suffered from a manic form of melancholy himself. In a dizzying back and forth, Burton exaggerates the fiction of the conventional retraction by retracting his retraction several times over, emblazoning the artificiality of the gesture and its claim to sincerity. He fears he has "overshot himself" and that he has accused wrongly. He acknowledges the irony that he is apologizing for precisely those qualities in his writing that will be the subject of the *Anatomy*. At the heart of his defense is the alibi that it is not Burton but Democritus Junior who speaks. He makes the problem of role-playing key to his defense, begging his reader to remember what it is to play a part:

> If I have overshot my selfe in this which hath beene hitherto said, or that it is, which I am sure some will object, too phantasticall, *too light and Comicall for a divine, too Satyricall for one of my profession*, I will presume to answere with *Erasmus*, in like case, 'tis not I, but *Democritus, Democritus dixit.* (1:110)

Burton's retraction draws attention to the artificiality not only of Burton's Democritean mask but the mask of the author and of authority itself: "you must consider," he says, "what it is to speake in ones owne or anothers person, an assumed habit and name; a difference betwixt him that affects or acts a Princes, a Philosophers, a Magistrates, a Fooles part, and him that is so indeed" (1:110). He claims he is compelled to play the fool, lacking freedom to speak plainly, that his very choice to write a cento is a tactic of evasion, but the excuse is undermined by repeated and retracted disavowals. He leaps from feigned timidity to contempt, calling his satire the tart, if comic, *apéritif* to the textual feast that follows, reminding the reader that "one may speake in jest, and yet speake truth," which he calls "somewhat tart," but good for the palate, as "sharpe sauces increase appetite" (1:111).

Just as swiftly as he says this, Burton retreats again, taking cover, quite literally, under the shield of his namesake, but with swashbuckling bravado: "Object then

---

Adagia 2.9.53. On this phrase as humanist commonplace, see Raymond Waddington, *Aretino's Satyr: Sexuality, Satire and Self-Projection in Sixteenth-Century Literature and Art* (Toronto, ON: University of Toronto Press, 2004), 96–102.

and cavill what thou wilt, I ward all with *Democritus* buckler, his medicine shall salve it, strike where thou wilt and when: *Democritus dixit, Democritus* will answere it" (1:111). The buckler here invokes a popular figure in Neostoic writing for spiritual imperturbability (Du Vair's *De La Constance* was translated into English as *A Buckler against Adversity*). Unlike Zisca's speaking skin drum, to which he compares his book at the beginning of the Preface, and which we shall consider more directly in the next chapter, the buckler is a mute and solid prop among alibis that include the alibi of triviality associated with leisure:

> It was written by an idle fellow, at idle times, about our *Saturnalian* or *Dionysian* feasts, when as hee said *nullum libertati periculum est*, servants in old *Rome* had liberty to say and doe what them list. When our countrymen sacrificed to their Goddesse *Vacuna*, and sate tipling by their *Vacunall* fires, I writ this and published this ουτις ελεγεν [no one was speaking], it is *neminis nihil*. (1:111–12)

Burton claims that the *Anatomy* is the product of "idle times," and is therefore not to be taken seriously.[94] However, the weight of the sentence leans in the opposite direction, suggesting that the substance of the book has gone unnoticed while *others* "sate tipling by their *Vacunall* fires." The pretense of anonymity and frivolity evokes the masquerade of court, as does the performance of courtly presumption that follows:

> The time, place, persons, and all circumstances apologize for me, and why may I not then be idle with others? speake my minde freely, if you deny me this liberty, upon these presumptions I will take it: I say againe, I will take it. (1:112)

Burton turns the buckler of his alibi into a virtual codpiece that he grabs in an aped gesture of invulnerability, daring the reader to object: "If any man take exceptions, let him turne the buckle of his girdle, I care not. I owe thee nothing, (Reader) I looke for no favour at thy hands, I am independent, I feare not." This manic performance of fear and fearlessness, deference and indifference, underscores the theme of care, real and feigned, with which the Preface is so thoroughly preoccupied. It undermines the definition of melancholy as excessive fear or fear without grounds, ennobling worry in comparison with a Stoic invulnerability equated with aristocratic arrogance.

Burton's manic oscillation between deference and indifference echoes the book's outlying problem of discerning care from carelessness, conscientious regard for one's actions and the well-being of others from hollow exercises of self-examination. He pantomimes the formulaic examinations of conscience prescribed by contemporary spiritual hygienists with a litany of *mea culpas* for sins of impropriety that include the examination or "anatomization" of his own folly: "I have overshot my selfe, I have spoken foolishly, rashly, unadvisedly, absurdly, I have anatomized mine own folly." He apologizes for his self-examination and for

---

[94]   Perhaps, as editors of the Clarendon edition suggest, it was written during the Christmas holidays (4:167).

his apology, claiming temporary insanity, from which he was "awaked as it were out of a dream":

> I have had a raving fit, a phantasticall fit, ranged up and down, in and out, I have insulted over most kinde of men, abused some, offended others, wronged my selfe, and now being recovered, and perceiving mine errour, cry with *Orlando, Solvite me*, pardon (*o boni*) that which is past, and I will make you amends in that which is to come; I promise you a more sober discourse in my following Treatise. (1:112)

But if the Preface has been a phantasticall or raving fit, it is less exceptional than paradigmatic of what is to follow. Burton will wildly dilate and digress from his course in a manner that calls the virtue of such consistency and its suggestively concomitant "constancy" into question. Indeed, he names the risk of such methodical single-mindedness, especially for the anatomist, whose cut is sometimes too deep, he says, and sometimes wayward.

Burton pleads the ingénue to seek pardon in advance for his slippery hand and the wounds that may ensue from his satire. He apologizes for his inconsistency with a defense taken from Juvenal. It's hard not to write satire, he says: "*Difficile est Satyram non scribere*, there be so many objects to divert, inward perturbations to molest" (1:113). The elusive fantasy of rhetorical and methodological consistency stands in here for the Neostoic fantasy of imperturbability and tranquility. Neither are possible or just responses to a world as filled with troubles as ours. Burton follows this defense of inconsistency with the Pauline argument that offense is taken in one's guilty recognition of the self as offender: "I hope there will no such cause of offence be given; if there be, *Nemo aliquid recognoscat, nos mentimur omnia*.[95] Ile deny all (my last refuge) recant all, renounce all I have said, if any man except, and with as much facility excuse as he can accuse." The "all persons fictional" clause lifted from the pseudo-Plautan comedy, *Querolus sive Aulularia*, or *The Moaner*,[96] is addressed both by and to no one, as the *Anatomy* is "ουτις ελεγεν, neminis nihil," nothing by "Nobody." Burton hopes to evade the myopic censure of his critics the same way that Odysseus escaped the Cyclops' revenge, by claiming anonymity as his *nom de guerre*. At the same time, the disclaimer "*Nemo aliquid recognoscat*" addresses the reader *as* Nobody, rendering any offense here taken the result of a hapless slinging by a one-eyed (or winking) satirist. Burton closes the Preface with an exaggerated appeal to the reader's generosity that

---

[95] From the prologue to *Querolus sive Aulularia*, attributed to Plautus. "Let no one take anything personally, all we say is lies" (4:168).

[96] Marcia Colish offers a persuasive reading of the play as a satire of Stoic fatalism (Marcia L. Colish, *The Stoic Tradition from Antiquity to the Early Middle Ages: Stoicism in Christian Latin Thought Through the Sixth Century*, vol. 2 [Leiden: Brill, 1990], 96). It seems likely that the play appealed to the anti-providentialist sentiments of late humanists. A longer version of the quote from the prologue that Burton cites prefaces the 1624 edition of the *Encomium Moriae* published by Andreas Cloucquium, under the Dutch imprint *Lugundi Batavorum* in Rotterdam.

poignantly contrasts the canting courtesy of the courtier's mannered grace (that both denies offense and refuses censure) and the grace displayed by the true giving and receipt of honest correction. If the reader takes exception, he says, recanting one last time, "Ile deny all (my last refuge) recant all, renounce all I have said ... and with as much facility excuse, as he can accuse." But the retraction is notably conditional. He would rather proceed out of "an assured hope and confidence" in the "good favour and gratious acceptance" of his book by his "gentle reader" (1:113). With this appeal to the reader's care and discernment, Burton concludes the epic preface to his book about the cares (or complaints) of melancholy and the empathic care that underwrites its effective cure.

Chapter 2
Heroic Hypochondria and the Sympathetic Delusions of Melancholy

A curious exchange in Middleton and Rowley's *The Changeling* makes reference, in quick succession, to Lipsius, Ovid, and the extraordinary list of melancholic delusions with which this chapter will be principally concerned. Lollio, the assistant keeper of a fictionalized Bethlem hospital, has been charged by the impotent Alibius (a likely parody of the real keeper of Bedlam, physiologist Helkiah Crooke) to keep his young bride, Isabella, chaste by locking her up out of sight.[1] Languishing in her cage, Isabella pleads for distraction, and Lollio lets her out to view the madmen. Among the lot are two young men who have been admitted on false pretense: one feigning idiocy, the other insanity in hopes of gaining access to Alibius's jealously guarded wife. Isabella's tour gives the men their chance at last. When Lollio discovers Antonio, the false idiot, courting Isabella in high verse as he angles in for a kiss, he quips: "How now, fool, are you good at that? Have you read Lipsius? He's past *Ars Amandi*."[2] The insinuation that Antonio has turned "lipsy" puns not only on his forwardness but also his sudden eloquence—for when Antonio first arrived at the hospital, his friend told the keeper that Antonio was barely able to "creep but on all four / Towards the chair of wit" (1.2.101–2). Lollio's learned joke suggests that the fool has made some quick gains as a scholar, having graduated from Ovid's amatory counsel to Lipsius's popular Neostoic work, *On Constancy*.[3]

The joke is almost lost amidst the din of madmen rehearsing off stage for the show they have been hired to perform that evening. The masked and costumed madmen burst upon the scene just as Antonio gets a little too friendly with the warden's wife. The hot and bothered would-be lover demands to know "what are these" creatures that have so intruded upon his suit. Isabella replies that they are

---

[1]   On the Alibius/Crooke connection, see Patricia Allderidge, "Management and Mismanagement at Bedlam, 1547–1633," in *Health, Medicine and Mortality in the Sixteenth Century*, ed. Charles Webster (Cambridge: Cambridge University Press, 1979), 141–64.

[2]   Thomas Middleton, *Five Plays*, ed. Bryan Loughrey and Neil Taylor (London: Penguin, 1988).

[3]   Antonio is described in the dramatis personae as the play's titular "changeling," and therefore the reference to Lipsius is doubly ironic as it refers both to the changeling's inconstancy and the popular accusation of the author's ironic inconstancy, having changed his confessional and political loyalties as circumstances seemed best to warrant. See Christopher Brooke, *Philosophic Pride: Stoicism and Political Thought from Lipsius to Rousseau* (Princeton, NJ: Princeton University Press, 2012), 68.

"Of fear enough to part us," and proceeds to give a more elaborate gloss of these changeable creatures, this "school of lunatics":

> Suiting their present thoughts; if sad, they cry;
> If mirth be their conceit, they laugh again.
> Sometimes they imitate the beasts and birds,
> Singing, or howling, braying, barking; all
> As their wild fancies prompt them. (3.1.176–83)

These peculiar and changeable conceits have both an ancient pedigree and renewed currency in late Renaissance medical writing, which we shall examine at length in this chapter. But before we do so, it begs noting that the false-fool, Antonio, frustrated in his attempt at cuckolding Alibius (he's literally "cock-blocked" by madmen in bird costumes who are summoned on stage by the call, "Cuckoo, cuckoo!") rejects Isabella's elaborate explanation, retorting that "these are no fears" (3.1.184), but a mere pretense or excuse to deter his love-making.

Isabella's highly aestheticized description of the madmen draws upon an ancient catalogue of melancholic delusions so established in the classical medical literature as to constitute a topos: a list of dysmorphic fantasies and conceits suffered by people who imagine they have been "sympathetically" transformed into animals or inanimate objects (such as glass, bricks, or corpses) with which they psychically identify. The list has its roots in antiquity, was elaborated in the writings of Galen, Rufus, Aretaeus, and Avicenna, and appears to have experienced a revival in the late sixteenth century.[4] In the earliest surviving examples, the delusions are treated as symptoms of a physiological disorder, typically of the hypochondriac organs housed below the ribs (*hypo chondros*), and are therefore regarded as symptoms of "hypochondria," or hypochondriacal melancholy. The modern definition of hypochondria as an imagined state of disease bears little overt relation to this early understanding of a mainly digestive disorder.[5] However, the rhetoric surrounding

---

[4]   See Rufus of Ephesus and Peter E. Pormann, *On Melancholy* (Tübingen: Mohr Siebeck, 2008), 33–5; Stanley Jackson, *Melancholia and Depression: From Hippocratic Times to Modern Times* (New Haven, CT: Yale University Press, 1986), 39–40; Galen, *On the Affected Parts*, trans. Rudolph E. Siegel (New York: Karger, 1976), 92–4. See the selection from Avicenna, "On the Signs of Melancholy's Appearance," in *On Black Bile and Melancholy*, from *Canon of Medicine*, in Jennifer Radden, *The Nature of Melancholy: From Aristotle to Kristeva* (Oxford: Oxford University Press, 2002), 77–8. On the revival of this topos in the Renaissance and for a list of representative examples, see Stuart Clark, *Vanities of the Eye: Vision in Early Modern European Culture* (Oxford University Press, 2007), 57–8; 74n99. See also Winfried Schleiner, *Melancholy, Genius, and Utopia in the Renaissance* (Wiesbaden: Otto Harrassowitz, 1991), chap. 4. Two of the most comprehensive versions of this list are found in Simon Goulart, *Admirable and Memorable Histories Containing the Wonders of Our Time*, trans. Edward Grimeston (London, 1607), 370–84; and Malachias Geiger, *Microcosmus hypochondriacus sive de melancholia hypochondriaca tractatus, cum curatione hujus affectus* (Monaco: Straub, 1652), 481–95.

[5]   For an incisive review of the problems of historical continuity/discontinuity of hypochondriacal diagnoses, see Yasmin Haskell, "The Anatomy of Hypochondria:

the description of these delusions attributed to disorders of the hypochondriacal organs (especially the liver and spleen) seems even in the most ancient sources to associate hypochondria with disease of a psychic or spiritual nature.

We find in Galen a striking mix of pathos and disdain for melancholics suffering from delusions of mimetic or sympathetic transformation that include "one patient [who] believes that he has been turned into a kind of snail and therefore turns away from everyone he meets" for fear of being crushed, and another who "is afraid that Atlas who supports the world will become tired and throw it away and he and all of us will be crushed and pushed together."[6] Galen remarks that there are "a thousand other imaginary ideas," characterizing melancholy as (paradoxically) copious in its variety of morbid fascinations, even as its sufferers share a common quality of fearfulness and despondency that causes misanthropy. These patients "hate everyone whom they see, are constantly sullen and appear terrified, like children or uneducated adults in deepest darkness."[7] Not quite a century earlier, the physician Aretaeus of Cappadocia similarly remarked on the antisocial character of delusional melancholics. His definition of melancholy as a kind of fear without cause provides one of the earliest instances of the moralized diagnosis of melancholia's psychosomatic and affective symptoms: "Patients are dull or stern, dejected or unreasonably torpid, without any manifest cause."[8] However, it is not the absence of cause but the unpredictability of disposition that makes the disease so treacherous. Melancholics, says Aretaeus, "are prone to change their mind readily; to become base, mean-spirited, illiberal, and, in a little time, perhaps, simple, extravagant, munificent, not from any virtue of the soul, but from the changeableness of the disease."[9]

While the association between melancholy and misanthropy (or, at the very least, associability) is present as early as the first century and continues to be found in medieval *practica* such as Bernard de Gordon's *Lilium Medicinae*, it seems not to be until the late sixteenth century that the classic examples of mimetic, melancholic conceit come to be treated as evidence of spiritual degeneracy.[10] In the lists that appear in late sixteenth- and early seventeenth-century hygiene manuals, those afflicted are routinely described as obstinately deluded. The treatments they

---

Malachias Geiger's *Microcosmus Hypochondriacus* (Munich 1652)," in *Diseases of the Imagination and Imaginary Disease in the Early Modern Period*, ed. Yasmin Haskell (Turnhout: Brepols, 2011), 275–300; Susan Baur, *Hypochondria: Woeful Imaginings* (Berkeley: University of California Press, 1989), 21–5.

6   Galen, *On the Affected Parts*, 93.

7   Ibid.

8   Jackson, *Melancholia and Depression: From Hippocratic Times to Modern Times*, 39.

9   Ibid.

10   Schleiner observes that the causal connection between personality, profession, and a person's delusional conceits appears not to have been systematic until the seventeenth century. He points to Tobias Tandler's *De melancholia eiusque speciebus* (Wittenberg, 1608) as a first example (*Melancholy, Genius, and Utopia in the Renaissance*, 155).

receive are related as merry anecdotes celebrating the ingenious correction of stubborn fools—merry both in the physician's approach to correction and in the mirth these stories are assumed to provide the reader.[11] This chapter will showcase the subtle but striking differences between Burton's lyrical presentation of the delusions of melancholy and the presentations we find of these classic cases in late Renaissance medical and spiritual hygiene books. I will suggest that, for Burton, these figures and their fantasies of sympathetic mimesis attest to the positively transformative powers of the imagination. But beyond this recognition of their purpose for Burton, the present chapter seeks to understand the appeal of these figures for early modern spiritual hygienists and physicians. I argue that the discourse surrounding the melancholic's mimetic delusions illuminates key tensions within the period's contradictory pathologies of melancholy as both the excess and deficit of impressionability and resolve, compassion and imperviousness, and, finally, faith and despair. In order to foreground the significance of these tensions *vis-à-vis* the historiography of melancholic hypersensitivity, a condition that modernity has come to refer to idiomatically as a thinness of skin, I begin with a brief discussion of the skin as we are invited to meditate on it in the opening pages of the *Anatomy*.

I. Thin-Skinned

In the Preface to *The Anatomy of Melancholy*, Robert Burton compares his book to the drum of the infamous Hussite warrior, John Zisca, who, according to legend, requested that his skin be made into a battle drum after his death so that he would continue to terrify his enemies in death as he had in life on the battlefields. Burton tells us that he hopes his book will have a direct medicinal potency of the same kind, warding off melancholy in the sounding out of its passages.[12] The comparison to Zisca's skin drum at the outset of the *Anatomy* presents the book to us not so much as a flayed effigy of the author's suffering repurposed for the reader's benefit but a speaking instrument whose voice is only made audible through the reader's

---

[11]   See, especially, Tomaso Garzoni, *The Hospitall of Incurable Fooles* (London, 1600), 15–22. For a more sympathetic account of these delusional figures and the means by which they were treated, see Pedro Mexia and Antoine Du Verdier, *The Treasurie of Auncient and Moderne Times*, ed. and trans. Thomas Milles (London, 1613), 476–9. Schleiner observes that Luther seems to have taken a charitable view of the delusions of melancholy. He argues that the versions of these stories that Luther presents in the *Colloquia* showcase the salve of company and the danger of faith in justification by merit (*Melancholy, Genius, and Utopia in the Renaissance*, 152–7).

[12]   Robert Burton, *The Anatomy of Melancholy*, ed. Thomas C. Faulkner, Nicolas K. Kiessling, and Rhonda Blair, Introduction and Commentary by J.B. Bamborough and Martin Dodsworth, 6 vols. (Oxford: Clarendon Press, 1989–2000) 1:6. Unless otherwise indicated, all references to the *Anatomy* along with bibliographical notes and translations of Burton's non-English passages refer to the Clarendon edition, hereafter cited parenthetically by volume and page number.

direct contact with it.[13] The drum yields its sound at the point of contact between the skin of the drummer and the hide of the drum. Burton's analogy renders the reader as the percussor who releases the "skinned" voice of the author through the striking of its passages in a remarkably physical rendering of the encounter between reader and text that draws on the resemblance between the lined surface of the reader's body and the inscribed surface of the parchment or paper text.

Of course, the analogy between skin and book is hardly a novel trope. The production of books has long depended on the use of skins and on the analogy between imprinted skins and their hide bindings: the material resemblance, that is, between the body's interior and exterior. Steven Connor has shown how bookmakers throughout modern history have played on this relation. He cites examples of medical and dermatological texts made of hanged criminals whose tanned skins bind their own execution reports and of lovers who bequeath their skins to their beloved by binding poems in their own hides.[14] Still, Zisca's skin drum is an especially compelling figure for Burton to select as a totem for his book, not only for its suggestion that the *Anatomy* will serve as an amulet, or for its promotion of the ethical powers of the melancholic's mimetic imagination (as I will emphasize in this chapter), but because the very form of his book, the porous tissue of living skin, is less a solid surface than a composite organ that receives, transmits, and registers impression. As we have seen in the previous chapter, Burton's *cento* is nothing short of an elaborate experiment in the registry of textual influence, and his art lies precisely in the weaving of its textile fragments. The playfulness of the cento represents the "master" text as a scissile surface and in so doing suggests that the authority vested in it is only "skin deep." Indeed, this modern cliché ironizes the association between skin and surface by making skin the sign not merely of shallowness but of the suspicion with which we regard objects—and persons—of inscrutable depth.

In *Skin: On the Cultural Border Between Self and the World*, Claudia Benthien offers a history of skin as "the central metaphor for separateness," arguing that it is only at this boundary that subjects are able to "encounter one another."[15] Benthien follows Didier Anzieu's reasoning that, since the Renaissance, Western epistemology (modeled on the "penetration and uncovering" of bodies in Vesalian anatomy) has been predicated on the notion that "knowledge of what is essential means breaking through shells and walls in order to reach the core that lies in the innermost depths."[16] According to Benthien, it is only with the development

---

[13]   Mary Ann Lund commences her study of the *Anatomy* by remarking on Burton's reference to Zisca as a statement of the direct and curative effect that he hopes his book will have on the reader (*Melancholy, Medicine and Religion in Early Modern England: Reading "The Anatomy of Melancholy"* [New York: Cambridge University Press, 2010], 2–3).

[14]   Steven Connor, *The Book of Skin* (Ithaca, NY: Cornell University Press, 2004), 42–5.

[15]   Claudia Benthien, *Skin: On the Cultural Border Between Self and the World* (New York and Chichester: Columbia University Press, 2004), 1.

[16]   Ibid., 7.

of modern psychoanalytic discourse that we have come to recognize the skin's ontological destabilization of interiority and exteriority.[17] That the skin is or has been at various periods in Western history "the place where boundary negotiations take place" is indisputable.[18] How the limits of the "skin boundary" are drawn, and whether the skin has always been the site of such symbolic differentiation, is, however, a matter of much greater complexity.

Whereas modern English refers to the skin as a single surface, early modern English imagines skin as a plural entity.[19] We still retain this sense in the Greek and Latin medical terms, *derma* and *cutis*, which describe layers of skin, but lay English has all but lost its earlier sense of the thickness of skin—the idiomatic sense that there are skins both beneath and within skins. Organs inside the body were, in early modern medical writing, described as being cased in skins. Skin referred to tissues in the brain, chest, or wrapping the heart. Indeed, the word tissue is, along with "superficies," a frequently occurring synonym for skin in early modern medical treatises such as Helkiah Crooke's *Mikrokosmographia* (1615). For Crooke, the skin has equally important retaining and transmissive functions: it both "knitteth the whole body together" and is punctured throughout by large *foramina* or orifices and an infinite number of small pores: "It is an unseamed garment covering the whole bodie, yet hath it certaine breaches made by Nature for her ease and reliefe."[20] Crooke identifies three principle layers of skin: an uppermost (creamy) cuticle, then the "scarfe-skin," and lastly, the "true and genuine skin."[21] This complex of skins may be exceedingly thick or exquisitely fine, as in the skin of one's lips. He gives the curiously exotic example of the thick-skinned elephant, which "can by the corrugation or wrinkling of his skinne, kill the flies that molest him."[22] If the skin is of such indefinite and relative thickness that it can be so rare as to be transparent to the blush of flesh beneath the lips or so thick as to crush a fly with a mere twitch, how can one say where the skin becomes

---

[17]   Echoing Anzieu, Benthien writes that neurophysiology "has had to come to terms with the paradox that even the brain is a rind—and the human 'center' is actually situated at the periphery" (Benthien, *Skin*, 7).

[18]   Ibid., xi.

[19]   Steven Connor makes an analogous point about the plurality of air as understood by most ancient cultures and reflected in their languages. See *The Matter of Air* (London: Reaktion, 2010), 15.

[20]   Helkiah Crooke, *Mikrokosmographia: A Description of the Body of Man* (London, 1615), 72.

[21]   This "true" skin is problematized by the etymology Crooke provides for it. The Greeks called this "true skin" *dermis*, he says, precisely "because it may be excoriated or flayed off." The "true skin" is true only insofar as it is removable. Moreover, it lacks the protective and sensitive qualities of the more superficial layers. If the true skin is stripped of its cuticle, it "cannot distinguish between one Temper and another; because the very gentlest touch of the bared skin breedeth paine, and the sensation is confused" (ibid., 71).

[22]   Ibid.

part of the flesh, or where it becomes so rare as to be indistinguishable from the atmosphere or from the bodies of others?

The prevailing view amongst contemporary literary historians has been that the porosity of the early modern body (both of the fine, dermal surface and the larger, foraminous "holes" or orifices) posed a grave threat to its integrity. According to this reading, the more open the body, the greater its potential risk of penetration and likelihood of both literal and figural incontinence. Women, then, were deemed to be more vulnerable not only to physical but spiritual penetration. The softer, more porous bodies of women made them more susceptible to impression, as evidenced by the expectant mother's ability to imprint information perceived from "outside" her body onto her unborn child.[23] As Nancy Caciola has illustrated, the porosity of the late medieval female body made women more vulnerable to demon possession. But the same porosity, she notes, also made women more open to divine and spiritual inhabitation.[24] This potentiality has received far less attention in recent criticism than the abject impressionability of the vulnerable female (or feminine) body, mind, and spirit.

Giving her account of the emergent disciplines of self-mastery in early modern hygiene books, Gail Kern Paster reminds that "solubility," or physiological openness, was "the sine qua non of bodily health" in Hippocratic medicine, but understands this necessary indeterminacy between the body's "internal and external economies [as] potentially fraught with peril."[25] Michael Schoenfeldt has attempted to qualify this "anxious reading" of early modern solubility by drawing attention to the regimens of care associated with regulating as opposed to sealing the pores and orifices, regimens that attended vigilantly to what goes in as well as out of the body: the quality and kinds of food taken, the frequency and properties of excretion, etc.[26] This provocative work continues, however, to cast a view of the relationship between the interior and exterior of the body as perilous and the skin continues to be construed as the battered precipice between a putative "inside" and "outside" of the body, obscuring other physical and psychical locations where the boundary between self and other was discursively wrought. In what follows, I will suggest that the site of such discriminating functions in the *Anatomy*, as in much of the period's spiritual and medical literature, is not the dermal surface of the body so much as the imagination, and that it is in this context that the sympathetic delusions of (hypochondriacal) melancholy resonate as profoundly as they do.

---

[23] According to Jan Baptist van Helmont, such fetal imprinting is the result of a woman's seduction by "vitious humors" (*A Ternary of Paradoxes: The Magnetick Cure of Wounds*, trans. Walter Charleton [London, 1650], 84).

[24] Nancy Caciola, *Discerning Spirits: Divine and Demonic Possession in the Middle Ages* (Ithaca, NY: Cornell University Press, 2003), chap. 3.

[25] Gail Kern Paster, *The Body Embarrassed: Drama and the Disciplines of Shame in Early Modern England* (Ithaca, NY: Cornell University Press, 1993), 9.

[26] Michael Carl Schoenfeldt, *Bodies and Selves in Early Modern England: Physiology and Inwardness in Spenser, Shakespeare, Herbert, and Milton* (Cambridge: Cambridge University Press, 1999).

II. The Hypochondriacal Imagination and the Power of Conceit

On the heels of invoking Zisca's skin drum, Burton warns that reading the descriptions of melancholy detailed in his book could worsen the symptoms of a reader who, "by applying that which hee reads to himselfe, aggravating and appropriating things generally spoken, to his owne person (as Melancholy men for the most part doe)," is wont to experience these conditions themselves (1:24). Burton regards the melancholic reader as someone who experiences the pains of others as his or her own. Modern psychiatry refers to such mimetic assimilation as hypochondria and has retained the later seventeenth century's more pronounced suspicion of appropriated pain while at the same time obscuring what was, in earlier accounts, a keener sense of the physical excruciations of the disease. André du Laurens writes that hypochondriacal melancholy "holde[s] the partie with such pangs, as the[y] thinke to dye euery moment."[27] Du Laurens likewise emphasizes the severity of the perceived pain, not the incommensurability between its perception and cause. Melancholic hypochondria was in this way still largely associated with somatic experience in the late sixteenth and earlier seventeenth centuries. Along with the fears and delusions classically associated with hypochondria, those afflicted typically experienced a rumbling or swilling in the stomach, shortness of breath, "biting" or "burning" pain in the sides, palpitations ("extraordinary and violent kinde of mouing of the heart"), cold sweats, irregular pulse, general "wearisomnes and feebleness," and weight loss.[28] These symptoms were deemed to be the result of some obstruction or compromising of the mesenteric organs (pancreas, duodenum, liver, and spleen).[29]

Physical pathology notwithstanding, the delusions classically associated with melancholic hypochondria come to bear a closer resemblance, in early modern accounts, to modern representations of hypochondria as an imaginary illness. But whereas modern psychology has predominantly understood hypochondria as a kind of primary narcissistic injury,[30] Renaissance hygienists and spiritual physicians understood the same symptoms to be characteristic of the melancholic personality. André du Laurens gives the following "liuely" portrait of this "abased and corrupted" condition:

> The melancholike man properly so called ... is ordinarily out of heart, always fearefull and trembling, in such sort as that he is afraid of euery thing, yea and

---

[27]   André du Laurens and trans. Richard Surphlet, *A Discourse of the Preservation of the Sight* (London, 1599), 128–9.

[28]   Ibid., 129.

[29]   Ibid., 125–6.

[30]   See Sigmund Freud, "On Narcissism: An Introduction," in *Standard Edition of the Complete Psychological Works of Sigmund Freud*, vol. 14 (London: Hogarth Press, 1961), 67–104. For contemporary feminist challenges to this reading, see, especially, "The Lesbian Phallus and the Morphological Imaginary," in Judith Butler, *Bodies That Matter: On the Discursive Limits of "Sex"* (New York: Routledge, 1993); E.A. Grosz, *Volatile Bodies: Toward a Corporeal Feminism* (Bloomington: Indiana University Press, 1994), 77–78.

maketh himself a terror vnto himself, as the beast which looketh himself in a glasse; he would runne away and cannot goe, he goeth always sighing, troubled with the hicket, and with an vnseperable sadness, which oftentimes turneth into dispayre; he is always disquieted both in bodie and spirit, he is subiect to watchfulness, which doth consume him on the one side, and vnto sleepe, which tormenteth him on the other ... . To conclude, hee is become a sauadge creature, haunting the shadowed places, suspicious, solitarie, enemie to the Sunne, and one whom nothing can please, but onely discontentment, which forget vnto it selfe a thousand false and vaine imaginations.[31]

Readers will recognize in this picture the mold after which so many iconic Renaissance melancholics appear to be fashioned, from the solitary Romeo and melancholy Jaques to the ghosted Hamlet who will not cast his "knighted color off," feeling that he is "too much in the sun" (1.2.67–8). The ironies of the melancholic diagnosis of each of these literary figures may be partially illuminated by the dogmatic purposes to which Du Laurens puts this portraiture, calling it a warning "Against Atheists which think the soule to be mortal." For Du Laurens, the melancholic's gloom constitutes a rejection of God's light and of man's obligation to live in His image. This rejection renders man a brute. However, he warns the reader not to mistake the transformative power of melancholy to have any "essential" effect on the soul: "I would not haue thee (O thou Atheist whosoeuer thou art) hereupon to conclude that the soule of man suffereth any thing in his essence ... it is neuer altered or changed, neither can it suffer any thing, it is his instrument that is euill affected." Like the sun that may be clouded or eclipsed, the soul is never diminished by its melancholic obscuring.[32] Herein lies the paradox of melancholy for early modern spiritual physicians. Melancholy is a diagnostic sign of the present health and not of the ultimate fate of the soul, but the relationship of the one to the other is nonetheless, at the very least, a quasi-instrumental one. Melancholy may only be a passing shadow but its temporary darkness may lead to deadly sin, and to the sin of despair especially.

Against this view, which we see distributed throughout the literature of early modern spiritual hygiene, Burton seems to suggest that melancholy tenderizes the spirit and does so specifically through a torrent of fears that may be viewed as extremes of compassion rather than false projections of a diseased imagination. The dyspeptic, hypochondriacal "hicket" or hiccup to which Du Laurens's melancholic is disposed becomes, in Burton's analysis, a more prominent feature of melancholy in general. While the partitions and divisions of the *Anatomy* maintain a traditional, etiological distinction for hypochondria, Burton repeatedly rejects the feasibility of isolating hypochondria from other types of melancholy.[33] At the

---

[31]   Du Laurens, *A Discourse of the Preservation of the Sight*, 82.

[32]   Ibid.

[33]   "It is a hard matter, I confesse, to distinguish these three Species [of head, body, and hypochondriacal melancholy] ... . I could give instance of some that have had all three kindes, *semel and simul* & some successively. So that I conclude of our melancholy Species, as many polititians doe of their pure Formes of Commonwealths, Monarchies,

same time, he suggests both a kind of ubiquity and special status associated with this form of the disease, intimating that the universal melancholy that the *Anatomy* treats is emblematized by the windy one figured so prominently on the engraved title page. In this image (Figure 2.1), Hypocondriacus sits at the edge of a hard wooden chair. Apothecary pots lie at his feet and glass vessels line the shelf above him, with medical recipes strung beneath them. His posture, head in hand, mimics both the reclining figure of Democritus as he is pictured in the top and center frame (see Figure I.2) and the more recognizable image of Melancholy in Dürer's famous engraving (Figure 2.2), but Burton's Hypocondriacus wears a gentler expression than Dürer's winged scholar. She sits low to the ground surrounded by objects and symbols of occult and humanistic study. Her clenched fist supports a head transfixed by thought, the intensity of which is suggested by a fierce and distant gaze. In her other hand, Dürer's Melancholy holds a compass with which she is drawing an unseen object. Burton's Hypocondriacus, by contrast, appears to be burdened by thought into inaction. He props his head up with a soft, open hand, fingers pressed into his temple and brow, while the other hand is set akimbo. The verse "Argument of the Frontispiece" explains:

> Hypocondriacus *leanes on his arme,*
> *Winde in his side doth him much harme,*
> *And troubles him full sore God knows,*
> *Much paine he hath and many woes.*
> *About him pottes and glasses lye,*
> *Newly brought from the Apothecary,*
> *This* Saturnes *aspects signify,*
> *You see them portraid in the skye.* (1:lxii)

We will return to these pots and glasses later in this chapter in our examination of the delusions of brittleness associated with these objects (and will consider the windy theme of Burton's melancholy in Chapter 4). What warrants noting here is that Burton casts Hypocondriacus as the literal bearer of the sign of Saturn, the very model of melancholy with all its pains and woes.

While he maintains a nosological separation between hypochondriasis and the "Terrors and Affrights" associated more broadly with melancholy, Burton explains that the fearful melancholic is unable to experience the pains of others or the horrors of the world as separate from his or her own body:

> Many cannot endure to see a wound opened, but they are offended; a man executed, or labour of any fearfull disease, as possession, Apoplexies, one bewitched: or if they read by chance of some terrible thing, the symptomes alone of such a disease, or that which they dislike, they are instantly troubled in minde,

---

Aristocracies, Democracies, are most famous in contemplation, but in practise they are temperate and usually mixt … . In such obscurity therefore … how difficult a thing is it to treat of severall kindes apart; to make any certainty or distinction among so many casualties, distractions, when seldome two men shall be like affected *per omnia*?" (1:170–1).

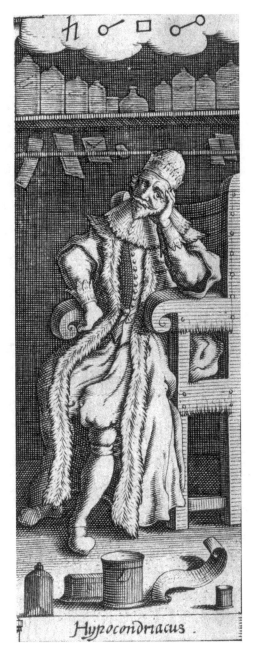

Figure 2.1   Detail of "Hypocondriacus." Christoph Le Blon, engraved title
page to Robert Burton, *The Anatomy of Melancholy*, 1632 (first
printed in the 1628 edition). Division of Rare and Manuscript
Collections, Cornell University Library.

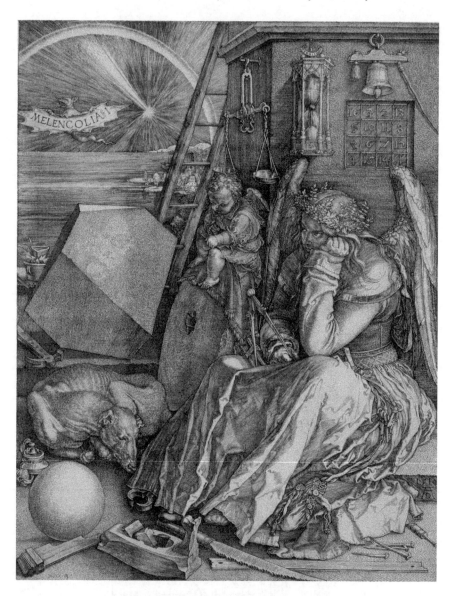

Figure 2.2   Albrecht Dürer, "Melencolia I," 1514. Princeton University
               Art Museum.

agast, ready to apply it to themselves, they are as much disquieted, as if they had
seene it: or were so affected themselves. *Hecatas sibi videntur somniare*, they
dreame and continually thinke of it. (1:335)

The power of "conceit" to move a body into a state of physical distress is proof
not only of the body's ability to contract disease by power of the imagination
but to move thereby from affliction to health. In other words, it is through this
same capacity to receive impression that melancholia can be abated: "As some
are so molested by phantasie; so some againe by Fancy alone, and a good conceit,
are as easily recovered" (1:253). In everyday experience of this phenomenon,
Burton tells us, we see "Tooth-ache, Gout, Falling-sicknesse, biting of a mad
Dog, and many such maladies, cured by Spells, Words, Characters and Charmes"
(1:253–4). Like Thomas Browne and Francis Bacon, Burton attributes these
transformations not to the inherent "vertue in such Charmes, or Cures, but a strong
conceit and opinion alone."[34] However, unlike Browne and Bacon, he does so
not to demystify transformations by force of imagination but to marvel at their
extraordinary efficacy.[35]

The same powers of the imagination that communicate symptoms from one
body to another are responsible for the more spectacular fantasies of transformation
of form, shape, sex, species, and substance:

> *Agrippa supposeth* ... that some are turned to wolves, from Men to Women, and
> women againe to Men (which is constantly beleved) to the same Imagination:
> or from Men to Asses, Dogges, or any other shapes; Wierus ascribes all those
> famous transformations, to Imagination; that, in *Hydrophobia* they seeme to
> see the picture of a Dog, still in their water, that melancholy men and sicke
> men, conceave so many phantasticall visions, apparitions to themselves, and
> have such absurd apparitions, as that they are Kings, Lords, Cocks, Beares,
> Apes, Owls; that they are heavy, light, transparent, great and little, senselesse
> and dead ... can bee imputed to naught else, but to a corrupt, false and violent
> Imagination. (1:252)

Burton's use of the word "false" here underscores the discrepancy between
external cause and the concrete, physiological manifestation of "imaginary"
effect. The imagination may be violent and "false," but its effects are indisputable.

---

[34]   See Thomas Browne, *Pseudodoxia Epidemica, or, Enquiries into very many
received tenents and commonly presumed truths* (London, 1646), 44; 327; Francis Bacon,
Sylva Sylvarum, or, A Naturall Historie in Ten Centuries (London, 1627), chap. 10.

[35]   I am not arguing, as earlier historiographers have, that these writers were dismissive
of the powers of the imagination. Rather, along with Julie Solomon and Todd Butler I
see them (Bacon especially) as profoundly interested in the study of these powers for the
sake of their better control and manipulation. See Julie Robin Solomon, *Objectivity in the
Making: Francis Bacon and the Politics of Inquiry* (Baltimore: Johns Hopkins University
Press, 2002), 44; Todd Wayne Butler, *Imagination and Politics in Seventeenth-Century
England* (Burlington, VT: Ashgate, 2008), 17–18.

So-called "normal" transmissions and reception of bodily sensation (the curious way in which we catch a yawn, or clench our jaws at the thought of sour foods or the sound of a scraped plate) are but quotidian examples along a spectrum of behaviors that illustrate the ways in which we communicate and transfer sensorial and somatic experience:

> So diversely doth this phantasie of ours affect, turne and winde, so imperiously command our bodies, which, as another *Proteus, or a Camelion, can take all shapes; and is of such force* (as *Ficinus* addes) *that it can worke upon others as well as our selves.* How can otherwise bleare-eyes in one man, cause the like affection in another? Why doth one man's yawning, make another yawne? One mans pissing provoke a second many times to doe the like? Why doth scraping of trenchers offend a third, or hacking of flies? (1:254)

The infectiousness of bodily impulse and sensation serves as proof of the body's capacity to be moved involuntarily to mimic other bodies: The sight of watery eyes will make one's eyes water; the sound of a person urinating will provoke the urge in another. The perceived symptom infects the perceiver with the impulse to reproduce observed behavior (rubbing one's "bleare-eyes," urinating, scratching), regardless of the authenticity of the example. The witness' eyes will water, his bladder will ache, and his skin will bristle at phantom flies. The observer will be moved to respond at the sight of a performance that might well be feigned or misperceived. Such is the mimetic force of the imagination.

These seemingly innocuous examples of "infectious" behaviors serve as the basis for far more spectacular transformations of the body under the persuasion of the imagination, which can be impressed upon by other bodies. Burton goes on to consider (in the same vein and of a kind) the influence of "forcible imagination" upon carcasses that bleed in the presence of their murderers, the "fascination" of children by witches, the alteration of climate, and the ability to "move bodies from their places" (1:254). Rather than caution the reader against the vulnerability of the body to such influence by proxy, however, Burton is clearly stirred by the body's capacity to be "moved" from without. On the one hand, he de-emphasizes the verifiability of these extraordinary occurrences, citing them as varieties of popular belief whose implausibility is outweighed by the good sense it registers. On the other hand, he leaves the reader with a lasting impression of the meteorological and cosmological powers of the imagination, a faculty capable of changing the weather and teleportation.[36] Suggestively, the subsection ends not with the horror of witches and corpses but with a kind of cosmic optimism that recalls both the Agrippan view of the powers of the imagination and the reformed Neoplatonism of Paracelsian medicine. Burton concludes that "this strong conceit or imagination"

---

[36]   Compare with Henricus Cornelius Agrippa, *Three Books of Occult Philosophy*, trans. John French (London, 1651), 65–6; Marsilio Ficino, *Platonic Theology*, ed. James Hankins and William R. Bowen, trans. Michael J.B. Allen and John Warden, vol. 6, I Tatti Renaissance Library (Cambridge, MA: Harvard University Press, 2001), chap. 13.

is not the corrupter of the senses and the seat of disorder, but rather our anchor to the stars, "*astrum hominis*, and the rudder of this our ship," even as he cautions that this ship, "overborne by phantasie," is "often overturned" (1:254).[37]

Burton returns to the indisputable physiological effects of the power of the imagination in preface to his discussion of "precendent" causes of melancholic fear and sorrow. He gives Petrus Bayerus's example of a person who may walk across a low bridge without any trouble. But, he says, "*if the same planke be laid over some deepe water, in steed of a bridge, hee is vehemently moved, and 'tis nothing but his imagination*, forma cadendi impressâ, *to which his other members and faculties obey*" (1:420).[38] The glands and organs take their cue from the imagination, not an "outside cause." By this logic, Burton argues that the inward or perceived experience trumps the very idea of an objective one for the melancholic. The distinction between inward and outward, objective and subjective, itself does not hold, and with it collapses the clinical utility of defining melancholy as "*a kinde of dotage without a feaver, having for his ordinary companions, feare, and sadnesse, without any apparent occasion*" (1:162).[39]

The comparison between the man who walks over a plank suspended high above deep water and the other who only thinks he does (when unbeknownst to him he is quite safe) is used to illustrate the material irrelevance of discerning true from "false" causes of melancholic fear:

> Yea, but you inferre, that such men have a just cause to feare, a true object of feare, so have melancholy men an inward cause, a perpetuall fume and darknesse, causing feare, griefe, suspition, which they carry with them, an object which cannot bee removed; but stickes as close, and is as inseparable as a shadow to a body. (1:420)

The ineffectiveness of rational tactics for the dissuasion of irrational fears renders them unethical; as he says: "You may as well bid him that is sicke of an ague, not to bee adry; or him that is wounded, not to feele paine." The final phrase is particularly poignant in its ambiguity as to whether Burton refers here to physical or imaginary wounds. The point, of course, is that it doesn't matter, and the

---

[37]   Burton refers the reader here to a long list of contemporary authorities on the malignant powers of the imagination: Johann Weyer, Francisco de Vallés, Marcellus Donati, Levinus Lemnius, Girolamo Cardano, Cornelius Agrippa, Phillip Camerarius, Hieronymus Nymann, André du Laurens, and Thomas Feyens. We may glean a sense of Burton's resistance to and departure from this more phobic approach in his comment that Feyens's resounding denunciation of the powers of the imagination is "*instar omnium*," and so may stand for all the others on the subject.

[38]   Pietro Biero, to whose *Tractatus de peste* Burton refers in this passage (5:59).

[39]   As the Clarendon editors point out, this is Surphlet's translation of Du Laurens (4:195). Along with Du Laurens, Burton cites Nicolas Le Pois, Marcello Donati, Donato Altomare, Leonarto Giachini, Muhammad ibn Zakariyā Rāzī, Francisco de Vallés, and Leonhard Fuchs as examples of authorities who give this "common definition" of melancholy, "approved by most" (1:162).

ethical implications of this for the way in which we are to view melancholy and "irrational" suffering are, as we will see, quite profound.

III. Delusional Melancholy and Spiritual Hygiene

Burton's positive appraisal of the sympathetic powers of the melancholic imagination truly comes into focus in comparison with appraisals by contemporary medical writers such as André du Laurens. While the two may both be said to share a common goal of alleviating the stigma associated with melancholy, they do so in quite opposite ways. Burton elaborates the uniquely transformative powers associated with the melancholic imagination, whereas Du Laurens takes an approach more typical of the hygienists, undermining the notion of melancholic exceptionality and arguing instead that the melancholic's bizarre fixations are merely intensifications of common concupiscible and irascible (desiring and repudiating) passions. The ambitious melancholic who dreams of being a king and the melancholic lover who "will do nothing but plot the purchase of his loue" are examples, for Du Laurens, of melancholics whose behaviors, while "irrational," are motivated by self-preservation or promotion. Nonetheless, Du Laurens concedes that these irrational conceits have a motive power of intent that may be quite effective. Like a huntsman who visualizes the fall of the beast before he looses his arrow, "the melancholike person, by the forwardness of his imagination, doth oftentimes see that which must come to passe, as though it were present before him."[40] Those fixed ideas that accompany appetitive desires or self-preserving repulsions therefore constitute a normative category of melancholic fantasy. On the other hand, fantasies that do not support manifestly logical appetites or aversions are deemed abnormal or "strange imaginations." It is to this latter, aberrant category that Du Laurens ascribes the list of hypochondriacal delusions passed down from antiquity with which we are concerned.

Having "described all the accidents which haunt those who are properly to be tearmed melancholike persons," Du Laurens claims that it "behoueth (to the end I may somewhat delight the reader) to set down some examples of such as haue had the most fantasticall and foolish imaginations of all others."[41] These "improper" melancholics are designated as a separate type and set forth in their idiosyncratic impropriety expressly for the reader's delight. He begins with Galen's case of the "melancholike man which tooke himself to bee a pitcher, and prayed all that came to see him, not to come neere vnto him, least they should dash him in peeces." The list continues in close keeping with classical catalogues: "Another imagined himselfe to be a cocke, and did crow when he heard other cockes crow, and bet his armes, as the cockes doe clap their wings. Another melancholike man was greatly perplexed in himself, fearing that Atlas in the end would be wearie of bearing vp heauen, and so might let it fall down vpon him." But Du Laurens's chief interest lies in the "cunning" by which such unusual conceits were remedied:

---

[40]   Du Laurens, *A Discourse of the Preservation of the Sight*, 98.
[41]   Ibid., 101–2.

Aetius writeth of one, which thought himselfe to haue no head, and did speake it openly euery where, that there was one which had cut it off for his tyrranous dealings. This man was cured very cunningly, by the skil of a Phisition named *Philotimus*. For he caused a skull of yron waying very heauie to bee put vpon his head: and he thereupon crying that his head did grieue him, was by and by confirmed by all them that stood by, which also cried: then you haue a head; which hee acknowledged by this meanes, and so was freed from his false imagination.[42]

In addition to Aetius, the story of Philotimus' ingenious cure is mentioned by the sixth-century physician Alexander of Tralles and the medieval Arab physician Ishaq ibn Imran,[43] but the insinuation that the cure takes its effect at least in part through punishment appears to be an innovation of the Renaissance hygienists, as does the increasingly suspicious view of these conceits and their association with spiritual melancholy and despair.[44]

The Swiss professor of medicine Felix Platter gives what might be the least sympathetic Renaissance portrayal of the classical conceits associated with melancholy, which he, like Aretaeus, defines as mental alienation and fear without cause: "For they cannot adduce any certain cause or grief or fear except a trivial one or a false opinion which they have conceived as a result of disturbed apprehension."[45] The first and most prominent example Platter gives of such derangement is, tellingly, spiritual anguish: those who "persuade themselves that they are damned, abandoned by god, and are not predestined, even though they had been religious and faithful" all their lives. Platter calls "this frightful melancholy, which often drives men to despair," the most common form of the disease, lamenting that he has been "very much impeded" in his own efforts to cure those afflicted. Interestingly, Platter does not distinguish spiritual melancholy from other varieties of melancholy by name. He instead seems to suggest that this changeable disease has many forms that are rather like moods of a single disorder. All those who suffer melancholy are therefore, by Platter's account, wont to experience despair and its concomitant ideations of extreme violence, such as his own patients report: "When seized by this [despair], they have felt themselves driven toward blaspheming God ... toward laying violent hands on themselves, killing their husbands or wives or children or neighbors or rulers."[46] These outbursts are not motivated by jealousy or envy "toward them, whom they

---

42   Ibid., 101.

43   Ephesus and Pormann, *On Melancholy*.

44   See Du Laurens, *A Discourse of the Preservation of the Sight*, 101–2.

45   See Felix Platter, *Praxeos seu de cognoscendis praedicendis, praecauendis, curandisque, affectibus homini incommodantibus* (Basel, 1602), 100–101. English translation from Oskar Diethelm and Thomas F. Heffernan, "Felix Platter and Psychiatry," *Journal of the History of the Behavioral Sciences* 1, no. 1 (1965): 15.

46   Oskar Diethelm and Thomas F. Heffernan, "Felix Platter and Psychiatry," *Journal of the History of the Behavioral Sciences* 1, no. 1 (1965): 15.

rather fondly love," but rather from an "involuntary compulsion" that is all the more terrible for its apparent dispassion.[47] At the same time, this "involuntary compulsion" is associated with extreme conscience and the conviction of one's exclusion not only from the grace of God but the good opinion of one's worldly superiors. Platter lists side by side the melancholic who fears he has lost God's favor with those who fear they have lost favor with human authorities: "They falsely imagine they are in bad grace with princes and magistrates and that they have done something wrong and are being summoned to punishment."

It is highly suggestive that Platter's discussion of the classical melancholic delusions appears here in the immediate context of his account of spiritual melancholy as a deficit of social confidence and resilience. Platter explains that whereas some melancholic types imagine their social or spiritual reprobation, "Others deceive themselves with some other nonsense conceived in and impressed on their minds":

> like the man who thought he had become an earthenware vessel and gave way to everyone and everything he met, fearing that he would collide with them. Thus some believe they are turned into brute animals. Likewise, someone who thought he had a long nose did not rid himself of that opinion until a surgeon by pretending to cut and then showing him some flesh deceived him into believing that he had amputated part of the nose. Likewise, there was a woman who was remarkably upset over being obliged to put her clothes on every day and take them off again. Another woman suffered these symptoms whenever she thought that her husband would take another wife after her death. Others talk foolishly that they have devoured serpents or frogs and are breading them alive in their bodies, or have other delusions; they talk foolishly of many marvelous things. With great pity and amazement, and sometimes not without laughter, I have listened to their disturbed and painful narrations of these things.[48]

In Platter's description, delusional melancholics are as changeable as their conceits are absurd. They sometimes "show the marks of sadness and fear with an abundance of continual tears," but at other times may be "indolent and quiet," seeking out solitude and "flee[ing] the company of men." Tearful melancholics may turn into raving lycanthropes "if out of hatred of light they seek the darkness and the forests and hide in coverts and caves (as the sacred writings testify about Nabuchodnosor)." Whereas for Burton the diversity of kinds and the commonness of the disease underscores the universality of melancholy as a human experience, this same diversity renders it more horrible for Platter, who describes melancholy as a nefarious form of possession that "does not produce the same effects in all" but keeps "a continual hold on those whom they have invaded" in periods of "remission" and "aggravation" alike.[49]

---

[47] Ibid.

[48] Ibid.

[49] Ibid. Curiously, Platter distinguishes hypochondria, with its perpetual and local pains in the region below the ribs, as a disease apart because those who suffer it know themselves

Like Platter, the English hygienist Thomas Walkington emphasizes the mercurial or changeable quality of melancholy, but draws in so doing on the ancient view of the disease as a kind of possession that could be divine in origin but is more likely to be demonic:

> The melancholick man is said of the wise to be *aut Deus aut Daemon*, either angel of heauen or a fiend of hell: for in whoseoeuer this humour hath dominion, the soul is either wrapt vp into an *Elysium* and a paradise of blesse by a heauenly contemplation, or into a direfull hellish purgatory by a cynicall meditation ... .[50]

Beyond this frightful polarity, those born under Saturn are disposed to illness and premature death: "leaden, lumpish, or an extreame cold and dire nature, which cuts in twaine the threed of his life long before it be spun." Walkington's depiction of the "unfortunate" melancholic as the walking dead moreover suggests that their inanimateness portends damnation: "Hee may rightly say with *Hecuba*, though she spoke of a liuing death ... I am dead before the appointed time of death."[51]

This ominous account of melancholy might seem somewhat surprising, given that Walkington at first appears to praise melancholy, citing Plato, Seneca, and Aulus Gellius on the popular association between melancholy and genius, but he goes on to call this association a fallacy:

> They conclude that melancholike men are endowed with the rarest wittes of all: but how shallow this their reason is, he that hath waded into any depth of reason may easily discerne: They mought prooue an Asse also of all other creatures most melancholike, and which will bray as if hee were horne madde to bee exceeding witty, they might say this as well, that because *Saturne* is the slowest Planet of all so their wits are the slowest of all.[52]

Like Shakespeare's Claudius, Walkington is less concerned with the melancholic's reputed genius than with the inscrutable and assumedly malignant intent that lurks behind the meditative, melancholic pose: "Oftentimes the melancholicke man by his contemplatiue facultie by his assiduitie of sad and serious meditation is a brocher of dangerous matchiauellisme an inventor of stratagems."[53] Whereas melancholy is scorned for its association with secrecy and scheming, sanguinity is favored not for its transparency but its decorum. The blush, for instance, becomes a courtesy that acquiesces to the demand for affective legibility that

---

to be truly ill: "*Est & species illius alia quam Hypochondria cam melancholiam à loco affecto denominant: in qua accidentia enarrata saepius, saepeque eodem die intermittunt, rursumque repetunt & qui ea laborant, quoties ad se redeunt, secus atque alii (qui nisi aliud quid accedat, de capitis tantum dolore, vel grauedine aliquando conqueruntur) se vere aegrotare agnoscunt*" (*Praxeos*, 100–101).

[50] Thomas Walkington, *The Optick Glasse of Humors* (London, 1607), 64v.

[51] Ibid., 65r–65v.

[52] Ibid., 66r–66v.

[53] Ibid., 66v.

melancholic pallor seems to refuse.[54] Walkington associates the sanguine humor with spontaneity and social grace:

> But for a nimble dextericall, smirke, praegnant, extemporary inuention, for a suddain ... pleasant conceit, a comicall ieast, a witty bourd, for a smug neat stile, for delightsome sentences, garnished phrases, quaint and gorgeous eloqution, for an astounding Rhetoricall veine, for a liuely grace in deliuery, hee can neuer bee aequiualent with a sanguine complection, which is the paragon of all.[55]

The sanguine speaker's "gorgeous eloquence" is clearly not "natural." It suggests, rather, the agreeability of one who proves able to assimilate rhetorical training into the art of pleasing and delighting others.

We will return to consider the mystification of sanguinity and social and spiritual grace in the final section of this chapter. I raise it here to note how the melancholic person is seen to transgress against certain rules of sociability whose infraction may help to explain the pleasure taken in the stories of their "merry" correction. These ancient examples are related as jokes that ridicule the earnestness and foolishness of the deluded:

> There was one possest with this humour, that tooke a strong conceit, that he was changed into an earthen vessell, who earnestly intreated his friends in any case not to come neare him, lest peraduenture with their jostling of him, he might be shakt or crusht to peeces. Another sadly fixing his eye on the ground, and hurckling with his heade to his shoulders, foolishlie imagined that *Atlas* being faint and weary with his burthen, would shortly let the heauens fall vpon his head and break his cragge.[56]

The denouement of these jokes in both Walkington and Du Laurens's accounts comes with the revelation of the physician's good guile, his ability to cure by turning the melancholic's conceit against itself. A doctor cures a woman who is convinced she has swallowed a snake by giving her an emetic and then surreptitiously tossing serpents into a basin as she vomits. A young scholar "taken with a strange imagination" that "his nose was so gret and so long, as that he durst not stirre out of his place, least he should dash it against something" is cured by feigned surgery in the following way: the doctor,

> Hauing taken a great peece of flesh, and holding it in his hand secretly, assured him that hee would heale him by and by, and that he must needs take away

---

[54]   In his *Disputatiuncula de taedio*, Erasmus similarly associates pallor with anger: "Eagerness goes with love only in the same way that pallor goes with anger, blushing with shame, laughter with joy, tears with sorrow," but he emphasizes that these "are outward signs, not causes, and are extrinsic to the emotions they betoken" ("A Short Debate Concerning the Distress, Alarm, and Sorrow of Jesus," in *Collected Works of Erasmus*, ed. J.W. O'Malley, vol. 70 [Toronto, ON: University of Toronto Press, 1998], 48).

[55]   Walkington, *The Optick Glasse of Humors*, 66v.

[56]   Ibid., 69v.

this great nose: and so vpon the suddaine pinching his nose a little, and cutting the peece of flesh which he had ... made him beleeue that his great nose was cut away.[57]

Du Laurens mentions that in some severe cases of melancholy, where patients "thinke themselues dead, and would not eate anything ... Phisitions haue used this sleight" to cure them:

> They cause some one or other seruant to lie neere vnto the sicke partie, and hauing taught him to counterfeite himself dead, yet not to forsake his meate, but to eate and swallow it, when it was put into his mouth: and thus by this craftie deuise, they perswaded the melancholike man, that the dead did eate as well as those which are aliue.[58]

Walkington relates a version of this story (one of the most frequently cited classical examples of delusional melancholy and its imaginary cure) with much added detail, coupling it with many more of his own examples of those who imagine they have been transformed into fragile, inanimate, and easily extinguished objects such as the "snuffe" of a candle.[59]

In Walkington's retailing, these cases become increasingly suggestive of a spiritual melancholy whose malignancy is thinly veiled beneath the veneer of comedy in which they are cast. We see this in his anecdote of the melancholic who mistakes his worldly wealth for spiritual riches and imperils his immortal soul as a consequence of his greed:

> Another vpon his death bed, greatly groned and was vexed within himself aboue measure with a phantasie, who being demaunded why he was so sorrowfull and bidden withal to cast his mind vpon the heauens; answered that he was well content to die, and would gladly be at heauen; but he durst not trauaile that way, by reason of a many theeues which lay in wait & ambush for him in the middle region, among the cloudes.[60]

Walkington appears to be drawing on antipuritanical stereotypes in this depiction of the melancholy pietist who jealously guards his soul in the same way that a

---

[57] Du Laurens, *A Discourse of the Preservation of the Sight*, 101–2. See similar descriptions of these two examples in Goulart (*Admirable and Memorable Histories*, 375) attributed to and based closely on the versions given by Levinus Lemnius. See *The Touchstone of Complexions*, trans. Thomas Newton (London, 1576), 150v–151r.

[58] Du Laurens, *A Discourse of the Preservation of the Sight*, 102.

[59] Garzoni gives the following version of the candle-snuff delusion, which he includes in a lengthy list of "modern examples": "But what shall we say to *Nicoletto* of Gattia, who possessed with this indisposition of the braine, thought one day that he was become the snuffe of a candle, and therefore he willed euery one to blowe vpon him before, behind, and on each side, fearing he shoulde burne so much while he were all consumed?" (*The Hospitall of Incurable Fooles*, 18).

[60] Walkington, *The Optick Glasse of Humors*, 70v.

fool guards his gold. The analogy underscores the murkiness of the proprietary relationship between the soul and the ensouled in predestinarian theology and seems to warn of the potential abuse whereby a person may "covet" their soul with over-preciseness. Other "merry" examples in Walkington's account seem to relate the punishment of a spiritual pride that manifests in fantasies of monstrous aggrandizement. The story of the scholar's imaginary monstrous nose is given a much more violent rendering in Walkington's account than in Du Laurens's: "They rased his skinne with a rasour till the bloud thrilled downe, and whiles hee cried out vehemently for the paine, the Physicion with a jirke twitcht it from his face, and threw it away."[61] Walkington follows this anecdote with another that seems to allegorize the punishment of pride in the story of a man who thought himself dead and would not eat.[62] He glosses this ancient example with another version of the tale, describing a patient who refused food because he thought he was a god and was fed only incense and aromas until he confessed his hunger and frailty.[63]

The hubristic fantasies in Walkington's catalogue contrast sharply with the conceits of fragility that characterize other hypochondriacal delusions that Walkington is obliged by tradition to include in his survey. He curates these by emphasizing their bathetic rather than pathetic nature, dwelling on cases such as the man with imaginary glass buttocks who "neuer durst sitte downe to meat, lest hee should haue broken his crackling hinderparts, nor euer durst walk abroad lest the glazier should haue caught hold on him & haue used him for quarreles and paines."[64] He reserves the chief and last place in his list "of all conceited famous fooles" for the man "that choos'd rather to die than let his urine go," being persuaded that he would unleash a deluge that would drown the world. This story, he says, is "most worthy to bee canoniz'd in the chronicles of our memory":

> They inuented this quirke, to wit, to set an old ruinous house forthwith on fire, the Physicions caused the bels to bee rung backeward, and entreated a many to runne to the fire, presently one of the chiefe inhabitants, of the town, came running post hast to the sickeman, and let him vnderstand the whole matter, shewing him the fire: and withal desired him all fauours very earnestly and with counterfeit teares to let go his vrine and extinguish this great flame, which otherwise would bring a great indamagement to the whole towne, and that it will burne also the house vp where hee did dwell: whoe presently not perceiuing the

---

[61]   Ibid., 70v–71r.

[62]   The most elaborate version of this tale that I have been able to find in the contemporary literature is in Milles's *Treasurie* (477–8). On the elusiveness of Milles's sources, both for his plot details and his note that the story was performed as a play for Charles IX, see Karen L. Edwards, "Thomas Browne and the Absurdities of Melancholy," in *"A Man Very Well Studyed": New Contexts for Thomas Browne*, ed. Kathryn Murphy and Richard Todd (Leiden: Brill, 2008), 215–17.

[63]   Walkington adds another example of prideful melancholic delusion in a tale borrowed from Athenaeus of a doctor who mistook himself for God on account of his ability to heal the sick (*The Optick Glasse of Humors*, 71v).

[64]   Ibid., 72r.

guile, and moued by the mans pittifull lament and outcry, sent forth an aboundant streame of vrine, and so was recouered of his maladie.[65]

The anecdote recalls Rabelais's depiction of a young and truant Gargantua who climbs a steeple to piss on the Parisians below, unleashing such a torrent "that he drowned two hundred and sixty thousand, four hundred and eighteen, besides the women and little children."[66] The tale of the man who held his water reflects contradictory impulses to self-abandonment and self-restraint, which suggests that part of what we are seeing in the hygienists' accounts of melancholic conceit is a reaction to the moralization of hygiene and physiological etiquette in early modernity. Whereas the unreformed Gargantua "dunged, pissed, spewed, belched, cracked, yawned, spitted, coughed, vexed, sneezed, and snotted himself like an archdeacon" the man who held his water would have literally preferred to die than so transgress.[67]

The hygienists present their catalogues of melancholic conceits as momentary reprieves from the heaviness of their subjects. As such, they are necessarily cut short. Walkington concludes his excursus on the delusions of melancholy, following his relation of the story of the man who held his water, by remarking that "divers other pleasant examples are recited of ancient writers: but our short breathing pen hastens to the races end."[68] Burton will pantomime this conventional use of the *occupatio* by concluding his own list of melancholic conceits with the protest: "*Sed abundè fabularum audivimus*" (1:403).[69] Unlike the hygienists, Burton does not return to his designated purpose but concludes the subsection there and then, leaving the reader to meditate not only on the contents of his list but the conspicuousness of this uncharacteristic full stop, the strangeness that Burton, who typically undercuts the gravity of his source texts with humor and levity, is here profound where they are jocund.

Another important difference between Burton's treatment of these conceits and those of his contemporaries is that Burton calls them products of mixed-humor melancholy, "the severall combinations of these foure humours, or spirits" (1:402). We might, considering the prominence of hypochondria in the frontispiece and its explanatory poem, regard them as the very emblems of Burton's *omnium gatherum*, his summa on the human melancholic condition. Burton's discussion of hypochondriacal melancholy seems at first to return to the more neutral tone of the classical accounts but it is distinguished by a profound sense of pathos conveyed

---

[65]   Ibid., 72r–72v.

[66]   François Rabelais, *Five Books of the Lives, Heroic Deeds and Sayings of Gargantua and His Son Pantagruel*, trans. Thomas Urquhart and Peter Motteux (London: A.H. Bullen, 1904), 61.

[67]   Ibid. On Rabelais and the discourse of hygiene, see Michel Jeanneret, *A Feast of Words: Banquets and Table Talk in the Renaissance* (Chicago: University of Chicago Press, 1991).

[68]   Walkington, *The Optick Glasse of Humors*, 72v.

[69]   "But we have heard quite enough of such stories" (5:50).

in part by its lyricism and in part by the suggestive way in which he renders them familiar to the reader. The delusional melancholics, as he describes them, exhibit inherently recognizable fears about their own imagined vulnerability or, worse, invulnerability. Some suffer imagined heaviness, others complain of unbearable lightness. Some cannot feel their own heads and there are those who feel so light and untethered to the earth that heavy irons must be set to their feet. He presents a slew of dysmorphic fantasies of great size and diminution, strength and weakness:

> One thinks himselfe a giant, another a dwarfe; one is heavy as lead, another is light as a feather. *Marcellus Donatus* … makes mention out of *Seneca*, of one *Seneccio*, a rich man, *that thought himselfe and everything else he had, great: great wife, great horses, could not abide little things, but would have great pots to drinke in, great hose, and great shooes bigger than his feet.* Like her in *Trallianus*, that supposed *shee could shake all the world with her finger,* and was afraid to clinch her hand together lest shee should crush the world like an apple in peeces: or him in *Galen,* that thought he was *Atlas,* and sustained heaven with his shoulders. Another thinks himselfe so little, that he can creepe into a mousehole: one feares heaven will fall on his head: a second is a cock; and such a one *Guianerius* saith hee saw at *Padua,* that would clap his hands together and crowe. Another thinkes he is a Nightingall, and therefore sings all the night long; another hee is all glasse, a pitcher, and will therefore let no body come neere him … and one amongst the rest of a Baker in *Ferrara,* that thought hee was composed of butter, and durst not sit in the sunne, or come neere the fire for feare of being melted: of another that thought hee was a case of leather, stuffed with winde. Some laugh, weepe, some are mad, some dejected, moped, in much agony, some by fits, others continuate, &c. Some have a corrupt eare, they thinke they heare musicke, or some hideous noise as their phantasie conceaves, corrupt eyes, some smelling: some one sense, some another. (1:402)

Burton assembles this congeries of somatic conceits by listing them through additive devices ("like her," "or him," "one," "a second"). These intensify the theme of resemblance as the passage progresses ("another" and "another") and resemblance turns to repetition of the same, with his "some … some … some" at the end. He amplifies melancholy through a *synathroesmus* that mimics the melancholic's assimilative imagination. The expansiveness of Burton's rhythm is contracted, however, by the morbid preoccupations of the delusions themselves. The melancholic hypochondriac attaches him- or herself to the object metonymically associated with mythological narratives of cosmic collapse: a stream of urine will unleash a second flood in an act of destruction that will undo the divine separation of the waters above and below; a woman's hand trembles for fear it will crush the world like that mortalizing apple offered up by the world's first lady.

The hygienists, by contrast, repeatedly draw attention away from the pathos of these figures to the manner by which their false conceits are "corrected." As in Du Laurens's account, in Walkington's version of the Philotimus story, the doctor treats the patient by fixing a "heauy steele cap" to his head, "which weighed so heauy and pincht him so grievously, that he cried amain his head ak't," at which the doctor triumphantly declared, "Thou hast then a heade belike."[70] The word "pinch" comes into use in the late sixteenth century as a synonym for suffering imposed or inflicted on a subordinate, as in Prospero's oppressive pinching of his slave, Caliban.[71] It also appears regularly in Protestant devotional writing to describe the pangs of conscience.[72] The hygienist's mocking tone implies that the melancholic hypochondriac is unworthy of the reader's compassion. On the one hand, these narratives about pinching cures seem to offer the reader a kind of smug pleasure or satisfaction in the meting of an imaginary cure for an imagined disease. At the same time, the appeal of these cures seems to lie less in their punitive than obliquely compassionate character. A certain care is shown in the physician's willingness to condescend to his patient's irrational conceit. If only by pretense, the physicians in these stories acknowledge the phantom disease and are thereby able to resolve its pinch. Such indulgence of "false belief" was unavailable to those in whose charge spiritual melancholia and cases of conscience fell. The discrepancy between the compassionate unreason used to treat the so-called "natural" melancholic suffering from a deemed physical ailment and the rational dissuasions employed to console the spiritual melancholic is precisely what these accounts of delusional melancholy bring into focus, and they do so to such a degree as to fundamentally unsettle the distinction between physical and spiritual melancholy, despite the efforts of spiritual hygienists to the contrary.[73]

Timothie Bright attempts to differentiate humoral melancholy from spiritual affliction in an effort to convince his "melancholick friend, M," that his symptoms do not prove his reprobation. "The minde," he says, "seemeth to be blame worthy: wherein it is blamelesse."[74] But the association between spiritual and physical melancholy is not so easily dissolved, not least because of the complex relationship between physical and divine spirit in late Renaissance faculty psychology. Bright distinguishes the blameless noncorporeal "minde" from the natural or physical spirits, which he calls "thinges corporall and earthly" that cause melancholy but,

---

[70]   Ibid., 70r. Walkington's list takes a more mocking tone as he recounts the tale of a man who "was constrained ... to pish among the strangers legges vnder the table" whenever he heard a lute played. He notes that this case belongs to the category of antipathetic delusions but includes it here before returning to examples of sympathetic (or mimetic) conceits that include: the man who thought he was made of butter, a king who came home from a bullfight convinced that he'd grown horns, and one who believed he was the "snuffe of a candle, wherefore he entreated the company about him to blow hard, lest he should chaunce to go out" (70r–70v).

[71]   *Oxford English Dictionary Online*, s.v. "pinch," v., I.4 and II.12, accessed November 19, 2012, http://www.oed.com/view/Entry/144068?rskey=PqiPRU&result=2& isAdvanced=false.

[72]   Ibid., II.11.b.

[73]   See Jeremy Schmidt, *Melancholy and the Care of the Soul: Religion, Moral Philosophy and Madness in Early Modern England* (Aldershot, UK: Ashgate, 2007), chap. 3.

[74]   Timothie Bright, *A Treatise of Melancholie* (London, 1586), 36.

being gross rather than divine, carry no prognosticating weight with regard to the fate of the soul.[75] At the same time, the physical spirits residing in the body are "an effectual, and pregnant substace" imbued with the spirit of God, and "bred in all thinges."[76] Bright labors to distinguish melancholy from conscience by differentiating their seats in the body. Conscience, he says, "first precedeth fro the mindes apprehension" and melancholy "from the humour." Finally, he argues that diseases of conscience are spiritual rather than physical less on etiological grounds than by method of treatment. Whereas "no medicine, no purgation, no cordiall" will "assure the afflicted soule," melancholic patients have recourse to simple and effective cures: "the vayne opened, neesing powder or bearefoote ministred."[77]

While Bright insists that there can be no physical help for cases of conscience, this in no way argues for their reprobation. On the contrary, he condemns those who "with a Stoicall prophanes of Atheisme" dismiss cases of conscience as mere melancholy and "skoffe at that kinde of affliction, against which they themselues labour to shut vp their hard heartes." Indeed, one finds the evidence of spiritual defect more readily in those who are rather too hard than soft, too thickly rather than thinly skinned. It shows an "obstinacie of stomach to beare out that whereof" those afflicted by conscience "tremble with horror," whereas a "pricked conscience" is the "refuge" of the soul. Those who lack such havens of feeling "passe ouer the sense with a desperat, & most flinty harted gallants of the world."[78] Such imperturbability contradicts the example of Christ, who "passed vnder these feares" of conscience and "sanctified them to his redeemed ... according to his example."[79] In other words, the torments of an afflicted conscience attest not only to God's loving husbandry but also to a pious mimicry of Christ's own melancholy that has been sanctified to the elect.

At the same time that melancholy is thus ennobled, the hygienists warn that it may imperil the soul as it "increaseth the terror of the afflicted minde, doubling the feare & discouragement, & shutteth vp the meanes of consolation," engendering "distrust of Gods mercy, & pardon."[80] Since the brain and heart are the "gates & enteraunce vnto the soule," says Bright, "As they be affected" they will either "ayd, or hinder" salvation. A distressed conscience that falls into "a melancholy state of body" closes itself off from consolation and "therby receiueth delay of restoring." Such imperviousness is contrasted with the open heart that invites "the grace of God, & his mercy, his comfortable spirit, & gracious fauor" to "restore the minde thus distressed which liethe equally open to the kind of cure, eue as it lay

---

[75]   Ibid.

[76]   Ibid., 45. This paradoxical representation of spirit as both earthly substance and divine emanation betrays the uneasy assimilation by Christian physicians of Greek accounts of *pneuma* that lay at the heart of Galenic medicine. See Introduction.

[77]   Ibid., 189.

[78]   Ibid., 188.

[79]   Ibid., 192.

[80]   Ibid., 196.

to the wound."[81] This ambivalent representation of the power of conscience that both wounds and cures is key to our understanding of the problem of melancholy in early modern England and the contradictory exhortations to sensitivity and insensitivity by which the faithful were instructed to avoid it.

IV. Unbearable Lightness

Because cases of conscience compounded by melancholy were seen to induce or aggravate fears and doubts associated with despair, both medical and spiritual physicians warned against adopting too severe habits and consistently urged their readers to cultivate a light and joyful demeanor. In fact, exhortations to temperance in the literature of spiritual hygiene moderated ascetic impulses almost as much as indulgence. One finds a curious homonymy in these treatises between divine grace and gracefulness expressed by an easy and cheerful manner of comportment. The Dutch physician Levinus Lemnius depicts the excessively severe personality as one that rejects the munificence of God's grace.[82] Such joylessness suggests ingratitude and pusillanimity that will show through in lapses not from temperance to license but in reversions from license to asceticism. Lemnius warns the reader not to be fooled by men who may put aside "their seueritie and Stoycal precysenes" long enough to "shak[e] their legges, and [foot] it as roundly as the best," only to recourse to their "Olde Nature, wanted manners, and accustomed grauity" when the "meery conuocation" is past.[83] Such recalcitrant, congenital hardness betrays a smallness of spirit thinly disguised by temporary and "counterfeit" cheer.

Lemnius's admonitions against severity find a close cousin in the soteriological reasoning of the *Thirty-Nine Articles*, which teaches that "curious and carnall persons have continually before theyr eyes, the sentence of Gods predestination," whereas those who "feele in themselves, the working of the spirite of Christe" are likely to comport themselves in such a way that reflects the sweetness, pleasantness, and "unspeakable comfort of this doctrine."[84] Grace, in other words, is likely to manifest in a cheerful aspect and pleasant, even charming disposition.

---

[81] Ibid., 197.

[82] "Thus haue I my selfe knowen some, and that of no meane callinge, who (eyther through inclynation of their Nature or custome of lyfe) cleane geeuen from all companye, lookinge wyth face and countenaunce grimrae and seuere, wyth browes knyt together & frowninge, wyth eyes sullen, sterne, terrible, glauncing asyde and eskāted, ynough to make such as meete them afrayde to loke vppon them" (Levinus Lemnius, *The Touchstone of Complexions*, trans. Thomas Newton [London, 1576], 138 v–139r).

[83] For such inveterately severe types, Lemnius prescribes "mery compaignyes," "Nuptiall society," and "pleasaunt conferences" so that they might "acquainte themselues wyth curtesye & familiar humanitye, discontinuinge and abandoning that their former counterfeite and disguysed seuerity" (ibid., 139r).

[84] Church of England, *Articles ... accordyng to the Computation of the Churche of England, for Thauoydyng of the Diuersities of Opinions, and for the Stablyshyng of Consent Touchyng True Religion* (London, 1563).

Lemnius writes that "there appeareth a kinde of heroicall grace and amyablenes, insomuch that the very viewe & sighte thereof, allureth and draweth euery one by a certayne secrete sympathie or cosent of Nature to loue it, wythout any hope of profite or commodity thereby to bee reaped or receyued."[85] These graces are reflected in the body's "physiognomy":

> The body is decently made & featly framed, conteyninge an absolute construction and comely frame of al the parts together. The head not aslope cornered, but rounde and globewyse fashioned, the hayre of fayre aburne or chesten colour: the forhead smoth, cheerefull and vnwrynckled, beautifyed wyth comely eyebrowes, and greatly honoured wyth a paire of amyable eyes, not holow, but delightfully standinge out. The colour freshe, sweete and pleasaunte. The cheekes and the balles therof steygned and dyed in a perfect hew of whyte and redde, and that naturally, speciallye in the lusty yeares of Adolescencie.[86]

Lemnius's emphasis, however, is not on congenital features, not even those that seem to have been understood in early modern physiology to be humoral or, to use Mary Floyd-Wilson's term, geohumoral, in origin.[87] His portrait of a graceful physiognomy is rather almost wholly concerned with the manner in which one signals amiability through posture, gait, and, especially, speech:

> The porte & state of the body bolt vprighte, the gate or goinge framed to comelynes, not nycely affected nor curiously counterfaicted, as it were Players & disguysed Masquers, who by a kinde of vpstarte & stately gate, hopeth the rather to winne credite, estimation and authority, and to be made more accompte of, amonge the common people. The tongue prompt and ready, distinctly and sensibly able to pronounce and deliuer out his meaning, in wordes of gallant vtteraunce.[88]

Lemnius makes eloquence a sign of grace much in the same way that Walkington will idealize sanguine wit. For both, the putatively innate quality of grace is manifested in outward signs that are easily counterfeited and only discerned as genuine on the basis of their *apparent* naturalness. This makes the soteriological interpretation of affect difficult work indeed. It also helps to explain why melancholy is treated with such suspicion, as its supposed unnaturalness (its unholiness as well as its potential artificiality) undermines the naturalness of what is deemed to be goodly and godly cheer.

Melancholy contrasts with a godly amiability that is neither severe nor luxurious but rather, in the popular idiom of Christian Neostoicism, "tranquil." The spiritual hygienist Robert Bolton depicts tranquility as a state of internal repose expressed

---

[85] Lemnius, *The Touchstone of Complexions*, 36v.

[86] Ibid.

[87] Mary Floyd-Wilson, *English Ethnicity and Race in Early Modern Drama* (Cambridge: Cambridge University Press, 2003).

[88] Lemnius, *The Touchstone of Complexions*, 36v.

in a pleasant aspect that closely resembles the cheer commended by Lemnius, who writes: "Let the earth be moued, and let the mountaines fall into the middest of the sea: yet his heart is ioyfull, patient, resolute, and contented."[89] The implicitly soteriological problem of discerning real from feigned tranquility troubles Bolton in a similar way that the problem of affected cheer and wit unsettles Lemnius, Walkington, and Bright. Bolton cautions that "Sweetnesse of nature, louelines of disposition, fairenes of conditions ... affability in cariage, and conuersation; an vnswaied vprightnes in ciuill actions" all "make a goodly shew." These signs on their own may mean much or little, but combined with "an accession of profession of the Gospell, of outward performance of religious exercises, of some correspondence with the seruants of God," he says with an oddly morbid twist of phrase, "the matter is strike dead."[90]

Bolton's vision of tranquility is pleasurable rather than ascetic and is distinctly worldly. Spiritual joy is tied to earthly life and its fleeting temporality. Bolton warns, in *Instructions for a Right Comforting*, that the window of opportunity for storing up joyful helps for the spirit is short: "Let every one of us ... in this short Sommers Day of our abode on earth, and in this glorious Sunn-shine of the Gospell, and pretious seasons of grace, imploy all meanes, improve all opportunities, to gather in, with all holy greedinesse, and treasure up abundantly much spirituall strength, and lasting comfort against the *evill Day*." He urges melancholy readers to protect their souls by making a "wise, and happy treasuring up, of heavenly hoards, and comforts of holinesses aforehand," in order to "allay the bitternesse and smart of that heavinesse and sorrow: of those fearefull amazements, and oppressions of spirit" which are not merely "naturally incident to times of trouble," but clearly associated with the acute sensitivities of conscience encouraged by the spiritual physicians.[91] Bolton's counsel thereby raises and leaves unresolved difficult questions concerning the nature of grace: whether it is fixed or not, whether its quantity or quality can be increased or diminished.[92] The terms in which late sixteenth-century English physicians and hygienists speak of the spirits may have offered some, albeit contradictory, way around the strict determinism of predestinarian theology in this matter. Election may be predetermined but the complex relationship between divine and vital spirit makes one's "spiritual" condition patently subject to alteration. At the same time that grace seems to inhere in the fullness or repletion of vital spirit, it can be depleted by sadness. Grief, Bolton warns, "grates most upon the vitall spirits, dries up soonest the freshest marrow in the bones; and most sensibly suckes out the purest, and refinest bloud

---

[89]   Ibid.

[90]   Robert Bolton, *A Discourse about the State of True Happinesse* (London, 1611), 14.

[91]   Robert Bolton, *Instructions for a Right Comforting of Afflicted Consciences* (London, 1631), 20.

[92]   As Paul Cefalu has observed, accounts of the "complete and unalterable nature of the sanctified agent" are frequently contradicted by the remarks of English Calvinists "on the gradualist and perfectionist nature of sanctification" (*Moral Identity in Early Modern English Literature* [Cambridge: Cambridge University Press, 2004], 59.

in the heart." Joy replenishes spirit, whereas bitterness destroys it, transfiguring a graceful countenance into one that portends degeneracy. "All the Objects of lightsomenesses, and joy, are drowned in an heauy heart," says Bolton, "even as the beauty of a Pearle, is dissolved in vineger."[93]

The crux of this contradictory instruction in what we might, borrowing a term from Teresa Brennan, describe as a kind of Puritan affective "entrainment" is a theological problem concerning the limits of *caritas*.[94] This problem becomes even more apparent in the practical divinity of later seventeenth-century divines such as Richard Baxter. In his 1682 sermon, "The Cure of Melancholy and Overmuch Sorrow," Baxter warns that because "a hardened Heart is so great a part of the Malady and Misery of the unregenerate, and a *soft* and *tender Heart* is much of the *New Nature* promised by Christ, many awakened Souls under the work of Conversion think they can never have Sorrow enough."[95] Put plainly, good Christians risk melancholic disease by feeling too much. With this belief that "their danger lies in hard-heartedness," he warns, "they never fear *overmuch sorrow* till it hath *swallowed them up*." Baxter skirts the tension between charitable obligation and self-preservation in his definition of excessive sorrow. "*Sorrow* is *overmuch*," he says, "when it is fed by a mistaken cause: All is too much where *none* is due; and great sorrow is too much when the Cause requireth but less."[96]

Baxter's tautological definition of sorrowful excess contradicts the sacrificial ethic of Christ's passion. "Sorrow," he says, "is overmuch when it hurteth and overwhelmeth Nature itself, and destroyeth bodily Health or Understanding."[97] Grace, on the other hand, "is the due qualification of Nature," which would not have us harm ourselves for our spiritual betterment: "God will have mercy and not sacrifice; and he that would not have us kill or hurt our neighbour on pretense of religion, would not have us destroy or hurt ourselves, being bound to love our neighbour but as ourselves."[98] Baxter deems charity excessive not only when it would seem to exceed its warrant, and not because the preservation of the self takes precedence over others, but seemingly because prevenient grace renders charity superfluous to salvation. The distinction between "good works" that are "pleasing and acceptable to God in Christ" and supererogative acts—"voluntary workes" that go "over and above Gods commandmentes" and "can not bee taught

---

[93]   Bolton, *Instructions for a Right Comforting of Afflicted Consciences*, 20.

[94]   Teresa Brennan, *The Transmission of Affect* (Ithaca, NY: Cornell University Press, 2004).

[95]   Baxter, "The Cure of Melancholy and Overmuch-Sorrow by Faith and Physick," in *A Continuation of Morning-Exercise Questions and Cases of Conscience Practically Resolved by Sundry Ministers in October, 1682*, ed. Samuel Annesley (London, 1683), 265.

[96]   Ibid.

[97]   Ibid., 266.

[98]   The emphasis of Baxter's rhetoric throughout his sermon is on self-governance as civic duty and Christian life as social contract: "As civil, and ecclesiastic, and domestic government are for edification and not for destruction, so also is personal self government" (ibid.).

without arrogancye and impietie"—remains most tenuous in Baxter's practical divinity.[99] The paradoxical value accorded to sufficient rather than excessive good works parallels the affective problem made prominent by Baxter's practical advice. One must be sufficiently softhearted to recognize the pangs of conscience but hard enough to withstand the pathos that threatens, to use his preferred phrase, to "swallow us up."[100] Unlike earlier spiritual physicians, Baxter suggests that physical melancholy, that is, melancholy caused by "distemper, weakness, and diseasedness of the body" is "less sinful and less dangerous to the soul than spiritual melancholy," though "nevertheless troublesome but the more."[101]

Whereas spiritual melancholy could serve earlier English Protestants as a sign of God's loving reproof (and possibly as a sign of grace itself), Baxter regards the condition as a potential cover for sectarian enthusiasm. He infantilizes the melancholic and rejects Bolton's argument that spiritual melancholy may precede physical or natural melancholy but that the reverse is impossible. He writes that the "natural temper" of those predisposed to spiritual melancholy "is a strong disease, of troubling sorrow, fear and displeasedness." If not yet melancholy, they are "of so Childish, and sick, and impatient a temper, that one thing or other is still either discontenting, grieving, or affrighting them." Their impressionability renders them vulnerable to all manners of disturbance. They are "like an Aspen leaf, still shaking with the least motion of the air."[102] Such persons are childish not because they are fearful (the godly, after all, should fear) but because, like Burton's hypochondriacal readers, they appropriate all perceived suffering to their own condition. These fragile creatures become spiritual hypochondriacs because of their unbridled impressionability: "A word, yea, or a look, offendeth them; every sad story or news or noise affrighteth them."[103] Baxter characterizes this mimetic excess as childish cupidity, "as children must have all that they cry for before they will be quiet," suggesting that the work of Christian discipline involves the sublimation of empathic impulses. At the same time, he tells us that the spiritual melancholic's appetite for sorrow is beyond his or her control. The misery of their condition is that "*what they think, they cannot choose but think.*"[104] Baxter very nearly quotes Burton as he continues:

> You may almost as well persuade a man not to shake in an Ague, or not to feel when he is pained, as persuade them to cast away their self-troubling thoughts,

---

[99]   Church of England, *Articles ... accordyng to the Computation of the Churche of England, for Thauoydyng of the Diuersities of Opinions, and for the Stablyshyng of Consent Touchyng True Religion.*

[100]   Baxter, "The Cure of Melancholy and Overmuch-Sorrow by Faith and Physick," 266.

[101]   Ibid., 269.

[102]   Ibid.

[103]   Ibid. Compare with Richard Greenham, *Paramython: Two Treatises of the Comforting of an Afflicted Conscience* (London, 1598), 34–5.

[104]   Baxter, "The Cure of Melancholy and Overmuch-Sorrow by Faith and Physick," 269.

or not to think all the enormous, confounding thoughts as they do, they cannot get them out of their heads night or day: tell them that they must forbear long musing, which disturb them, and they cannot: tell them that they must cast out false imaginations out of their minds, when Satan casts them in, and must turn their thoughts to something else, and they cannot do it: Their thoughts, and troubles, and fears, are gone out of their power, and the more, by how much the more, melancholly and crased they are.[105]

The melancholic's obliviousness to his or her own unreason serves as reason why their "revelations" and "prophesies" are not to be credited. Still, the "sadder, better sort" recognize that their affliction is caused from without, suggesting a residually preferential treatment of sadness in Baxter's soteriology, at least as compared with enthusiastic frenzy.[106]

V. Brittle—Glass Delusions and Despair

The delusional figures in the catalogues of conceits studied by Du Laurens, Platter, Walkington, and Burton represent what we might call the threat of psychic rupture under the pressure of competing affective demands in popular piety and hygiene scripts. They represent either the inability or refusal to suffer the contradictory demands to appear both cheerful and grave, confident and meek, imperturbable and compassionate. It is in this context that delusions of gigantism and diminution, heaviness and lightness, vulnerability and invulnerability seem to have resonated most profoundly. These contradictions are perhaps most suggestively illuminated in the glass delusions that appear in early modern medical descriptions of melancholic delusion as well as in more literary elaborations such as Cervantes's *El licenciado vidriera*.[107] This novella tells the story of a young peasant named Tomas, a rising star at the University at Salamanca, who travels across Europe before settling down to practice law. During his travels he is encouraged to enlist in the army but refuses on point of conscience, regarding the paid soldier's life as a mercenary one. Upon his return to Salamanca, he unwittingly wins the heart of an older woman who nearly kills him with a botched love potion.[108] When he awakens from his stupor he is convinced that he is made of glass and, like similar delusional melancholics in classical and neoteric medical literature, lives in terror of being accidentally broken by anyone who comes near him. Tomas becomes a vagabond philosopher, gaining fame for his piercing social commentary, a

---

[105] Ibid., 270. Compare with Burton at 1:420.

[106] Ibid.

[107] The novella was first published in Cervantes's collection of short stories, *Novelas ejemplares*, in 1613.

[108] Cervantes may have been alluding to the legend told by Jerome that Lucretius was given a madness-inducing love potion by his wife in order to discredit the poet's materialist heresies. See George Depue Hadzsits, *Lucretius and His Influence* (New York: Longmans, Green and Co., 1935), 5.

talent that emerges as a response to the abuses he suffers in his newly fragile and paranoid condition. He fires off witty retorts while dodging stones flung by boys who claim to test whether he is really made of glass. Tomas eventually recovers but is unable to earn a living as a lawyer because his audiences have come to expect the sharper counsel he was famous for while delusional. He quits the law in fear of starvation and, in a poignantly ironic twist, has no recourse but to join the army he once disdained, "avail[ing] himself of the strength of his arm since he could not avail himself of the powers of his intellect." He is, as Cervantes eulogizes, finally remembered not for his brilliance as the glass scholar but for "having been a prudent and very valiant soldier."[109]

Timothy Reiss discusses the story in a lengthy chapter of *Mirages of the Selfe*, titled "Essences of Glass, Histories of Humans." Reiss calls the glass delusion a fantastic desire to have one's innermost thoughts made plain to others.[110] Gill Speak, whose essay on the glass delusion remains the only one on this particular subject (and the most sustained reading of any of the melancholic conceits), writes that Tomas's fear "must have been connected with the notion that his body was, not fragile, but transparent," like Donne's fear that "Tis much that Glass should bee / As all confessing, and through-shine as I."[111] The interest of Cervantes's story seems to me, however, to lie in the contrast between Tomas's delusional fragility and incisive wit. His vulnerability enables him to reflect hypocrisy and injustice with unmitigated honesty and clarity. Until his "madness," the lowborn scholar is deferent and submissive. The sudden onset of his irrational fear renders him an unabashed expositor of social hypocrisy.

Reiss reads the glass delusion as a fracture of the mirage of embodiment. He quotes numerous references to early modern representations of the mind and soul as being cased in glass. These include Walkington, who wrote that the mind needs tending like a "christall glass to saue it from cracking"; Luisa Sabuco, who described the eyes as "two glasses or windows of the soul"; Guillaume du Bartas, who wrote that God set the soul in an "earthen vase, More fluid than water, more brittle than glass"; and Vives, who depicted the mind as a prisoner in a house with no openings but for a glass window prone to clouding.[112] To these examples I would add the glass souls of women that are perpetually at risk of being "blown

---

[109]   Miguel de Cervantes, *Exemplary Stories*, trans. Lesley Lipson (Oxford: Oxford University Press, 1998), 130.

[110]   This yearning for the vulnerability afforded by transparency, he suggests, could only have been a "privilege" for monarchs. For the rest of humanity, "to live in the world was ever to experience this brittle fragility" (Timothy J. Reiss, *Mirages of the Selfe: Patterns of Personhood in Ancient and Early Modern Europe* [Stanford: Stanford University Press, 2003], 32).

[111]   Gill Speak, "An Odd Kind of Melancholy: Reflections on the Glass Delusion in Europe (1440–1680)," *History of Psychiatry* 1, no. 2 (1990): 202. Speak sees these contents/ vessel delusions as variants of body/soul fixations that disguise fears of death and longing for immortality.

[112]   Reiss, *Mirages of the Selfe*, 36–7.

up" in Webster's *The Duchess of Malfi*,[113] a play whose structural opposition of hard- and softheartedness is echoed in contrasting images of other hard and soft things (diamonds, for instance, and melancholy birds) and the somatized conceit of lycanthropy—being "hairy on the inside" as a consequence of forced unfeeling.

Reiss surmises that the glass delusion represented, on the one hand, adustion (the heating and rarefication of black bile being comparable to the process of making glass from sand) and a literalized assimilation of a popular metaphor for the embodiment of the soul that aptly "caught the sense of teetering between solidity and brittleness, between the mind grounded on earth, 'safely' lodged in matter, and one whose walls had given way … to 'shaping fantasies.'"[114] In these remarks, he seems to echo scholars who have been quick to regard such images of fragility as projections of anxious vulnerability. He offers a somewhat different insight, however, by suggesting that the cultural resonance of the glass delusion may have had more to do with the fantasy of undermining than of bolstering the ego: that the glass delusion "forbad belief in separable *self*."[115] Early modern sufferers of delusions of hardness recognize this adamantine condition as the chief obstacle to their redemption. Like Hamlet, they worry not for their too-soft but their too-solid flesh, and like the many belated penitents of the Renaissance stage, from Lear to Bosola, they bid their hearts to break, but too late.

Unsurprisingly, Renaissance depictions of the hypochondriacal "conceits" of melancholy, of which the glass delusion becomes a chief example, bear strong resemblance to popular accounts of spiritual melancholy. Both seem to have appealed to readers for their symbolic exposition of Protestantism's contradictory exhortations to charitable engagement and tranquility, empathy and apathy, faith and doubt. The best-known and most illustrative case for this comparison is found in the legends surrounding Francis Spira, but reports of spiritual melancholy and despair litter the devotional and medical literature of the period. These accounts highlight the extraordinarily public and theatrical nature of "private" spiritual crisis. Nathaniel Bacon writes that "multitudes of all sorts" came daily to see Spira, "some out of curiositie only to see and discourse: some out of a pious desire to try all meanes that might reduce him to comfort again, or at least to benefit themselves, by such a spectacle of misery and of the justice of God."[116] Spira's prominence as a lawyer and public figure made his case especially public, but other records (from the more private diary of Elizabeth Isham written in the 1620s to the more polemical *Mrs. Drake Revived* in the 1640s and the later *Narrative of Mrs. Hannah Allen*) foreground the public face of private doubt and the communal response it seemed to command.[117]

---

[113] John Webster, *The Duchess of Malfi and Other Plays*, ed. René Weis (Oxford: Oxford University Press, 2009), 4.2.78–9.

[114] Reiss, *Mirages of the Selfe*, 40.

[115] Ibid.

[116] Nathaniel Bacon, *A Relation of the Fearefull Estate of Francis Spira in the Year, 1548* (London, 1638), 36–7.

[117] See Schmidt, *Melancholy and the Care of the Soul*, chaps. 3 and 5.

William Perkins and Robert Bolton both transcribe their conversations with melancholy parishioners such as Spira and Allen. They do so, purportedly, to demonstrate techniques for their consolation, but the technique of reproduced dialogue has the effect more often than not of showcasing the insufficiency of the pastor's response to his parishioner's overly zealous but undeniably pious interpretation of Reformation theology. Where these men and women err they err in affect, failing to meet the harsh decree of predestination with good cheer. To accuse them of being too precise or excessively conscientious is to accuse them, in a sense, of being too great imitators of Christ. Spira is tormented by pangs of conscience not for his own sin but all sin. To Spira, all sins resemble one another; all are part of the collective burden Christ assumed on our behalf: "thus guiltie of one guiltie of all. And therefore it is no matter whether my sinnes be great or small, few or many; they are such as Christ's bloud, nor Gods mercie belongs to mee."[118]

It is only in the certainty of his exclusion from redemption that Spira's piety flounders. In his misbegotten humility he betrays his suspicion, if not outright rejection, of the idea of gratuitous salvation. Spira is unable to recognize himself as the recipient of a gift of which he insists he is undeserving. Similarities in the covert hostility toward the delusional melancholic and spiritual melancholic suggest that the overweening sense of one's reprobation constitutes not only an inverse pride but a claim to exceptionality that disavows him or her of the insoluble debt of grace. This disavowal would have registered not only as a repudiation of the doctrine of justification by faith alone but as a rejection of the sociability of credit that was a key ideological prop for early English capitalism.[119] A maligned rhetoric of wishful reciprocity pervades the account of Spira given by England's early glossator, Thomas Beard, in his 1597 *The Theater of God's Judgments*. Beard writes that Spira believed he would be denied clemency because he denied Christ. He rebukes the son "that opened his mouth to make him swallow some food, to sustaine him; saying, Since he had forsaken his Lord and maister, all his creatures ought to forsake him."[120] This arithmetical reasoning is key to the uneasy depiction of the "overly precise" spiritual melancholics of the late sixteenth and early seventeenth centuries.[121] It bespeaks a specific kind of pusillanimity (the

---

[118]   Nathaniel Bacon, *A Relation of the Fearefull Estate of Francis Spira in the Year, 1548*, 54.

[119]   On the sociability of credit in early modern England, see Craig Muldrew, *The Economy of Obligation: The Culture of Credit and Social Relations in Early Modern England* (New York: St. Martin's Press, 1998).

[120]   Thomas Beard, *The Theatre of Gods Iudgements: Or, A Collection of Histories out of Sacred, Ecclesiasticall, and Prophane Authours, Concerning the Admirable Iudgements of God Vpon the Transgressours of His Commandments* (London, 1597), 64.

[121]   I refer to the term "preciseness" as Theodore Bozeman draws attention to it, in the propaganda both supporting and undermining the Antinomian backlash of the early seventeenth century. Bozeman does not however consider the relationship I am drawing between the accusation of preciseness or moral stringency and the radical view of irrational grace. See *The Precisianist Strain: Disciplinary Religion and Antinomian Backlash in Puritanism to 1638* (Chapel Hill: University of North Carolina Press, 2004).

opposite of the naturally gracious person's extravagance) that is beguiled by and even hostile to the irrational economics of grace stressed by Luther and Calvin.[122] Spira's refusal to accept the possibility of his salvation may have registered as a refusal to be beholden for a debt he was incapable of repaying, a refusal of the gift itself.

The fame of the desperate Francis Spira could not have been unaided by the providential irony of his name. While the Italian name, "Spiera," by which Francis was known in the early accounts, derives from the verb *spierare*, to spy, the Italian homonyms for Francis's anglicized name would have invoked the double irony of both the possessive Francis *de* Spera (Francis *of* hope) and the privative Francis *de*spera, Francis, of no hope, or even Francis De-spair.[123] I would suggest a further resonance. The name Spira, a common variation of the name Shapiro (associated with the Jews of Speyer, Germany), may well have intimated an inherited, racial obduracy and antipathy to Christian faith. Spira repeatedly attributes his despair to a natural hardness of heart: "*O here is the knot (said Spira) I would I could believe; But I cannot.*"[124] He takes this obduracy as chief evidence of his reprobation,[125] and characterizes this defect as a failure of imagination: "You thinke it an easie matter to perswade a man to believe ... but this is the hell to mee, my heart is hardned, I cannot believe."[126] The lesson of Spira's suffering is in no small part that faith requires disbelief in the improbability of one's own redemption. It requires that one imagine an abundance of God's love that is greater than one's iniquities and, more difficult still, to accept that one should receive this love without warrant.

The appeal of irrational melancholic delusions for Renaissance readers might have rested precisely in their capacity to anthropomorphize God's inscrutable favor and make plausible the implausibility of God's irrational love. This would offer us a new way of reading the depiction of lovesickness in the period and of Burton's infamous treatment of erotomania in *The Anatomy of Melancholy*. The melancholic lover becomes a spectacle of renewed curiosity and rhetorical pleasure in this same period that recasts the delusional melancholic as a figure of pathological impressionability and the spiritual melancholic as a figure of pathological obduracy, exhibiting unmovable conviction or "faith" in his or her own damnation. The lover's irrational devotion, by contrast, offers a compelling allegory for grace.

---

[122]   Contemporary theologians associated with the Radical Orthodoxy movement (John Milbank, Catherine Pistock, Graham Ward) have sought to redeem precisely this quality of radical indebtedness as a principal tenet of Reformed Christian faith. See, especially, John Milbank, *Being Reconciled: Ontology and Pardon* (New York: Routledge, 2003).

[123]   Bacon puns a final admonitory message in his concluding address to the reader that capitalizes on the homonymic significance of Spira's name: "I bid thee farewell, and hope well, while the space of Grace lasteth, *Dum spiras spera:* so mayest thou take good and no hurt, by the reading of this terrible example" (*A Relation of the Fearefull Estate of Francis Spira in the Year, 1548*, 134).

[124]   Ibid., 76.

[125]   Ibid., 62.

[126]   Ibid., 83.

Burton's portrait of erotomania attenuates spiritual suffering by reversing the position of the pursuer and pursued. Man becomes the fickle and elusive object of God's incorrigible devotion. The lover, Burton says, "will not change fortune with a Prince" though he lives and dies by the favor of his inconstant lady. Whilst he is pleasing to her, "the *Persian* Kings are not so Joviall as he is" (3:151), and when she hides her favor, he despairs:

> I am undone,
>> *Neque virgo est usquam, neque ego, qui è conspectus illam amisi meo,*
>> *Ubi quaeram, ubi investigem, quem percuncter, quam insistam viam?*
> The virgin's gone, and I am gone, shee's gone, shee's gone, and what shall I doe? (3:152)

If she frowns at him "*he is instantly tormented,* none so dejected as he is, utterly undone, a castaway ... a dead man, the scorn of fortune, a monster of fortune, worse then naught, the losse of a kingdome had bin lesse" (3:152). Burton is here quoting from Terence's *Eunuch,* a play about a lovelorn soldier who disguises himself as a eunuch in order to serve in the household of his beloved.[127] This degradation would have reminded Christian audiences of Christ's sacrificial incarnation, his willingness to become flesh in order to serve mankind. The soldier's pleas, "Ubi querem, ubi investigem ..." ("Where shall I seek her? Where shall I find her? Whom shall I ask? What way, what course shall I take? What will become of me?") in Burton's joint consolation of love and spiritual melancholy furthermore recalls God's allegorical pursuit of his beloved people in the Song of Songs.

The allegory of the lover illustrates God's irrational but nonetheless constant devotion. Having chosen us once, God will choose us again. Likewise the lover:

> If once therefore enamored, he will goe, runne, ride, many a mile to meet her, day and night, in a very darke night, endure scorching heat, colde, wait in frost and snow, raine, tempests, till his teeth chatter in his head, those Northerne winds and shoures cannot coole or quench his flames of love. (3:171)

Considered in this way, Burton's notorious parading of medieval antifeminist arguments for the abjectness of the beloved's body does not serve up the misogynistic feast identified as such by many contemporary scholars so much as an allegory for human abjection:

> though she bee very deformed of her selfe, ill favored, wrinkled, pimpled, pale, red, yellow, tan'd, tallow-faced, have a swolne Juglers platter face, or a thin, leane, chitty face, have clouds in her face ... crooked, dry, bald, gogle-eied, bleare-eyed, or with staring eyes, she looks like a squis'd Cat, hold her head still awry, heavy, dull, hollow-eyed ... hooke nosed, have a sharpe fox nose, a redde nose, *China* flat, great nose ... a nose like a promonotory, gubber-tushed, rotten teeth, black, uneven, browne teeth, beetle browed, a Witches beard, her breath stinke all the roome, her nose drop winter and summer, with a *Bavarian* poke

---

[127]   Terence, *Eunuch,* 560.

under her chin, a sharpe chin, lave eared, with a long cranes necke, which stands awry too ... *dugges like two double jugges*, or else no dugges, in that other extreame ... a rotten carkasse, a crooked backe, she stoops, is lame ... her feet stinke, she breed lice, a meere changeling, a very monster ... whom thou couldst not fancy for a world, but hatest, loathes, and wouldst have spit in her face ... a dowdy, a slut, a scold, a nasty, ranke, rammy, filthy, beastly queane ... if hee love her once, he admires her for all this, he takes no notice of any such errors, or imperfections, of body or minde ... (3:164)

The delight of this notorious *contreblazon* for Burton and his melancholic reader resides in its celebration of irrational love and, by analogy, grace. Like the foul mistress, we are loathsome, and God loves us still. We are endeared to the absurdity of erotomania for its hopeful suggestion that if we can love undeservedly, so too might we be loved.

The delusional melancholic paradoxically serves as a champion of the irrationality of faith even as his or her morbid preoccupations might be seen to lack faith in the supreme good, possibly even to reject indebtedness out of suspicion for the gratuity of grace. The hope for the spiritual melancholic lies precisely in his or her acute feeling of God's absence: a point the Puritan divines repeatedly make, arguing that one cannot miss what one has never known.[128] This assurance, however, exposes a further point of contention and a crucial point for Burton: faith necessitates a suspension of belief in one's own unworthiness of redemption. The man who walks a plank across a great chasm feels no less terror, Burton reminds, than the blindfolded man who walks the same plank suspended only inches above the ground and merely believes he's hovering over the abyss (1:420). Biero's anecdote does more than simply illustrate the somatic powers of the imagination. It intimates that faith, like fear, resides in the imagination.[129] The question the anecdote raises then is whether it is better to be fearful and cautious or trusting and steadfast. The despairer's conviction in his or her reprobation is not rational, but neither is the certainty they reject. To this question, despite his levity, Burton famously answers by choosing melancholy. It is "better to be sad than merry," to be "wise and still vexed," and to be "miserable than happy." "Of two extreames," he says, "it is the best" (2:207). The melancholic's delusional brittleness warns against the consequences that ensue from delusions of imperviousness and imperturbability cultivated in the name of good spiritual hygiene.

---

[128] See conclusion to "An excellent Treatise of Comforting suche as are troubled about their Predestination," appended to William Perkins, *A Golden Chaine, or, The Description of Theologie Containing the Order of the Causes of Saluation and Damnation* (London, 1591).

[129] This idea of faith, or belief, and its opposite, despair, as functions of the imagination is expressed by Paracelsus. See Heinz Schott, "Paracelsus and Van Helmont on Imagination," in *Paracelsian Moments: Science, Medicine, & Astrology in Early Modern Europe*, ed. Gerhild Scholz Williams and Charles D. Gunnoe Jr. (Kirksville, MO: Truman State University Press, 2002), 139.

Chapter 3
Exhilarating the Spirits:
Study as Cure for Scholarly Melancholy

In "Exercise Rectified of Body and Mind," Burton praises the "many flourishing Commonwealths" that prescribe "labour and exercise to all sorts of men" to "prevent those grievous mischiefs that come by idlenesse."[1] It is to the cause of idleness that Burton attributes "this feral disease of melancholy" that "so frequently rageth ... amongst our great ones."[2] And for this reason, he says, *"there can be no better cure, then continuall businesse, as Rhasis holds, to have some employment or other, which may set their minde aworke, and distract their cogitations"* (2:68). Of all such distracting employments, he says, "there is none so generall, so aptly to be applyed to all sorts of men, so fit & proper to expell Idlenesse and Melancholy, as that of *Study*" (2:84). This advice would seem to contradict the Aristotelian view of melancholy as a highly unstable humor that could produce a frenzied state of genius if overheated, which, Aristotle's commentators argued, was more likely to occur through mental overexertion. Modern scholars have therefore tended to regard Burton's own elaborate study either as an unwitting propagation of the disease it seeks to alleviate or an ironic illustration of the way that scholarly melancholia endlessly perpetuates itself through more and more study. This chapter hopes to show how Burton subtly elides pathological explanations of melancholia while at the same time revising the grounds on which the physiological relation between melancholy and genius had historically been drawn. He regards the intense concentration required to produce adust brilliance as a hazard for the melancholic, for whom he sees no better cure than diversion. He is adamant on this point: treatment of melancholic dishumor demands recreation of the spirits. He lists many ways by which this may be accomplished but considers study the best by far (2:90). The regimen of diverse and diverting study that Burton breathlessly describes in "Exercise Rectified of Body and Mind" and models in the "Digression of the Ayre" has led scholars to characterize the *Anatomy* as the work of an amateur who moves across too great a

---

[1] Robert Burton, *The Anatomy of Melancholy*, ed. Thomas C. Faulkner, Nicolas K. Kiessling, and Rhonda Blair, 6 vols. (Oxford: Clarendon Press, 1989), 2:67. Unless otherwise indicated, all references to the *Anatomy* are to this edition, hereafter cited parenthetically in text by volume and page number.

[2] Burton's copy of Pietro Pomponazzi's *De naturalium effectuum causis* (1556) is heavily marked throughout, although none of the marks appear to be in his hand but one: "mens torpet otio," or "idleness dulls the mind" (Ch f.8.45[1], sig +3r). See Nicolas K. Kiessling, *The Library of Robert Burton* (Oxford: Oxford Bibliographical Society, 1988), 239.

surface without plumbing any particular subject with sufficient depth.[3] The intent of this chapter will be to consider the therapeutic value that Burton accords to studies weighed not in terms of depth or gravity but rather for their capacity to elevate and recreate the spirits. I argue that Burton's ecstatic study aims to induce wonder as a salubrious alternative to spiritual rumination and that it does so by appealing directly to the transformative powers of the imagination as accessed primarily through rhetorical evocation.

To the degree that Burton's rhetorical performance has been assessed for its therapeutic qualities, it has been subject to mainly instrumental analyses that have overlooked the powers accorded by premodern psychology to the irrational and prerational faculties and the powers of suggestion by which melancholics were understood to be cured as well as afflicted. Angus Gowland and Mary Ann Lund have illustrated the rhetorical and intellectual contexts for what is now generally recognized as Burton's antipathy to Calvinism and his unorthodox spiritual counsel.[4] However, the complementarity of Burton's rhetorical style and spiritual counsel has only recently begun to attract scholarly attention.[5] The present analysis hopes to recouple the psychic and somatic aspects of Burton's spiritual counsel by

---

[3]   This characterization is not entirely inaccurate. Indeed, the description of Burton's study as *amateur* recalls historical connections between two of Burton's favorite subjects, scholarly and love melancholy, and reminds us of the close relationship between the status of melancholy and the status of pleasure or *delectatio* in their complexly interwoven discursive histories. For an account of the slippage between the two as a matter of "linguistic coincidence," see Noel S. Brann, *The Debate Over the Origin of Genius During the Italian Renaissance* (Leiden: Brill, 2002), 25.

[4]   See Angus Gowland, *The Worlds of Renaissance Melancholy: Robert Burton in Context* (Cambridge and New York: Cambridge University Press, 2006); Mary Ann Lund, "Reading and the Cure of Despair in *The Anatomy of Melancholy*," *Studies in Philology* 105, no. 4 (Fall 2008): 533–58; and Mary Ann Lund, *Melancholy, Medicine and Religion in Early Modern England: Reading "The Anatomy of Melancholy"* (New York: Cambridge University Press, 2010).

[5]   In a recent article, Gowland describes the *Anatomy*'s counsel as a kind of humanist "cognitive and imaginative therapy" rooted in classical and Christian traditions of *cura animi* ("Consolations for Melancholy in Renaissance Humanism," *Societate Și Politică* 6, no. 11 [2012]: 25). However, he emphasizes the Stoic contexts for Burton's consolations (which he regards as rational inducements to tranquility) whereas I am foregrounding the therapeutic effects of Burton's rhetorical performance itself and its *irrational* remediation of melancholy through the inducement of curative and contrary passions. In an earlier article, Gowland described Burton's rhetorical performance as being instrumental as an epideictic revelation or "showing forth" of the author's own melancholy ("Rhetorical Structure and Function in *The Anatomy of Melancholy*," *Rhetorica: A Journal of the History of Rhetoric* 19, no. 1 [2001]: 1–48). Lund describes Burton's spiritual counsel as bibliotherapeutic in its readerly address, but does not give extended consideration of its informing physiology or the roles of the imagination assumed by early modern rhetorical theory (*Melancholy, Medicine and Religion in Early Modern England*, 13). Gowland is somewhat more elaborate on this ("Consolations," 23–4).

considering the direct, material physic purveyed by his rhetorical performance in general and his promotion of study in particular.

The first section of this chapter situates Burton's understanding of imaginative instrumentality in the contexts of Renaissance faculty psychology, rhetorical theories of affect, and the pneumatic account of the spirit advanced, in particular, by the Renaissance Neoplatonists. I follow by evaluating the rhetorical and psychological impact of Burton's opposition between scholarly melancholy and studious delight. In the final section, I illustrate how Burton's catalogues of curiosities and recommended studies sonically induce wonder as sympathetic medicine for scholarly withdrawal and a powerful antidote against religious despair. I begin, however, with a brief summary of the historical association of melancholy with genius in order to identify the maneuvers whereby Burton promotes the melancholic's ability to be cured by study.

Background: Genius and Melancholy

In their highly influential study, *Saturn and Melancholy*, Klibansky, Panofsky, and Saxl trace the history whereby, over the course of two thousand years, the Platonic frenzies associated with heightened spiritual sensitivity became the wellspring of a theory of melancholic genius. They begin with *Problem XXX*, attributed to Aristotle, wherein the question is posed: "Why is it that all those who have become eminent in philosophy or politics or poetry or the arts are clearly melancholic, and some of them to such an extent as to be affected by diseases caused by black bile?"[6] They explain the significance of *Problem XXX* as the first work to attribute a natural and physiological cause for what was previously believed to be a state of demonic or divine possession. However, the relationship between melancholy and genius as expressed by *Problem XXX* is, at best, an unstable one, as it deems melancholics to be subject to extreme fluctuations in the temperature of their bile, which produces a wild variety of symptoms and behaviors. Cold bile could bring about paralysis or torpor. Heated bile had the somewhat ambiguous advantage of producing cheerfulness and song but also ecstasies and sores—the latter "erupting" from the same general process of internal combustion.[7] The argument that the melancholic temperament congenitally allowed for greater insight, intellectual aptitude, or artistic creativity was, according to most, late in the making and fraught with the implication that melancholy itself was understood, even by the author of *Problem XXX*, to be a waste product, the "dregs of the blood."[8]

---

[6] Raymond Klibansky, Erwin Panofsky, and Fritz Saxl, *Saturn and Melancholy: Studies in the History of Natural Philosophy, Religion, and Art* (New York: Basic Books, 1964), 18. The text is now widely attributed to Theophrastus. The standard citation for this re-ascription to Theophrastus is Hellmut Flashar, ed., *Problemata Physica* (Berlin: Akademie Verlag, 1962).

[7] Klibansky, Panofsky, and Saxl, *Saturn and Melancholy*, 23.

[8] The heightened intellectual or spiritual fervor that arose secondarily to melancholy was largely suspect in classical writing and would be associated in the later seventeenth

Physiological explanations of the melancholic's special aptitudes remained ambivalent at best at least until Ficino, or rather his interpreters, as Ficino himself gives a rather tentative appraisal of melancholic privilege:

> Melancholy or black bile is of two kinds: the one is called natural by doctors, the other comes about by adustion. The natural is nothing but a more dense and dry part of the blood. The adust, however, is divided into four kinds: it originates from the combustion either of natural melancholy, or of the purer blood, or of the bile, or of salty phlegm. Any melancholy which arises from adustion, harms the wisdom and the judgment, because when that humor is kindled and burns, it characteristically makes people excited and frenzied, which melancholy the Greeks call mania and we madness. But as soon as it is extinguished, when the more subtle and clearer parts have been dispersed and only a foul black soot remains, it makes people stolid and stupid; they properly call this disposition melancholy and also being out of one's wits and senselessness.[9]

The humoral concoctions of melancholy in Ficino's analysis are complex and infinitely various. Only natural black bile leads "to judgment and wisdom," says Ficino, "but not always."[10] Melancholy is the mercury of the humors, "Extremely hot, it produces the extremest boldness ... extremely cold, however, fear and extreme cowardice."[11] Ficino's explanation of how such an inconstant humor could be conducive to intelligence lay in the subtlety of the melancholic spirits themselves. The heat produced by the melancholic's intense concentration rarifies the spirits of black bile, making them brighter, quicker, and "more vigorous in action" as they are "squeezed" through the "narrow passages" of the brain. The spirits, "pouring forth continually from a solid and stable state," enable the mind to sustain its investigations: "Whatever it is tracking, it easily finds, perceives it clearly, soundly judges it, and retains the judgment long."[12] Ficino therefore attributes melancholic genius to an innate abundance of melancholic spirit, which may be refined by concentration to allow for heightened cognition.

---

and eighteenth centuries with *enthusiasm*, much as it had been associated in classical times with frenzy. This is the basis for Winfried Schleiner's correction to what he regards as the overemphasis on ennobling melancholy in the tradition of *Saturn and Melancholy*. See Winfried Schleiner, *Melancholy, Genius, and Utopia in the Renaissance*, Wolfenbütteler Abhandlungen Zur Renaissanceforschung (Wiesbaden: In Kommission bei Otto Harrassowitz, 1991).

[9]   Marsilio Ficino, *Three Books on Life*, ed. and trans. Carol Kaske and John Clark (Binghamton: Center for Medieval and Early Renaissance Studies, State University of New York Press, 1989), 117.

[10]   On its own, natural bile "beclouds the spirit ... terrifies the soul, and dulls the intelligence." If mixed with phlegm it makes one sluggish, hopeless, and weary even "to look at the dome of the sky," as he says, quoting Virgil, "*taedet caeli conuexa tueri,*" *Aeneid*, 4.451 (ibid.).

[11]   Ibid.

[12]   Ibid., 121.

The authors of *Saturn and Melancholy* attributed the elevated status of melancholic genius in the Quattrocento in large part to the humanist rehabilitation of the figure of Saturn and the transformation of melancholy from a congenital disposition or temperament to a mood.[13] However, they argue that the fifteenth-century promotion of melancholic genius was only possible in that same context that dismissed the medieval opposition of the contemplative and active life with a more classical understanding of humanistic inquiry as activity, "*vita speculativa sive studiosa.*"[14] In the first full-length reappraisal of Saxl, Panofsky, et al., Noel Brann offers a different account for the rise of melancholic genius in the Italian Renaissance. He ties the promotion of scholarly melancholy to the contemporaneous ennoblement of love melancholy on the basis of "a mere linguistic coincidence, arguing that Renaissance medical writers engaged in a word play that turned erotic love into heroic love, transforming *eros* into *hereos* simply by aspirating the letter *e*. Brann writes that this linguistic "accident" enabled medical theorists to transfer "the ravishing aspirations of the melancholy hero … to the philosophical lovers of wisdom and the poetic and artistic lovers of beauty."[15] This "heroic" love provided a common template for the coding and representation of amatory desire, religious ecstasy, and the scholar's passionate pursuit of knowledge.[16]

As numerous scholars have noted, Burton's summary of classical faculty psychology gives us little evidence of his genial view of melancholy, much less of the relationship between melancholy and genius.[17] He does not preface his study of melancholy by seeking to understand its relationship to artistic and intellectual achievement. Rather, when he broaches the question at the end of the

---

[13] Klibansky, Panofsky, and Saxl, *Saturn and Melancholy*, 217–18.

[14] Ibid., 245.

[15] The classical source for this linguistic "slip" was Plato's *Cratyllus*. Brann shows how Renaissance readers such as Mario Equicola drew on Plato to show the significance of the linguistic connection: "A man truly enamored, now with a superabundance of joy and now in a lowly sorrow … lives beyond the law of nature and surpasses all mediocrity …" (*The Debate Over the Origin of Genius During the Italian Renaissance*, 25). For more on this linguistic slip, see Marion A. Wells, *The Secret Wound: Love-Melancholy and Early Modern Romance* (Stanford: Stanford University Press, 2007), 22–4; Mary Frances Wack, *Lovesickness in the Middle Ages: The Viaticum and Its Commentaries*, Middle Ages Series (Philadelphia: University of Pennsylvania Press, 1990), 292.

[16] Brann, *The Debate Over the Origin of Genius During the Italian Renaissance*, 138–9.

[17] See Bridget Gellert Lyons, *Voices of Melancholy: Studies in Literary Treatments of Melancholy in Renaissance England* (Routledge & Kegan Paul, 1971), 128. Lyons notes that the "favorable aspect of curiosity that the Florentine Neoplatonists elaborated upon … is never present when [Burton] is talking about [melancholy] directly." Rather, as Mary Floyd-Wilson remarks, "the text's most direct link between melancholy and genius is Burton's own self-conscious commentary on the authorial production of the *Anatomy* itself" (Mary Floyd-Wilson, *English Ethnicity and Race in Early Modern Drama* [Cambridge: Cambridge University Press, 2003], 76).

first partition, he does so in the context of a more general inventory of classical and contemporary debates on melancholic etiology:

> Why melancholy men are witty, which *Aristotle* hath long since maintained in his Problems: and that all learned men, famous Philosophers, and Law-givers, *ad unum ferè omnes Melancholici*, have still beene Melancholy; is a Probleme much controverted. *Jason Pratensis* will have it understood of naturall melancholy, which opinion *Melancthon* inclines to … but not simple, for that makes men stupid, heavy, dull, being cold and dry, fearfull, fooles, and solitary, but mixt with the other humours, fleagme only excepted: & they not adust, but so mixt as that blood be halfe, with little or no adustion, that they be neither too hot nor too cold. *Aponensis*, cited by *Melancthon*, thinkes [melancholic genius] proceeds from melancholy adust, excluding all naturall melancholy, as too cold. *Laurentius* condemnes his *Tenent*, because adustion of humours makes men mad, as Lime burnes, when water is cast on it. It must bee mixt with blood, and somewhat adust, and so that old Aphorisme of *Aristotle* may bee verified, *Nullum magnum ingenium sine mixturâ dementiae*, no excellent wit without a mixture of madnesse. (1:421)

On the surface, Burton's summary is unremarkable. On closer examination, we may observe his subtle departure from the etiology of temperament on which Aristotle and his commentators relied. Burton lets Fracastoro, the early theorist of contagion, "decide the controversie," citing a table of temperaments borrowed from Fracastoro's dialogue, *Turrius sive de intellectione*:

> *Fracastorius* shall decide the controversie, *Phlegmaticke are dull: Sanguine lively, pleasant, acceptable, and merry, but not witty: Cholericke are too swift in motion, and furious, impatient of contemplation, deceitfull wits: Melancholy men have the most excellent wits, but not all, this humour may be hot or cold, thicke, or thinne; if too hot, they are furious and mad: if too cold, dull, stupid, timorous, and sad: if temperate, excellent, rather inclining to that extreame of heat, then cold.* This sentence of his will agree with that of *Heraclitus*, a dry light makes a wise mind, temperate heat and drynesse, are the chiefe causes of a good wit; therefore, saith *Aelian*, an Elephant is the wisest of all brute beasts, because his braine is dryest. (1:421–2)

Burton is likely having fun with his reference to the elephant's dry wits, painting a satirical picture not unlike the vapors and fumes of Swift's satire in *A Tale of a Tub* or the steaming undulations rising from Melville's head as he composes his "little treatise on Eternity," and which he compares to the canopy of vapor that crowns the contemplative whale.[18] The reference to "dry light" echoes the incandescence of heated bile that Ficino regarded as the source of melancholic genius. However, Burton seems to be seizing on the obscurity of cause and effect in *Problem XXX*

---

18   Herman Melville, *Moby-Dick, or The Whale*, ed. Harrison Hayford, Hershel Parker, and G. Thomas Tanselle (Evanston and Chicago: Northwestern University Press and the Newberry Library, 1988), 374.

(and Ficino's derivation thereof) in order to suggest, as he does throughout the *Anatomy*, that temperament can be entirely reconfigured through diet, exercise, atmosphere, and, above all, study.

I. The Study Cure in Context

Burton's faculty psychology at first appears to accord with the medieval ventricular arrangement, but closer attention reveals the greater emphasis he places on the powers of the imagination and the influence of Pico della Mirandola's argument that the phantasy is "one, single power of the sensitive soul."[19] According to the medieval scheme, *phantasia* is the first and least refined of the inner senses located in the *sensus communis* in the anterior ventricle of the brain. *Imaginatio* follows directly behind *phantasia*, either in the *sensus communis* or in the middle ventricle where information is passed for further evaluation. Burton departs from this scheme by folding the discrete, hierarchical functions of *phantasy* and *imaginatio* into a single power ("Phantasie, or Imagination, which some call *Aestimative*, or *Cogitative*") in a central processing faculty that "doth more fully examine the Species perceaved by common sense."[20] Phantasy, in Burton's scheme, plays a direct part in the production of intentions and hybrid images based on abstract relationship and resemblance. These "phantasms" do not simply combine new

---

[19] "The proposition of greatest way ... is that there exists a power of the soul which conceives and fashions likenesses of things, and serves, and ministers to, both the discursive reason and the contemplative intellect; and to this power has been given the name *phantasy* or *imagination*. For the opinion of Avicenna, whereby he separated the phantastic from the imaginative power, has long since been exploded, and that notion of his which attributed to phantasy supernatural powers of strength and efficacy has also been condemned by reputable philosophers" (Giovanni Francesco Pico della Mirandola, *On the Imagination*, trans. Harry Caplan [New Haven, CT: Yale University Press, 1930], 37).

[20] Burton's more direct source for this representation of the imagination, and his discussion of the internal and external senses in general, is Joannes Velcurio, *Commentarii in universam physicam Aristotelis* (Basel, 1543). The same redistributed hierarchy of the inward senses also appears in Daniele Barbaro's commentary on the power of rhetoric (*Aristotelis Rhetoricum libri tres*, 1544). On faculty psychology and Renaissance rhetorical theory, see Lawrence Green, "Aristotle's Rhetoric and Renaissance Conceptions of the Soul," in *La Rhétorique d'Aristote: Traditions et Commentaires de l'Antiquité au XVIIe siècle*, ed. Gilbert Dahan and Irène Rosier-Catach (Paris: Vrin, 1998): 283–98; and William Covino, *Magic, Rhetoric, and Literacy: An Eccentric History of the Composing Imagination* (Albany: State University of New York Press, 1994). On the decline of medieval ventricular arrangements in the later Renaissance and the consolidation of the imagination as a single, mediating power, see Stuart Clark, *Vanities of the Eye: Vision in Early Modern European Culture* (Oxford: Oxford University Press, 2007), 43–4. On pictorial representations of redistributed ventricular faculties and functions in the Renaissance, see Claudia Swan, "Eyes Wide Shut. Early Modern Imagination, Demonology, and the Visual Arts," *Zeitsprünge: Forschungen Zur Frühen Neuzeit* 7 (2003): 561–81.

data with stored information; they allow the brain to innovate by forming images of things unknown and never before seen. Burton's study cure draws upon the potency of the melancholic imagination to produce such phantasms. He is particularly faithful to his source, Joannes Velcurio, on the weakness that is also the strength of the melancholic imagination; it is "most Powerfull and strong, and often hurts, producing many monstrous and prodigious things" but, at the same time, in "Poets and Painters forcibly workes, as appeares by their severall fictions, Antickes, Images" (1:152).[21] He echoes Velcurio and, somewhat more distantly, Pico throughout the *Anatomy* by suggesting that the melancholic's vulnerability to fear, pain, and cupidity is a consequence of the same imaginative strength and agility that induces hope, joy, and love if so moved.[22]

Analyses of rhetorical function in the *Anatomy* have emphasized the role of Aristotelian *logos* as opposed to its use of Ciceronian, Longinian, and Quintilian techniques for engendering *pathos*, but Burton relies less heavily on rational than evocative tactics, especially *enargeia*, or vividness, to stir the imagination and alter the spirits.[23] Quintilian's discussion of *enargeia* was particularly important for Renaissance theorists of rhetorical affect. In the *Institutes*, he argues that the rhetor who wishes to move an audience must himself be moved, and he responds to the objection that this cannot be easily accomplished because "our feelings are not in our power" by offering the following method of imaginative inducement: "What the Greeks call φαντασίαι (*phantasiai*) we call *visiones*; images by which the representations of absent objects are so distinctly represented to the mind, that we seem to see them with our eyes, and to have them before us." Quintilian promises that "whoever shall best conceive such images will have the greatest power in moving the feelings" and assures that "this faculty may

---

[21]   Velcurio remarks that melancholics, cholerics, dreamers, drunks, and furious, frenzied, and feverish *phantasmoi* (φαντασμοι) who are both wonderfully strong (*mire valent*) and agile of imagination are also deeply and gravely affected by hope, joy, fear, pain, jealousy, love, etc. (*Commentarii in universam physicam Aristotelis* [Tübingen, 1544]; 217v). Adam Wood has prepared a partial English translation of Book 4 based on the 1588 London edition. See http://www.fordham.edu/mvst/awood/awoodtrans.html.

[22]   In Pico's argument, those who are prone to disorders of the imagination may also be cured by the powers of imagination. The disordered imaginations of spiritual melancholics, those who are plagued by images "of fire and brimstone, tortures, demons and the like," may be corrected by the light of faith. See Covino, *Magic, Rhetoric, and Literacy*, 39–40.

[23]   Debora Shuger and Wayne Rebhorn argue that historians have tended to overstate the rational Aristotelian focus of Renaissance rhetorical theory, obscuring more instrumental understandings of the sensuous and irrational powers of rhetoric. Shuger emphasizes the Hermogenean tradition in English Protestant ecclesiastical writing (*Sacred Rhetoric: The Christian Grand Style in the English Renaissance* [Princeton, NJ: Princeton University Press, 1988]). Rebhorn considers how classical techniques for moving the passions were developed by humanist rhetoricians such as Luis de Granada, Rudolph Agricola, Jacques Amyot, and Juan Vives (*The Emperor of Men's Minds: Literature and the Renaissance Discourse of Rhetoric* [Ithaca, NY: Cornell University Press, 1995]).

readily be acquired by ourselves if we desire it."[24] Wayne Rebhorn has shown how Renaissance rhetoricians identified such agility as a valuable technique for political persuasion and manipulation.[25] But the power of words to bend the will was of equal or greater importance for ecclesiastical rhetoricians such as John Rainolds, who delivered an impassioned argument against the Stoic denigration of *pathos*, arguing that emotion "is a natural commotion of the soul, imparted by God for following good and fleeing evil."[26] Burton's spiritual physic follows in this clerical tradition of engaging *pathos* for the purposes of bringing about spiritual transformation. His use of *enargeia* in the description of a study cure cultivates an imaginative agility in the reader by which he or she may replace melancholic thoughts and images with those that are, quite literally, more uplifting.[27]

In the Burtonian view, melancholia is not merely the byproduct of intellectual overexertion; neither is genius the activated potential of an abundance of melancholic spirit. Rather, by diverting the heaviness of melancholic spirit, the melancholic experiences a kind of physiological ecstasy through release. Burton departs somewhat from Galenic humoralists who defined passions "properly, and non-metaphorically, classif[ying them] ... as diseases affecting the functioning of the organism,"[28] drawing instead on a revised, post-Ficinian faculty psychology that privileges the role and impressionability of the imagination. He moves from the more limited view of imaginative causation offered by Aristotle toward more efficacious accounts developed both by the Neoplatonist philosophers Marsilio Ficino, Bernardino Telesio, and Tommaso Campanella and the Paracelsian and Helmontian medical reformers. As Leen Spruit details in his history of the intelligible species, the second half of the sixteenth century witnessed a profusion of radical departures from Aristotelian, Scholastic, and Platonic theories of perception. Impelled by recent discoveries in the study of anatomy and physiology, the New Philosophers, chief among them Giordano Bruno and Telesio, sought alternative models of perception and intellection based on evidence appropriable by the senses.[29] Telesio understood perception and sensation to be more active

---

[24]   Quintilian, *Institutes of Oratory*, trans. John Watson (London: Bell, 1907), 6.2.29–30.

[25]   See Rebhorn, *The Emperor of Men's Minds*, chap. 2.

[26]   John Rainolds, *Oxford Lectures on Aristotle's Rhetoric*, ed. and trans. Lawrence D. Green (Cranbury, NJ: Associated University Press, 1986), 143. Rainolds, who was one of the lead translators of the King James Bible, delivered these lectures in his position as Greek Reader at Corpus Christi College, where he would later serve as President.

[27]   On the use of contraries and substitutions in Renaissance psychological medicine and for an outline of the instrumental use of the passions and imagination in rectifying psychic disturbance, see Stanley Jackson, *Care of the Psyche: A History of Psychological Healing* (New Haven, CT: Yale University Press, 1999), pt. 5, "Healing and the Principle of Contraries."

[28]   Gowland, *The Worlds of Renaissance Melancholy*, 47.

[29]   Leen Spruit, *Species Intelligibilis: From Perception to Knowledge*, vol. 2 (Leiden: Brill, 1994), 198.

than in the Aristotelian model, which dictated that images sent out by perceived objects impressed only copies of themselves upon the percipient's internal senses. In Telesio's reformulation, perception became "the result of the impact of external objects touching the spirit in the extreme parts of the body." Telesio thereby translated a virtual assimilation of information into a physical one, arguing that sensation was "based on a real tactile 'passio,'" and that "all senses (with the exception of hearing) may be reduced to touch, which therefore has primacy over the other senses."[30] Campanella further developed this receptive model to stress that all perception takes place by "immutatio" or alteration of the percipient and does so by "emphasizing the identity between the knowing soul and known object."[31] For Campanella, knowledge is formed through a process of assimilation that, furthermore, requires the percipient to recognize him- or herself as having been altered by contact with the perceived object. It is by such a formulation that Burton seems best poised to suggest that melancholics are not, as Ficino had argued, congenitally inclined to genius but rather that they demonstrate a heightened imaginative agility and capacity for assimilative mimesis that causes them to become overburdened by the same studies in which they seem especially astute.

Campanella's model of conscious impressionability is of a kind with the willing credulity to which Burton credits the transformative powers of the imagination.[32] What we now only figuratively call the "open mind" was understood in this earlier model to represent a physiological openness necessary not only for the assimilation of knowledge but for empathy, as we saw in the previous chapter. According to Campanella's assimilative account of cognition, the mind inclines toward the object that it wishes to imitate. Studious "intent" sends the spirits in the direction of the object the mind has fixed upon. For this reason, Burton argues, the melancholic should not only avoid pondering heavy things but actively contemplate lofty and wondrous things, as you are what you study—what you literally put your mind to—as much as what you eat or breathe. Paracelsus understood the instrumentality of the mind's identification with the studied object in similar terms.[33] "Man," he said, "has a mind that flies out and does not remain in him; for mind is spirit. If he intends to experience heaven, his

---

[30]   Ibid., 2:199–200. Campanella furthermore ascribed a certain sentience to matter (varying in degree of intensity and subtlety with size and texture) as a kind of co-participant in this process of perception. See Germana Ernst, *Tommaso Campanella: The Book and the Body of Nature* (Dordrecht: Springer, 2010), 120–21.

[31]   Spruit, *Species Intelligibilis: From Perception to Knowledge*, 2:220.

[32]   See, especially, the subsection titled "Terrors and Affrights Causes of Melancholy" (1:333–6).

[33]   On Paracelsus's Neoplatonist inheritance, see Walter Pagel, *Paracelsus: An Introduction to Philosophical Medicine in the Era of the Renaissance* (Basel: Karger, 1982), 218–23 and 297–301. On the power of the imagination in Paracelsian chemical philosophy, see also Walter Pagel, *Joan Baptista van Helmont: Reformer of Science and Medicine* (Cambridge: Cambridge University Press, 1982); Allen G. Debus, *The English Paracelsians* (London: Oldburne, 1965).

spirit is in heaven, if herbs, his spirit is in herbs, also in air, also in water."[34] "To know," according to Paracelsus, "is to 'learn of,' to 'listen to,' to be 'taught by' the object ... not by the 'grasp of reason' but by the force of imagination."[35] Jan Baptist van Helmont, Paracelsus's chief disseminator, emphasized the power of the imagination as a force of magnetic attraction in a way that echoes the force of mimetic assimilation in Campanella's account. He argued that an object is "drawn into" the person who is exerting imaginative powers and then "impressed" on another person.[36] This magnetic impulse of the imagination explains the power of prayer to heal, of the mother's imaginings to imprint the unborn child and, of course, of the melancholic's somatized conceits. The magnetic force of sympathetic transmission also explains cures (and afflictions) transmitted by proxy and at great distances.

Renaissance Neoplatonists and Paracelsian writers alike described such seemingly invisible transformations as involving the transfer of minute bodies (corpuscles, atoms, and spirits) across a densely animated pneumatic medium.[37] They adopted this argument from the Stoics, who held that the universe is suffused with *pneuma*, the spirit-laden air or breath that is the originating and sustaining principle of life. In Stoic cognitive theory, the presence of pneuma in the body provides a sympathetic mechanism or "material bridge" by which information is physically received in the mind and properly recognized by the estimative faculties. This process is not a strictly internal one. Pneuma flows from the cognitive center (*hegemonikon*) to the sense organ, where it exits and interacts with the perceived object in the animate air that surrounds it and returns with a sense image formed on the basis of this extramental contact.[38]

---

[34] Pagel, *Joan Baptista van Helmont*, 30.

[35] Ibid.

[36] Pagel, *Joan Baptista van Helmont*, 122.

[37] John Sutton and Koen Vermeir have lamented the lack of attention to the role of air and pneuma in premodern cognitive theory. See Sutton, *Philosophy and Memory Traces: Descartes to Connectionism* (Cambridge: Cambridge University Press, 1998), chap. 2; and "Spongy Brains and Material Memories," in *Environment and Embodiment in Early Modern England*, ed. Mary Floyd-Wilson and Garrett A. Sullivan Jr. (New York: Palgrave Macmillan, 2007), 14–34; Koen Vermeir, "The 'Physical Prophet' and the Powers of the Imagination. Part I: A Case-Study on Prophecy, Vapours and the Imagination (1685–1710)," *Studies in History and Philosophy of Science Part C: Studies in History and Philosophy of Biological and Biomedical Sciences* 35, no. 4 (2004): 561–91. See also Carla Mazzio's discussion of air and affect in "The History of Air: Hamlet and the Trouble with Instruments," *South Central Review* 26, no. 1 (2009): 153–96.

[38] See Marcia Colish, *The Stoic Tradition from Antiquity to the Early Middle Age* (Leiden: Brill, 1985), 51–3. On pneuma and spiritus, see James Bono, "Medical Spirits and the Medieval Language of Life," *Traditio* 40 (1984): 91–130. The classical account of pneumatic theory in antiquity is Gérard Verbeke, *L'évolution de la doctrine du Pneuma: du stoicisme à S. Augustin* (Paris: Desclée de Brouwer, 1945). For a recent critique and reappraisal, see A.P. Bos, *The Soul and Its Instrumental Body: A Reinterpretation of Aristotle's Philosophy of Living Nature* (Leiden: Brill, 2003).

The appeal of this pneumatic reasoning for Burton, whose aim in the *Anatomy* is ultimately to attenuate the melancholic's experience of alienation, is especially evident through Campanella's elaboration. Wayne Shumaker writes that in Campanella's pneumatic universe, "human consciousness is less pitiably isolated, and human feelings can reach out towards, or shrink away from, a quasi-spiritual 'sense' that informs their physical environment."[39] In a world where bodies communicate with one another sympathetically along currents of sentient matter, we are, conceivably, never alone. Knowledge requires a conscious imitative assimilation of the information communicated through what Campanella calls a "conscious air." To demonstrate, Campanella gives the example of Zisca's drum (the same one Burton prominently alludes to in the Preface to the *Anatomy*), which reputedly scattered the dead warrior's enemies when its hide (made of Zisca's own flayed skin) was struck on the battlefield. The skin drum serves Campanella as an illustration of the power and range of sympathetic transmissions through an animate pneumatic medium.[40] He wonders, "if the sense of a magnet is drawn out as far as the (terrestrial) pole, who will doubt that the senses of other things can communicate through the air?"[41]

The vitality of air is also crucial to Ficino's understanding of sympathetic and occult transmissions and, in particular, his account of the power of music. Ficino writes that we are thoroughly penetrable by this ambient medium that enters us "on all sides" and "flourishes in the heart, into whose chambers it flows now steadily, now suddenly; thus straightway affecting the spirit according as it is itself disposed."[42] He suggests that we are better nourished by air than food, giving Democritus' *ars moriendi* as illustration of this point. When the philosopher, at 107 years of age, felt the hour of his death close upon him, he sustained himself for three days by holding freshly baked loaves to his nose in order to allow his sister to leave his bedside and participate in the festival of Thesmophoria. The story illuminates the Stoic ideal of self-sustenance not as ascetic self-denial but rather as a state of communion with the vital "ayre and dew of heaven" (1:309), a state that

---

[39]   Quoted in Wayne Shumaker, *Natural Magic and Modern Science: Four Treatises, 1590–1657* (Binghamton: Center for Medieval and Early Renaissance Studies, State University of New York Press, 1989), 100. See also Bernardino M. Bonansea, *Tommaso Campanella: Renaissance Pioneer of Modern Thought* (Washington, DC: Catholic University of America Press, 1969), chaps. 3–4.

[40]   See Chapter 2. Given the consonant ways that both invoke this story, it seems likelier that Burton borrows the legend from Campanella than from Foxe's *Acts and Monuments*, where it had earlier appeared.

[41]   From the fourth book of Campanella, *De sensu rerum et magia* (1590), cited in Shumaker, *Natural Magic and Modern Science*, 106.

[42]   Ficino, *Three Books on Life*, 223. Burton's description of his capricious compositional style that "runnes sometimes precipitate and swift, then dull and slow; now direct, then *per ambages*" (1:18) seems to echo Ficino's remarks about the permeability of the heart to ambient spirit more than Quintilian's depiction of the grand style orator in book 12.10.61, as Gowland suggests (Gowland, "Rhetorical Structure and Function in *The Anatomy of Melancholy*," 1–3; 47).

both facilitates and is facilitated by charity. Democritus' selflessness is precisely what allows him to be nourished by such subtle matter.[43]

Burton refers to Democritus' legendary sustenance on fragrance in his subsection on "Alteratives and Cordials" (2:253), one of many places where he discusses remedies that remediate air as a non-natural or "adjacent" cause of both illness and its cure. He discourses at length on the detriments of foul air and the benefits to be had by a change of air, especially by travel. This discussion of fair and foul air occurs exactly in between the "Digression of the Ayre" and his defense of study in "Exercise Rectified of Body and Mind." Noting this topical arrangement, Michael O'Connell asks, "What do the ample fields of knowledge [in the 'Digression'] have to do with the air we breathe?"[44] He suggests that the answer, implied but never explicitly stated, is in the analogy between atmospheric air and cosmic knowledge.[45] I would press the analogy further to consider the kinds and qualities of air in the *Anatomy* beyond the physical air that the body suspires and the ostensibly figurative air that suspends Burton's digressive flights. Whereas O'Connell suspects that Burton wishes to "compensate for the bookishness of his method and material" by offering us only the "illusion of speaking endlessly to the reader,"[46] I am suggesting that the company of Burton's voices and the healing he administers by them is more than merely symbolic. The pneumatic account of cognition provided Renaissance philosophers with the mechanics by which to explain sympathetic cures and other occult (invisible or hidden) forms of action at a distance.[47] It similarly informed Burton's understanding of the distant but nonetheless physically transformative contact in which scholars could engage with one another through study.

Burton's study cure invites the reader into spiritual commerce in the spirit-laden, conscious air to which it gains access by power of the imagination.[48]

---

[43] See C.C.W. Taylor, ed., *The Atomists, Leucippus and Democritus: Fragments: A Text and Translation with a Commentary* (Toronto, ON: University of Toronto Press, 2010), 58; 66.

[44] Michael O'Connell, *Robert Burton* (Boston: Twayne, 1986), 64.

[45] Ibid., 66.

[46] Ibid., 75. See chapter 4, "Words against Melancholy," for O'Connell's extended argument regarding the therapeutic quality of Burton's vernacular sound.

[47] See Ioan P. Culianu, *Eros and Magic in the Renaissance* (Chicago: University of Chicago Press, 1987), chap. 1; D.P. Walker, "The Astral Body in Renaissance Medicine," *Journal of the Warburg and Courtauld Institutes* 21 (1958): 119–33; D.P. Walker, *Spiritual and Demonic Magic: From Ficino to Campanella* (University Park: Pennsylvania State University Press, 2000); John Sutton, "Soul and Body in Seventeenth-Century British Philosophy," in *The Oxford Handbook of British Philosophy in the Seventeenth Century*, ed. Peter Anstey (Oxford: Oxford University Press, 2013); Vermeir, "The 'Physical Prophet' and the Powers of the Imagination. Part I," 580–85.

[48] See, especially, D.P. Walker, "Ficino's Spiritus and Music," *Annales Musicologiques* 1 (1953): 131–50. In addition to Walker, see Gary Tomlinson, *Music in Renaissance Magic: Toward a Historiography of Others* (Chicago: University of Chicago Press, 1993); and

His principal means of accomplishing this is by courting the mind's ear, which is to say, by the music of his prose. It was, of course, by air that music, the best-known cure for melancholy (for which "air" was a common early modern synonym) was understood to work its medicine.[49] Burton calls music "a roaring-meg against melancholy," quoting Levinus Lemnius in his explanation that music works by "*affecting not only the eares, but the very arteries, the vitall and animall spirits, it erects the minde, and makes it nimble*" (2:113). He acknowledges that "many men are [made] melancholy by music" but notes that this variety "is a pleasing melancholy" (2:116). Music is, for Burton, a synonym for pleasure and mirth, which is to be recommended for nearly all melancholics, except the "light *inamorato* … who capers in conceit all the day long, and thinkes of nothing else, but how to make Jigges, Sonnets, Madrigals, in commendation of his Mistresse" (2:116). Lest we take this dismissive caveat too seriously, it bears noting that in the roughly 1,500 words of his short treatise on the subject, Burton refers to no fewer than 50 sources that attest to the curative powers of music. There's none of his characteristic display of arguments for and against. The truth Burton takes as self-evident—that the vital spirits are most affectively moved by the ear—underscores the sonic power of suggestion in the *Anatomy*.

II. Scholarly Melancholy: The Hawk in his Mew

Our understanding of early prose reading has been so impoverished by modern reading practices that we routinely overlook the complex and sensuous character of rhetorical performance in texts we believe to have been read silently and in private.[50] Scholars regard the acoustic dimensions of Burton's prose as at best echoing or intensifying Burton's suasory intent. However, this approach subordinates the irrational power of sound (which, like air, has been anachronistically misconstrued as empty or insubstantial) to the rational power of

---

Penelope Gouk, *Music, Science, and Natural Magic in Seventeenth-Century England* (New Haven, CT: Yale University Press, 1999). That historians of music have observed the power of sound in early modern culture more readily than literary historians (especially historians of prose) says more about modern than early modern disciplinary bias.

[49]   See Tomlinson, *Music in Renaissance Magic*; Gouk, *Music, Science, and Natural Magic in Seventeenth-Century England*; Amanda Eubanks Winkler, *O Let Us Howle Some Heavy Note: Music for Witches, the Melancholic, and the Mad on the Seventeenth-Century English Stage* (Bloomington: Indiana University Press, 2006).

[50]   See Heidi Brayman Hackel, *Reading Material in Early Modern England: Print, Gender, and Literacy* (Cambridge: Cambridge University Press, 2005); Roger Chartier, "Leisure and Sociability: Reading Aloud in Early Modern Europe," in *Urban Life in the Renaissance*, ed. Susan Zimmerman (Cranbury, NJ: Associated University Press, 1989), 103–20. The work of historical phenomenologists of sound, such as Bruce Smith, has yet to make its full impact *vis-à-vis* the study of early modern private reading practices. Meanwhile, see D.R. Woolf, "Hearing Renaissance England," in *Hearing History: A Reader*, ed. Mark M. Smith (Athens: University of Georgia Press, 2004), 112–35.

"substantive" argument and renders the affective register of irrational arguments inaudible to the modern ear. Burton's seemingly contradictory statements about the pleasure of study and the misery of scholars are a case in point. His exhortations against the scholarly life are among the most vituperative passages in the *Anatomy* and as such are among the most frequently cited in evidence of his admonitions against study in general. Readers of these excerpted passages might consider the notion that Burton promotes study as a cure for melancholy to be absurd, but this impression mistakes Burton's indictment of the university for a censure of intellectual curiosity. Scholarly melancholy, as Burton describes it, is caused not by mental exertion but by the disparity between the scholar's labor and reward by recognition. The therapeutic value of a roving intellectual exercise is contrasted with the incarcerating conditions that make scholars miserable.[51] Nonetheless, the close proximity between Burton's scholarly complaints and his intellectual reverie calls attention to the way the latter emerges as an allopathic response (if only a fantastical one) to the study of divinity in early seventeenth-century Oxford.

Burton cites an arsenal of classical and Christian admonitions against intellectual *vanitas*, which are easily but mistakenly conflated with his complaints about the corruptions of institutional scholarship. He calls curiosity "that irksome, that tyrannising care ... an itching humor or a kinde of longing to see that which is not to bee seene, to doe that which ought not to bee done; to knowe that secret, which should not be known," and "to eat of the forbidden fruit" (1:363–4). He gives examples of the "superfluous industry about unprofitable things" that have consumed great men, leaving no field of study or labor immune to censure: "Be it in Religion, humanity, Magicke, Philosophy, policie, any action or study, 'tis a needlesse trouble, a meere torment ... . What fruitles questions about the Trinity, Resurrection, Election, Predestination, Reprobation, hell fire, &c. how many shall be saved, damned? ... What is most of our philosophy but a labyrinth of opinions, idle questions, propositions, Metaphysicall tearmes?" (1:364). To this long list of "superfluous" and "unprofitable" pursuits (of which theology notably reigns supreme), Burton adds the secular sciences: astrology, geography, physic, philology, and metaphysics:

> For what matter is it for us to know how high the *Pleiades* are, how farre distant *Perseus* & *Cassiopea* from us, how deepe the Sea, &c., we are neither wiser, as he followes it, nor modester, nor better, nor richer, nor stronger for the knowledge of it ... . what is Astrology, but vaine elections, predictions; all Magicke, but a troublesome error, a pernitious foppery? Physicke, but intricate rules and prescriptions? Philology, but vain Criticismes? Logicke, needlesse Sophisms? Metaphysicks themselves, but intricate subtilties, and fruitlesse abstractions? Alcumy, but a bundle of errors? To what end are such great Tomes? why doe wee spend so many yeares in their studies? (1:364)

---

[51] For a reading of Burton as an early modern sociologist of scholarly melancholy, see Douglas Trevor, *The Poetics of Melancholy in Early Modern England* (Cambridge: Cambridge University Press, 2004), chap. 5.

Burton declares ignorance preferable to these *end-less* examinations: "Much better to know nothing at all, as those barbarous *Indians* are wholly ignorant, then as some of us, to be so sore vexed about unprofitable toies: *stultus labor est ineptiarum*, to build an house without pinnes, make a rope of sand, to what end? *cui bono?*" But the parroted critique of *vanitas* ("searcheth every creeke, Sea, Citty, Mountaine, Gulfe, to what end? See one Promontory (said *Socrates* of old), one Mountaine, one Sea, one River, and see all") reminds readers how easily this reasoning can be abused to equate purpose, or "end," with a very specific kind of pragmatism (1:364).

The effect of all this grumbling is finally not wizened stoicism but conspicuously cantankerous complaint. Alchemists are swindlers or beggars, or both. Collectors and antiquaries are scavengers, mere busybodies who go clamoring after "news" (1:364–5). Burton is playing the cynic for whom all is vain: the philosopher, scientist, monarch, and tyrant are yoked together as examples of feckless ambition and intellectual pride: "*Aristotle* must find out the motion of *Euripus*; *Pliny* must needs see *Vesuvius*, but how sped they? One loseth goods, another his life. *Pyrrhus* will conquer *Africke* first, and then *Asia*; he will be a sole Monarch, a second immortall, a third rich; a fourth commands" (1:365). Burton sums up: "we runne, ride, take indefatigable paines, all up early, downe late, striving to get that which we had better be without, (*ardeliones* busie bodies as wee are)," and concludes that "it were much fitter for us to be quiet, sit still, and take our ease" (1:365).

We ought always to be suspicious when Burton takes a tally. The quiet life of repose might be the "*voluptas*, or *Summum bonum* of *Epicurus*" (2:99), but it isn't Burton's. On the contrary, it is precisely by meditating upon "*superfluous industry about unprofitable things*" (1:363) that Burton diverts his own melancholia and advises we do the same. In the subsection titled, "Exercise Rectified of Body and Mind," he writes: "Whosoever he is therefore that is overrunne with solitarinesse … I can prescribe him no better remedy then this of study, to compose himselfe to learning of some art or science" (2:90). So he lists them: astrology, physic, philology, logic, metaphysics, alchemy. The entire catalogue of "vain pursuits" decried in the first partition reappears as treatments for melancholic withdrawal in the second. He especially recommends travel to faraway places, the study of antiquities, and the viewing of collections and cabinets of curiosity. All the restless busy-making Burton previously (and we may guess theatrically) condemned is now heartily approved.

The motif that structures Burton's catalogue of vainglorious and blighted pursuits in the first partition is the repeated interrogative: "what matter," "to what end," "cui bono?" The question opposes the benefit of study with the most damning arguments against it. This rhetorical technique of refutation by anticipation is known as *procatalepsis*. George Puttenham describes both the utility and hostility of this preemptive attack, which he calls "presumption" insofar as it requires a certain "boldnesse to enter so deepely into another mans conceit":

> It serueth many times to great purpose to preuent our aduersaries arguments, and
> take vpon vs to know before what our iudge or aduersary or hearer thinketh, and
> that we will seeme to vtter it before it be spoken or alleaged by them, in respect

of which boldnesse to enter so deepely into another mans conceit or conscience, and to be so priuie of another mans mynde, gaue cause that this figure was called the [*presumptuous*] I will also call him the figure of *presupposall* or the *preuenter*, for by reason we suppose before what may be said or perchaunce would be said by our aduersary or any other, we do preuent them of their aduantage, and do catch the ball (as they are wont to say) before it come to the ground.[52]

Burton puts the device to great use throughout the *Anatomy*, but most prominently in his discussions of study and love. In both instances, he draws out the anticipated argument so extensively and at such a great remove from his eventual *volte-face* that some readers wonder whether Burton signifies anything other than mere equivocation or, more commonly, the equivocal quality of all learned opinions.[53] However, Burton's *procatalepsis* demands more scrupulous attention to the performative and affective logic of his giving such extended consideration to the discarded argument.

Burton uses *procatalepsis* (typically performed through borrowed speech in his *cento*) to indulge in a manner of self-ridicule that deflects as it discloses anticipated derision. His exposition of the anticipated counterargument exorcises the weaknesses of his own position in the unforgiving tones of a conjured opponent. He voices, or cites, the most vile and abject arguments against both love and the scholarly life only to grant both a conspicuously unadorned and undefended clemency. He does, in fact, offer explanation for why it is that the exercise of intellectual and sexual appetites makes a better remedy than their retention, but first he airs the opposition, or rather puts it on extended (one might say monstrous) display.[54] By foregoing rebuttal, Burton deflates the opponent's position by intimating that it warrants no defense. Like Cyrano goading his tormentors with insults of his own for his enormous nose, he supplies too ornate an argument against study. He makes the monstrosity of study (as he does elsewhere of women, cuckolds, and social climbers) suspect by denying it fair rebuke.

---

52   George Puttenham, *The Arte of English Poesie* (London, 1589), 194.

53   See Joan Webber, *The Eloquent "I": Style and Self in Seventeenth-Century Prose* (Madison: University of Wisconsin Press, 1968). Webber, with whose reading of the *Anatomy* I am mostly sympathetic, suggests that Burton's self-contradictions are intended to display the "universal mind" of "cosmic man" and that Burton "does not have a position in the same sense in which the authors whom he quotes do" (97). Rather, his "whole purpose is to include many different positions and possibilities" (87). Angus Gowland takes the representative view of late twentieth-century readers (following Fish) that Burton is "'ripping up' ... everything scientific written about melancholy, 'from the first to the last,' so that it may be 'descried'—discovered ... for the uncertainty it really is" (Gowland, "Rhetorical Structure and Function in *The Anatomy of Melancholy*," 36).

54   For a reading of the *Anatomy* as a monstrous disfigurement of the humanist enterprise, see Robert Grant Williams, "Disfiguring the Body of Knowledge: Anatomical Discourse and Robert Burton's *The Anatomy of Melancholy*," *ELH* 68, no. 3 (2001): 593–613.

At the same time, this theatrical aping of familiar abuse engenders pathos for the rhetor who uses this device to wince in public, drawing attention away from the monstrosity of the melancholy scholar and toward the causes and conditions of his suffering instead.

The exposition of melancholy caused "by Love of Learning, or overmuch study" promised by the title of this subsection is overwhelmed in force and scale by the "Digression of the misery of Schollers" that follows in the same subheading (1:302). Burton represents the authorities who discuss the melancholic affliction of students in less than one page and then moves on to itemize the social and institutional causes of scholarly misery for the succeeding 20. Whereas training in nearly every other trade enables the apprentice to sustain himself, there's no such guarantee for a scholar. Even a merchant has a one in four chance of his ship's return, he says, "only schollers, me thinks are most uncertaine, unrespected, subject to all casualties, and hazards." Burton laments the meager reward for a labor so few are fit to undertake, not for lack of ability but perseverance:

> not one of a many proves to be a scholler, all are not capable and docile, *ex omni ligno non fit Mercurius*: wee can make *Maiors* and officers every yeare, but not Schollers: Kings can invest Knights and Barons ... Universities can give degrees ... but he nor they, nor all the world, can give learning, make Philosophers, Artists, Orators, Poets. (1:307)

The rare few who have the intestinal fortitude, "*aeneis intestinis*," to endure it can only hope after 20 years of penury to "teach a Schoole, turn Lecturer or Curat" at a falconer's wages and do so only "so long as he can please his Patron or the parish," a crowd as fickle as "they that cryed *Hosanna* one day, and *crucifie* him the other" (1:308).

Burton tabulates the costs that scholars pay for the privilege of their servitude in a grim, if grandiose, manner that lampoons the heavy-handed parallelism of contemporary sermons. He borrows, or claims to borrow, much of his scholar's lament from a sermon delivered by John Howson:[55]

---

[55]   A one-time fellow student at Christ Church, Howson served as Bishop of Oxford, later Durham. His preference of liturgy over preaching and his perceived tolerance of both covert Catholics and Arminian teachings earned him suspicion and censure under George Abbot and promotion under William Laud, both archbishops of Canterbury (Nicholas W.S. Cranfield, "Howson, John [1556/7–1632]," in *Oxford Dictionary of National Biography*, ed. H.C.G. Matthew and Brian Harrison [Oxford: Oxford University Press, 2004]; online edition, ed. Lawrence Goldman, January 2008, http://www.oxforddnb.com/ view/article/14006 [accessed May 2, 2010]). It is conceivable that Burton invented this attribution to Howson. The STC has no record for a sermon by Howson on the date credited (November 4, 1597). Burton owned a copy of a sermon by Howson delivered December 4, 1597, but the material Burton cites is not found therein (Nicolas K. Kiessling, *The Library of Robert Burton* [Oxford Bibliographical Society, 1988], 159). It is of course possible that the sermon was either lost or never printed, but it would not be beyond Burton to credit his own theatrical invective to Howson under guise of misattribution.

> *If by this price of the expence of time, our bodies and spirits, our substance and patrimonies, we cannot purchase those small rewards, which are ours by law, and the right of inheritance, a poore Parsonage, or a Vicarige of 50l.* per annum, *but we must pay to the Patron for the lease of a life (a spent and out worne life) ... and that with the hazarde and losse of our soules, by Simony and perjury, and the forfeiture of all our spiritual preferments,* in esse *and* posse, *both present and to come.* (1:313)

Continuing in his "own" voice, Burton replaces Howson's sonorous parallelism with Democritus Junior's more characteristic *systrophe*: "fleeced by those greedy *Harpies* to get more fees, wee stand in feare of some precedent Lapse; we fall amongst refractory, seditious Sectaries, peevish Puritans, perverse Papists, a lascivious rout of Atheistical *Epicures* ... ." Burton's conspicuous alliteration or *paroemion* parodies Howson's melancholy reckoning and the dismal conclusions it compels:

> from a polite and terse Academicke, he must turn rusticke, rude, melancholise alone, learne to forget, or else, as many doe, become Maltsters, Grasiers, Chapmen, &c. (now banished from the Academy, all commerce of the Muses, and confined to a country village, as *Ovid* was from *Rome* to *Pontus*), and daily converse with a company of Idiots and Clownes. (1:324)

The complaint against the scholarly life concludes at last with more than a thousand words in Latin, by far the longest untranslated stretch in the book, in which he denounces too-easy access to the universities that have become breeding grounds for "*philosophastri*" and "*theologastri*," those charlatan scholars satirized in his own Latin comedy, *Philosophaster*. However, recalling the playful tone of Burton's remark that he had prostituted his muse by writing in English (1:16), we would be remiss to take Burton's recourse to Latin as uncensored revelation. He vacillates wildly between acrimony and apology (here, in Latin, much as he does in English in the Preface) and makes a spectacle of hyperbolic complaint that exorcises even as it parodies its own vexation.

Burton offers a brief but exquisite comment on the psychology of scholarly discontentment somewhat earlier in the subsection in his retelling of Plato's grasshopper fable. In the *Phaedrus*, Socrates says that before the time of the muses, grasshoppers were humans who were so ravished by music they forgot to eat and drink and consequently sang themselves to death. The muses honored them by returning them to life as grasshoppers, who feel neither hunger nor thirst and feast on air and music. In Burton's version, the grasshoppers were the "Poets, Rhetoritians, Historians, Philosophers, Mathematitians, Sophisters &c." who lived "before the *Muses* were borne ... without meat and drinke" and were transformed as punishment for the impudence of their self-sufficiency. He theatrically pines for this mythic time when scholars lived, like "those *Indian* birds of *Paradise*" (or the Stoic Democritus) on "the ayre, and dew of heaven ... for being as they are," meaning hungry, "their *Rhetoricke only serves them, to curse their bad fortunes.*" In Burton's rendition of the allegory, privation and lack of recognition breed contempt and turn the singing grasshopper, who once feasted on air and music, into a stinging wasp: "from Grasshoppers they turne Humblebees & Wasps, plaine Parasites, and make the *Muses*, Mules, to satisfie their hungerstarved panches, and get a meales meat" (1:309). The poet and scholar who would be sustained by books and philosophy are turned to parasites, groveling for meals and grumbling in a rhetoric that "serves them" only to sing in satire.

As Burton describes it, scholarly melancholy is the misery of servitude to fickle and unworthy masters. As such, it best resembles the melancholy Burton categorizes under the heading, "Loss of Liberty, Servitude, imprisonment." He suggestively uses the same phrase, "mewed up like hawkes" (1:307), to describe both the life of a scholar and "those *Italian* and *Spanish Dames*, mewed up like Hawkes, and lockt up by their jealous husbands" (1:343).[56] He plays on this resemblance in the anecdote of the keeper of the books at Leiden, who "was *mewed up*" (2:88) in his library for a year. And yet, despite this phrasing, Burton chastises the reader for mistaking the study for a prison:

> that which to thy thinking should have bred a loathing, caused in him a greater liking. *I no sooner* (saith he) *come into the Library, but I bolt the doore to me, excluding lust, ambition, avarice, and all such vices, whose nurse is idlenesse, the mother of Ignorance, and Melancholy her selfe, and in the very lap of eternity, amongst so many divine soules, I take my seat.* (2:88–9)

While he insists that the scholar in the library is not the hawk in his mew, structural echoes throughout the *Anatomy* make the resemblance more difficult to dismiss. Compared with other objects of his satirical vituperation (women, chastity, marriage), his invective against the scholarly life is not as easily overturned. There is undeniable tension between his complaints about scholarly confinement and freedom, and Burton appears to be more ambivalent than cleverly ambiguous about the relationship between the two, as we see in the following case.

As noted earlier, Burton suggests many kinds of recreation and diversion before coming to the lengthy topic of study. He heartily approves of games, dice, and cards, to which he says, "Many too nicely take exceptions" (2:80). He recommends chess, "*Dancing, Singing, Masking, Mumming, Stage-plaies*" (2:82), even the pranks and jests that great men play on the lesser, and gives a striking example. The Duke of Burgundy, while attending a winter wedding in Flanders, was prevented by weather from either hawking or hunting. Tired of cards, dice, and dancing, he would go walking about the town in disguise. Late one night he discovered a "country fellow dead drunke, snorting on a Bulke" and brought him back to the palace to be lavishly attired and attended (2:83), much like the unsuspecting Bottom in *A Midsummer Night's Dream*. The puzzled man was "served in state all the day … saw them dance, heard musicke, and the rest of those Court-like pleasures" (2:83), and when he fell asleep again (being "well tipled")

---

[56]   Indeed, Burton seems to be drawing on the pervasive trope, especially in Jacobean drama, of representing women as melancholy birds in cages.

the courtiers returned him to the place they discovered him. Burton explains that the point and pleasure of the jest was to witness the drunk man's astonished encounter with the luxuries to which the jesters were accustomed:

> Now the fellow had not made them so good sport the day before, as he did when he returned to himselfe, all the jest was, to see how he looked upon it. In conclusion, after some little admiration, the poore man told his friends he had seene a vision, constantly beleeved it, would not otherwise be perswaded, and so the jest ended. (2:84)

Burton notes that such tricks are not uncommon disport among royalty, known to wander anonymously among their subjects for pleasure. Antiochus, for instance, would "steale from his Court, and goe into Merchants, Goldsmiths, and other tradesmens shops, sit and talke with them, and sometimes ride or walke alone, and fall aboord with any Tinker, Clowne, Serving man, Carrier, or whomsoever he met first." Bored with the refinements of court, the king goes slumming like Prince Hal on the eve of Agincourt under the pretense of seeking honest company. But other motives come to light in the game Antiochus plays, quite similar to the duke's:

> Sometimes hee did *ex insperato* give a poore fellow mony, to see how he would looke, or on set purpose, loose his purse as hee went, to watch who found it, and withall, how he would be affected, and with such objects he was much delighted. (2:84)

Under cover of fatigue with privilege, the enervated aristocrats exercise a power available to them only in disguise, playing god with the fortunes of their subjects. This is not the pleasure of anonymous charity. Instead, as the duke's rather cruel story shows, the noble prankster seeks vicarious wonder at his own familiar privilege.[57]

Burton conspicuously relates these "harmless jests" as a preface to his recommendation of study as cure:

---

[57] There are innumerable examples of classical and biblical visitations by gods and angels in disguise who test the fidelity, piety, and hospitality of their subjects. The angels in Genesis 18 reward Abraham and Sarah for their hospitality with the conception of Isaac. Mercury and Jupiter spare the aged Baucis and Philemon from flood because of their hospitality in Ovid's *Metamorphoses* 8. But the courtly jest Burton remarks upon evokes a more cynical test, not unlike the wager between Satan and God in the Book of Job, or the test put to the shepherd Battus. Mercury steals Apollo's cattle, hiding them in a nearby wood. When he notices that Battus has witnessed the theft, he asks the shepherd to keep silent and Battus swears to be silent as a nearby stone. When Mercury disguises himself again and offers the shepherd double reward for the location of the cattle, Battus betrays him and Mercury turns Battus into that same stone, a punishment Ovid calls unfit and unfair: "*in durum silicem, qui nunc quoque dicitur index, inque nihil merito vetus est infamia saxo*" (*Metamorphoses*, 2.706–7).

> Many such tricks are ordinarily put in practise by great men, to exhilerate themselves and others, all which are harmelesse jests, and have their good uses.

> But amongst those exercises, or recreations of the minde within doores, there is none so generall, so aptly to be applyed to all sorts of men, so fit & proper to expell Idlenesse and Melancholy, as that of *Study*. (2:84)

Burton makes a curious exchange between the royal prank and the diversion to be had by scholarly pursuits. Several pages into his promotion of the study cure, he quotes oaths by mighty men who vowed they would trade whole empires to write a few lines of worthy poetry or spend their lives in a library. He reports that when King James came to Oxford and viewed Bodley's library, he "brake out into that noble speech, If I were not a King, I would be an University man; *And if it were so that I must be a Prisoner, if I might have my wish, I would desire to have no other Prison then that Library, and to be chained together with so many good Authors, et mortuis magistris*" (2:88). King James's remarks, phrased in the theatrical longing of the subjunctive mood, recall the fantasy of the aristocratic jest. The king's wish (*would that I were a scholar in his cell*) is somewhat less cynical, perhaps, than the fantasy of the royal prank: *Would that I could feast with a pauper's appetite, or know what it is to lack so that I might look on my riches with surprise*. But as a prelude to his discourse upon recreation by study, the anecdotes suggest their own resemblance to the intellectual flights of fancy Burton takes from the privilege of his library. He seems deliberately to be calling into question the opposition between the onerous labors of the mind and the pleasures that constitute scholarly delight.

In *Literature as Recreation in the Later Middle Ages*, Glending Olson studies late medieval justifications for the pleasure of reading. The recreation to which his title refers underscores the physiological benefit that such pleasure was understood to provide in restoring or "re-creating" the spirits. Reading is one of the many activities that physicians since antiquity had considered to be "restorative" diversions. Other recommendations typically included hunting, dancing, and singing: all activities that pertain to the *non-natural* "causes" of bodily health and disease.[58] The non-naturals referred to the body's six points of interaction with

---

[58]   Glending Olson, *Literature as Recreation in the Later Middle Ages* (Ithaca, NY: Cornell University Press, 1982), chap. 2, "The Hygienic Justification." For Renaissance views of the restorative effects of reading, see Katharine Craik, *Reading Sensations in Early Modern England* (Basingstoke, UK: Palgrave Macmillan, 2007), chap. 1. Scholarship on the physiology of reading as understood by early modern commentators has been spare and mainly focused on deleterious effects. See, for example, Michael Schoenfeldt, "Reading Bodies," in *Reading, Society and Politics in Early Modern England*, ed. Kevin Sharpe and Steven N. Zwicker (Cambridge: Cambridge University Press, 2003), 215–43. Adrian Johns explores the physiology of reading as it informed early modern bibliotherapy but mainly through the lens of later seventeenth-century writers (René Descartes, Jean-François Senault, and Thomas Willis) and their concerns (*The Nature of the Book: Print and Knowledge in the Making* [Chicago: University of Chicago Press, 1998], chap. 6).

and dependence upon its environment: air; food and drink; sleep and wakefulness; motion and rest; evacuation and repletion; and the passions of the mind/soul.[59] The adjacency of the "non-natural" to the "natural" underscores the indeterminate boundary between body, mind, and the external world in classical and Renaissance medicine. It is at this unstable boundary that the activity of reading was understood to excite the imagination, enliven the spirits, and consequently restore or transform one's disposition.

Olson pays particular attention to medieval accounts of the ways that literary delight restores the spirits. He notes the frequent repetition among such defenses of an apocryphal legend told by Cassian. A hunter reproaches the apostle John for absently petting a pheasant, asking what he means to gain by such trivial distraction. John, in turn, asks the hunter whether he goes about all day with his bow drawn and taut, explaining that in order to keep his mind in best condition, he needs to let it rest as well.[60] Medieval glosses of the legend argue that the value of delight is measured by the degree to which it enables the Christian mind to return to the more serious endeavors for which it was purposed.[61] Delight implied a momentary pause from which one returns to work again.[62] While the study he models in the "Digression of the Ayre" is presented as a moment of exceptional freedom, the diversionary injunction of Burton's cure follows from beginning to end. Burtonian study is not a temporary remedy for an acute condition; it is paradigmatic, which has led some scholars to surmise that its logic is also palliative. Martin Heusser finds Burton paradoxically optimistic about "the fundamental

---

[59]   For an overview of the complex history and varying interpretations of the non-naturals in Western medical literature, see Saul Jarcho, "Galen's Six Non-Naturals: A Bibliographic Note and Translation," *Bulletin of the History of Medicine* 44, no. 4 (1970): 372–7.

[60]   "If by a certain relaxation it did not occasionally lighten and loosen its taut tension, it would not be able to hearken to the power of the spirit when necessity demanded, since it would be weakened by its unrelenting exertion" (John Cassian, *The Conferences*, ed. and trans. Boniface Ramsey [New York: The Newman Press, 1997], 842).

[61]   Olson, *Literature as Recreation in the Later Middle Ages*, 91; 99. The sentiment is echoed in early modern recommendations by physicians such as Levinus Lemnius's for temporary restorative recreations: "Let a man taste of the delights of other studies at idle times, as for recreation and rest from labour, so that he return back to his wonted task and businesse, and that his mind may betake it self to those studies he hath intermitted for a time" (Levinus Lemnius, *The Secret Miracles of Nature: In Four Books* [London, 1658], 330).

[62]   The rising status of aesthetic pleasure as an end unto itself that begins to appear in Renaissance poetic theory in the later sixteenth century is witnessed in Jacopo Mazzoni's defense of Dante Alighieri. Poetry, he says, "is an art having the pleasure of man as its aim, in such wise that by means of pleasure it restores the energies grown weary in serious occupations; and when so considered it has no other function but to imitate human actions in a way to delight those who listen to them or who read them" (in Bernard Weinberg, *A History of Literary Criticism in the Italian Renaissance* [Chicago: University of Chicago Press, 1961], 26).

curability of melancholy" while at the same time painfully aware that if cured of the melancholy that inspires and authorizes his book he would be unable to write it.[63] However, this suggestion that Burtonian melancholy is the *felix culpa* of the text discounts Burton's sympathetic depiction of melancholy as a condition of heightened sensitivity that requires therapeutic management instead of cure. As his designated "best" therapy for chronic melancholia, Burton's study may require a different designation than "diversion," which suggests deflection away from melancholic dishumor, but toward what other end? The very question returns us to Burton's representation of study as both incarcerating and emancipating and to the parallelism between the scholar as "mewed hawk" bound by time and place and the hawk-in-flight who surveys a world of wonder in the "Digression of the Ayre."

III. Study as Cure: The Scholar's Delight

Still "giddy with roving about" (2:57), Burton makes his way in the "Digression of the Ayre" toward his exposition of a "roving cure" by punning an apology for going "off track": "But I rove: the sum is this, that variety of actions, objects, air, places, are excellent good in this infirmity, and all others, good for man, good for beast" (2:66). Shortly afterward, in "Exercise Rectified of Body and Mind," Burton catalogs the diverse forms of diversion one might undertake to cure melancholy, beginning with travel and sightseeing, or rather, with the *contemplation* of travel and distant marvels:

> What so full of content, as to read, walke and see Mappes, Pictures, Statues, Jewels, marbles, which some so magnifie, as those that *Phidias* made of old, so exquisite and pleasing to be beheld, that as *Chrysotome* thinketh, *if any man be sickly, troubled in mind, or that canot sleep for griefe, and shall but stand over against one of Phidias Images, he will forget all care, or whatsoever else may molest him in an instant?* (2:84)

For those who are moved by images, Burton recommends the viewing of "neat Architectures, Devices, Scutchions, coats of armes, read such bookes, to peruse old Coynes of severall sorts in a faire Gallery; artificiall workes, perspective glasses, old reliques, *Roman* Antiquities, variety of colours." He concedes that "artificiall toyes please but for a time," while insisting on the value of ephemeral diversion ("who is he that will not be moved with them for the present?") as a prophylactic against despair (2:84).

Burton points to Achilles, wracked with grief over the death of Patroclus but eased by delight at the scenes depicted on the buckler his mother brought to console him. This is the second buckler to which Burton introduces us in the *Anatomy*. The first is the Democritean buckler by which Burton protests his imperviousness to censure in the Preface. Achilles' buckler ironically undermines

---

    [63]   Martin Heusser, *The Gilded Pill: A Study of the Reader-Writer Relationship in Robert Burton's "Anatomy of Melancholy"* (Tübingen: Stauffenburg, 1987), 58.

Burton's earlier professed indifference,[64] underscoring for the reader that the book aspires to be the object of meditative and therapeutic delight. The scene depicted on Achilles' buckler, "in which were engraven Sunne, Moone, Starres, Planets, Sea, Land, men fighting, running, riding, women scolding, hils, dales, townes, castles, brooks, rivers, trees, &c. with many pretty landskips, and perspective peeces," bears striking resemblance to the survey Burton makes both of pleasurable studies and those objects Burton advises we "look upon" when he commends the viewing of galleries and cabinets of curiosity, where one may see a variety of "Pictures, old Statues and Antiquities" and, like Achilles, "landskips" and "peeces of perspective."[65]

Burton rhapsodizes on the pleasures of the gallery and cabinet in the infinitive mood that underscores his recommended program of spiritual allegrification:

> to see such variety of attires, faces, so many, so rare, and such exquisite peeces, of men, birds, beasts, &c. to see those excellent landskips, Dutch-works, and curious cuts of *Sadlier of Prage, Albertus Durer, Goltzius, Vrintes* &c. such pleasant peeces of perspective, *Indian Pictures* made of feathers, *China* workes, frames, *Thaumaturgicall* motions, exoticke toyes, &c. (2:85)

As the list of ponderable wonders and recreations turns to the pleasure of literature, he shifts from the infinitive to the vocative, addressing these apostrophically as the subjects of his praise:

> Who is hee that is now wholly overcome with Idlenesse, or otherwise involved in a Labyrinth of worldly cares, troubles, and discontents, that will not bee much lightned in his minde by reading of some inticing story, true or fained … . Who is not earnestly affected with a passionate speech, well penned, an elegant Poem, or some pleasant bewitching discourse … . *O argumenta! O compositionem!* I may say the same of this or that pleasing Tract … . For what a world of bookes offers it selfe, in all subjects, arts, and sciences, to the sweet content and capacity of the Reader? (2:85–6)

Burton goes on to recommend "*Arithmeticke, Geometry, Perspective, Opticke, Astronomie, Architecture, Scultpurâ, Pictura … Mechanicks* and their misteries, *Military matters*, Navigation, riding of horses, fencing, swimming, gardening, planting, great Tomes of husbandry, Cookery, Fawkonry, Hunting, Fishing, Fowling, &c. with exquisite pictures, of all sports, games, and what not? In *Musick, Metaphysicks, Naturall* and *Morall Philosophy, Philology,* in *Policy, Heraldry, Genealogy, Chronology, &c*" (2:86). The indiscriminate mixture of recreations both physical and intellectual reveals that, for Burton, the mind that ails is a body

---

64   See Chapter 1.

65   For more on Renaissance discussions of the medicinal benefits of viewing art, see Frances Gage, "Exercise for Mind and Body: Giulio Mancini, Collecting, and the Beholding of Landscape Painting in the Seventeenth Century," *Renaissance Quarterly* 61, no. 4 (2008): 1167–207.

that ails, and both may be cured by sensuous inducements to wonder, which may themselves be invoked by rhetorical force rather than lived experience.

The extended *zeugma* that begins "Who will not be affected?" carries the question across a vast panorama of diverting pursuits, including the contemplation of mechanical wonders ("that Geometirical Tower of *Garezenda*," "the steeple and clocke at *Strasburrough*," or "that Engin of *Archimedes* to remove the earth it selfe") that inspire admiration "at the effects of art" (2:86). At the end of this list are "rare devises to corrivate waters, musick instruments," whose sounds Burton imitates in his own description of the "Trisillable *Echoes*" that resound from such machines, "againe, againe, and againe, repeated, with miriades of such" (2:86).[66] With the exclamatory motif, "What so sure, What so pleasant … What so full of content … What vast tomes … What greater pleasure … What more pleasing," Burton folds the superlative into the serial (2:86–7). Each object becomes its own summit—a place one might stop to meditate for an eternity. But these are false resting places along a deliberately inexhaustible itinerary of studious pursuits, of which the "Digression" is an obvious demonstration.[67] Burton's study cure works not by propelling the reader from wonder to some more sober study but from one wonder to the next. The forward momentum privileges the yet-to-come and the out of reach. This is the momentum of the extended zeugmata through which Burton incants his hypothetical or wishful lists of things "to see," "to read," and "to learn."[68] He suggests that the studious inventory of what one might *yet* study does more good for the melancholic than a ruminating occupation with any one subject.[69]

---

[66]   The Clarendon commentators suggest that Burton may be drawing from Cardan (Girolamo Cardano), who described such machines in *De subtilitate*, bk. 1, and from Josephus Blancanus, who illustrates how one might arrange rocks to produce such echoes in his *Sphaera mundi seu cosmographia demonstrativa* (Bologna, 1620) (5:178).

[67]   Burton's copious additions over subsequent revisions swelled the "Digression" with evidence of his own voracious reading. See Robert M. Browne, "Robert Burton and the New Cosmology," *Modern Language Quarterly* 13 (1952): 131–48.

[68]   Giancarlo Maiorino observes this ecstatic view of the infinite in Michelangelo's art and more generally in what he calls the baroque aesthetic of the *nonfinito*: "From a baroque standpoint, the Copernican 'breaking of the circle' fostered exploration instead of nostalgia. Regrets about the 'Old Philosophie' aside, infinity set up the challenge of endlessness as a mental attitude striving to feel at home in a universe where discovery itself became a form of epistemological certainty … . The capacity-to-be made possibility more attractive than achievement" (*The Cornucopian Mind and the Baroque Unity of the Arts* [University Park: Pennsylvania State University Press, 1990], 3).

[69]   For a persuasive account of the expansiveness of Burton's recommended reading as a rejection of increasingly narrow studies at the Universities, see Emily Anglin, "'The Glass, the School, the Book': The *Anatomy of Melancholy* and the Early Stuart University of Oxford," *ESC: English Studies in Canada* 35, no. 2 (2009): 55–76. In a similar vein, Kathryn Murphy regards Burton's copious style as a late humanist response to the threats of a burgeoning culture of abbreviation, Ramism, and growing antipathies to scholarly *copia*. See Kathryn Murphy, "Robert Burton and the Problems of Polymathy," *Renaissance Studies* 28, no. 2 (2014): 291.

By extension, it might appear that the curative effects of study are better wrought through contemplation than practice.[70] Numerous scholars have observed the seeming paradox that Burton's studies, for all their emphasis on sensorial experience, are enacted in the admittedly stale air of the library.[71] Some have interpreted Burton's declaration that he "never traveled but in map or card" as evidence of his reactionary promotion of the *vita speculativa* over the *vita activa*. However, early modern cognitive theory made no absolute distinction between the two and neither does Burton.[72] The *Anatomy*, in fact, repeatedly insists that the body does not clearly differentiate real from imaginary experience. Burton gives Petrus Bayerus's example (discussed in the previous chapter) of a person who, when asked to walk across a plank over flat ground, can do so without trouble. But "*if the same planke be laid over some deepe water, in steed of a bridge, hee is vehemently moved, and 'tis nothing but his imagination,* forma cadendi impressâ, *to which his other members and faculties obey*" (1:420).[73] The glands and organs take their cue from the imagination, not an "outside cause." If the man imagines he is in peril, his body will respond accordingly. The example does more than simply illustrate the powers of the imagination; it argues against the utility of using rational persuasion as a means of abating melancholy. The inward perturbations cannot be dissuaded by pointing out their subjective quality: "you may as well bid him that is sicke of an ague, not to bee adry; or him that is wounded, not to feele paine" (1:420).

Burton illustrates this point throughout the *Anatomy* in the heaps of arguments by which one might disabuse a friend of his or her melancholic conceit. These arguments are recited one after another as alternatives to which one might recourse when the preceding one fails, and they become more outrageous as they accumulate. They are marvels in their own right that delight by their very improbability and humor, as is clearly the case with the disenchantment that Burton facetiously recommends (from Bernardus Gordonius) of curing the melancholic lover by waving a bloodied menstrual cloth in his face, proclaiming, "*talis est amica tua*" (3:214).[74] The therapeutic evocation is clearly not of the beloved's abjection but the friend's care, even the imagined sound of his belligerent and outrageous solicitations. Burton suspends this rhetorical effect throughout the *Anatomy*, offering the consolatory suggestion that the book is addressed not to the patient but

---

[70]   Mary Ann Lund argues that "Burton deliberately presents cures which are literally unachievable, but which reveal instead the therapeutic pleasures of reading" (*Melancholy, Medicine and Religion in Early Modern England*, 105).

[71]   For example, Liliana Barczyk-Barakonska, "'Never to Go Forth of the Limits': Space and Melancholy in Robert Burton's Library Project," *Journal of European Studies* 33, no. 3–4 (2003): 212–26.

[72]   See Michel de Montaigne's dismissal of this opposition in his essay "Of Solitarinesse."

[73]   This passage refers to Pietro Biero's *Tractatus de peste* (5:59).

[74]   "This is your beloved."

to the friend, whose very act of reading testifies to the melancholic reader that he or she is loved and cared for. The address to the "friend" is, of course, among the oldest of conventions in medical writing, but it is particularly effective in Burton's hands. Burton invokes the oral presence of the friend as an auditory image (or *audible species*) that works directly on the mind to attenuate solitude. The friend whom Burton presumes (and indeed plays) for the reader need not be present to offer the company prescribed in his concluding advice that we should "*Be not solitary, be not idle*" (3:445).[75] Burton's marvels and mysteries likewise need not be witnessed to produce their therapeutic effects. The evocative power of the imagination that Burton's study cure assumes does not prove his greater valuation of speculative over experiential knowledge; it underscores instead the inutility of this distinction within an epistemological tradition that regarded meditation as experience in its own right and inducements to wonder as valuable outside of their objective verifiability.

The aim of Burton's study cure is to excite the scholarly imagination. To wit, his evidence and examples are suggestive rather than conclusive. In order for an anecdote, rumor, meditative emblem, or conceit to enliven the spirits it must simply invoke lively presence. When Burton marvels at Jean de Lery's "accurate diaries" or "a well-cut Herbal ... expressed in their proper colours to the life," it is the verisimilitude or "accuracy" of the writer's or artist's mimetic reproduction that spurs his imagination to reap the benefits of travel and exotic encounter.[76] Legend and testimony, reputed phenomena and recorded experiment, both work together to invoke a therapeutic sense of intellectual community within the *Anatomy*. Burton uses *enargeia* or vividness to induce a kind of *metastasis* or *translatio temporum*, allowing the reader to feel not only present in the scenes depicted but the enlivening presence of those minds that depicted them.[77] The *Anatomy* is, in

---

[75] Jonathan Sawday regards Burton's excessive speaking as "both symptomatic and palliative" of the author's melancholy, made worse by the absence of a sympathetic friend or confessor: "So, the speaker-writer relieves himself against trees and pillars (or readers), or eases himself in the solitude of his study, and the result is the *Anatomy*—a waste product which is a substitute for speech" (Jonathan Sawday, "Shapeless Elegance," in *English Renaissance Prose: History, Language, and Politics*, ed. Neil Rhodes [Tempe, AZ: Medieval & Renaissance Texts & Studies, 1997], 191–2).

[76] Angel Day similarly praises the evocative quality of cosmographic description in his manual on letter writing: "Doeth not the learned Cosmographer in acquainting us with the unknown delights, scituation, plentie and riches of Countries which we never sawe, not happily may ever approch unto, ravish us oftentimes, and bring in contempt the pleasures of our own soyle: and many times a huge wonder of the unheard secretes never before reported of ... that our eies do almost witnes the same, and that our verie sences are partakers of every delicacie in them contained ..." (*The English Secretorie* [London, 1595], 23–4).

[77] See Ruth Webb's discussion of *metastasis* or *metathesis*, in *Ekphrasis, Imagination, and Persuasion in Ancient Rhetorical Theory and Practice* (Farnham, UK: Ashgate, 2009), chap. 4, "Enargeia: Making Absent Things Present."

this way, a metacabinet of curiosity contained in books about books and reports of marvels witnessed or relayed by others.[78]

Burton invokes Richard Hakluyt's thrill as a young boy, discovering the pleasures of a *mappa mundi* left open on a table:[79] "Me thinkes it would well please any man to look upon a Geographicall Map ... to behold, as it were, all the remote Provinces, Townes, Cities of the World, and never goe forth of the limits of his study, to measure by the Scale and Compasse, their extent, distance, examine their site" (2:86). As he elaborates, the boyish fantasy of the map's epistemological immediacy becomes an ode to mediation itself:

> What greater pleasure can there now bee, than to view those elaborate Maps, of *Ortelius, Mercator, Hondius,* &c. To peruse those bookes of Cities, put out by *Braunus,* and *Hogenbergius.* To read those exquisite descriptions of *Maginus, Munster, Herrera, Laet, Merula, Boterus, Leander Albertus, Camden, Leo After, Adricomius, Nic. Gerbelius,* &c. Those famous expeditions of *Chirstoph. Columbus, Americus Vesputius, Marcus Polus,* the *Venetian, Lod. Vertomannus, Aloysius Cadamustus,* &c. Those accurate diaries of *Portugals, Hollanders,* of *Bartison, Oliver à Nort* &c. *Hacluits* voyages, *Pet. Martyres Decades, Benzo, Lerius, Linschotens* relations, those *Hodaeporicons* of *Jod. à Meggen, Brocard the Monke, Bredenbachius, Jo. Dublinius, Sands,* &c. to *Jerusalem, Aegypt,* and other remote places of the world ... *to read Bellonius* observations, *P. Gillius* his survaies; Those parts of America, set out, and curiously cut in Pictures by *Fratres à Bry.* (2:86–7)[80]

---

[78] W.H.D. Rouse wrote that in "reading the *Anatomy of Melancholy* we are amazed at Burton's assiduity as a collector, but we are silenced by his genius as curator of his own museum" (*Burton the Anatomist: Being Extracts from the "Anatomy of Melancholy" Chosen to Interest the Psychologist in Every Man,* ed. G.C.F. Mead and Rupert Clift [London: Methuen, 1925], xxix).

[79] "I do remember that being a youth, and one of her Majestie's scholars at Westminster, that fruitfull nurserie, It was my happe to visit the chamber of Master Richard Hakluyt, my cousin, a gentleman of the Middle Temple, at a time when I found lying open upon his horde certeine bookes of cosmographie, with an universall mappe; he seeing me somewhat curious in the view thereof, began to instruct my ignorance, by showing me the division of the earth into three parts, after the olde account, and then, according to the latter and better distribution, into more ... ." Hakluyt, preface to the *Principal Navigations* (London, 1589).

[80] Burton's recommended "recreational" bibliography on geography, chorography, and travel literature here is both comprehensive and current: Jodocus Hondius (Joost de Hondt), engraver and mapmaker; Georg Braun and Franz Hohenberg, *Theatrum urbium praecipuarum mundi* (1595–1616); Abraham Ortelius, *Theatrum orbis terrarum* (1584); Gerard Mercator, *Atlas sive cosmographicae* (1595); Giovani Magini, *Atlante geografico d'Italia* (1620); Sebastian Munster, *Cosmographiae Universalis* (1572); Antonio de Herrera, *Historia general de ... las Indias Occidentales* (1601–1615); Jan de Laet, *Novus orbis, seu descriptionis Indiae occidentalis libri XVIII* (1633); Gaudenzio Merula, *De Gallorum Cisalpinorum antiquitate ac origine* (1538); Giovanni Botero, *Imperiorum mundi catalogus et descriptio* (1613); Leandro Alberti, *Descriptio totius Italiae* (1567); William Camden, *Annales rerum Anglicarum* (1615); Leo Africanus (Hasan ibn Muhammad al-Wazzan al-Fasi), *De totius Africae descriptione libri novem* (trans. 1556); Adricomius (Christiaan

This catalogue of titles and authors suggests that the secondhand quality of wonder obtained by reading about travel intensifies wonder by placing the reader and writer in imaginative contact and community, marveling together across time and space.

Burton yokes the mediated pleasure of geography and ethnography to the delights of natural history in a zeugmatic line that perpetually extends the promise of more knowledge by forestalling concentrated study of a single subject. Each one is held just long enough to light an idea of itself in the reader's mind before leaping to the next:

> To see a well cut Herball, Hearbs, Trees, Flowres, Plants, all vegetalls expressed in their proper colours to the life, as that of *Matthiolus* upon *Dioscorides, Dalecampius, Lobel, Bauhinus*, and that voluminous and mighty Herball of *Beslar* of *Noremberge*, wherein almost every Plant is to his owne bignesse. To see Birds, Beasts, and Fishes of the Sea, Spiders, Gnats, Serpents, Flies, &c. all Creatures set out by the same Art, and truly expressed in lively colours, with an exact description of their natures, virtues, qualities, &c. as hath been accurately performed by *Aelian, Gesner, Ulysses Aldrovandus, Bellonius, Rondoletius, Hippolytus Salvianus, &c. Arcana coeli, naturae secreta, ordinem universi scire, majoris felicitates & dulcedinis est quam cogitatione quis assequi posit, aut mortalis sperare.*[81] (2:87)

These studies take Burton from the great to the small, from the globe to the gnat. Each seems equal in wonder, or rather there is greater wonder in the smallest of objects and creatures whose study exposes intricate worlds hidden in the seemingly unremarkable.[82] The contemplation of these studies could go on forever, both in the depths to which one could penetrate a single subject if he or she were so inclined (*O to think upon a gnat for eternity*) and in the seemingly limitless arena of subjects and authors *still to come.*[83]

---

van Adrichem), *Hierosolymae* (1588); Nicolaus Gerbel, *Pro declaratione picturae sive descriptionis Graeciae Sophiani* (1550); Vertomannus (Ludovico di Bartema), *Itinerario de Ludouico de Varthema Bolognese* (1510); Oliver à Nort (Olivier van Noort), *Wonderlijcke voyagie* (1598); Peter Martyr (Pietro D'Anghiera, Pietro Martire), *De rebus oceanicis & orbe novo decades* (1533); Jean de Léry, *Historia navigationis in Brasiliam* (1586); Jan Huyghen van Linschoten, *Navigatio ac iternerarium* (trans. 1599); George Sandys, *A relation of a journey* (1615); and Fratres à Bry, *Peregrinationes in Americam* (1590).

[81] "To know the mysteries of the heavens, the secrets of Nature, and the order of the Universe, is a greater happiness and pleasure than anyone can think of, or any mortal hope to obtain." From Cardan, *De rerum varietate*, +3, as translated by the Clarendon *Anatomy* editors (5:179).

[82] For a provocative discussion of the fantasy of expanding (and exploding) microscopic worlds in Robert Hooke and Margaret Cavendish, see Mary Baine Campbell, *Wonder and Science: Imagining Worlds in Early Modern Europe* (Ithaca, NY: Cornell University Press, 2004), chap. 6.

[83] Kathryn Murphy similarly observes the therapeutic promise of infinite and diverse learning in this section despite Burton's lamentations elsewhere about the surfeit of books in a dizzying age of print. See Murphy, "Robert Burton and the Problems of Polymathy," 281.

Burton invokes the names and presence of the great natural historians in a cadence that sonically as well as substantively resists closure: "*Aelian, Gesner, Ulysses Aldrovandus, Bellonius, Rondoletius, Hippolytus Salvianus, &c.*" The rhyming endings of the Latin nominal case, anchored by the rhyming "couplet" of the fourth and eighth names, *Aldrovandus* and *Salvianus*, repeat and intensify the rhythm of the preceding list: "Birds, Beasts, and Fishes of the Sea, Spiders, Gnats, Serpents, Flies."

> – – ˘ – ˘ ˘ –
> Birds, Beasts, and Fishes of the Sea,
>
> – ˘ – – ˘ –
> Spiders, Gnats, Serpents, Flies

And:

> –˘˘ – ˘ –˘ ˘ ˘ ˘ – ˘
> *Aelian, Gesner, Ulysses Aldrovandus,*
>
> ˘ –˘˘ ˘ ˘–˘˘ ˘ –˘ ˘ ˘ ˘– ˘
> *Bellonius, Rondoletius, Hippolytus Salvianus*

A heavy-stressed English monosyllabic tetrameter in the first phrase is converted into Latin trochaic tetrameter in the second. The tetrameter continues through both phrases, but the syllable count per measure increases: first by a third with the addition of a half stress (Birds→Spiders); then doubled by another half stress (Spiders→*Aelian*); and again with the half stress (*Aelian*→*Bellonius*). In the second phrase, the metrical scheme can be scanned as follows: trochee, trochee, amphibrach, tertius paeon / amphibrach, tertius paeon, secundus paeon, tertius paeon, or AABC, BCDC.[84] The names of the authors extenuate the measure of the previous line, suggesting both that the object of wonder gives birth to its study and that study propagates the wonder of the object.

Ovid's well-known distinction between hexameter and pentameter sheds light on the emotional register of Burton's meter here. He reports that he set out to write the *Amores* in heroic verse, the proper meter of weapons and war, but claims that

---

84 Very little has been written on English oratorical prose cadence and its relationship to Latin meter since the early twentieth century. Key references from this period can be found in Albert C. Clark, *Prose Rhythm in English* (Oxford: Oxford University Press, 1913); Morris Croll, "The Cadence of English Oratorical Prose," *Studies in Philology* 16, no. 1 (1919): 1–56; Norbert Tempest, *The Rhythm of English Prose* (Cambridge: Cambridge University Press, 1930). These studies emerged in response to John Shelly's "Rhythmical Prose in Latin and English," *Church Quarterly Review* (1912). Shelly's study of Latin *cursus* in the English Prayer Book focuses on the parallelism between Latin and English clausulae. This emphasis on terminal cadence fails to account for the complexity of Burton's rhythm. There is some analogy, however, between Burton's nonperiodic meter and the "unitary phrase" in nonfinal endings studied by Croll in the third chapter of his article. For discussion of the decline of formal prose study, see my article, "The Forbidden Pleasures of Style," *Prose Studies* 34, no. 2 (2012): 115–28.

Cupid's arrow maimed him, stealing a "foot" from his line and leaving him to hobble in elegiac couplets that "rise in six beats and fall back in five": "*Sex mihi surgat opus numeris, in quinque residat: / ferrea cum vestris bella valete modis!*"[85] He bids a theatrical adieu to iron wars and their iron meters, proclaiming that this limping rhythm better suits a wounded lover, whose hopes repeatedly rise and fall back in despair. The sonic cure for melancholy calls for a rising rhythm, not the heavy sighs of iambic endings. The marching tetrameter of Burton's reading list, like the song-like hexameter of his prefatory poem, militates against the despondency of the elegiac couplet by moving the reader onward and forward.

Burton's meditations upon the "still to read" and "yet to know" substitute wonder at the infinite horizon of knowledge for despair over its perennial recession. Any study "that will ask a great deale of attention" will do well, he says, but Burton singles out algebra as being especially effective in this regard. "*Nothing,*" he says, "*can be more excellent and pleasant, so abstruse and recondite, so bewitching, so miraculous, so ravishing, so easie withal and full of delight*":[86]

> By this art you may contemplate the variation of the 23 letters, which may be so infinitely varied that the words complicated and deduced thence will not be contained within the compasse of the firmament; ten words may be varied 40320 severall waies: by this art you may examine how many men may stand one by another in the whole superficies of the earth, some say 148456800000000 ... and so may you demonstrate with *Archimedes* how many Sandes the masse of the whole world might containe if all sandy, if you did but first know how much a small cube as bigge as a Mustard-seede might hold, with infinite such. (2:92)

The pleasure of algebra ravishes not by reducing the vastness of the cosmos to human scale but by enabling one to meditate on this vastness in relation to the tangible and minute. Astronomy similarly rouses the spirit in wonder at a universe made more breathtaking because uncompassable, even as magnificent new tools enable us to glean its breadth: "what is there so stupend as to examine and calculate the motions of the Planets, their magnitudes, apogeums, perigeums, excentricities, how farre distant from the earth, the bignesse, thicknesse, compasse of the Firmament, each starre, with their diameters and circumferences, apparent *area, superficies,* by those curious helps of glasses, astrolabes, sextants, quadrants" (2:92).

The use of the word "stupend" in this passage is illustrative of the mode of wonder in which Burton's study cure operates. Stupend, from the verb *stupere*, "to be astounded," and *stupor*, the state of insensibility from which the word "stupid" is derived, are false cousins. The association between stupendous wonder and stupor does not occur frequently in English until the early decades of the seventeenth century and then does so mainly in Protestant spiritual writing to

---

[85]   Ovid, *Amores*, 1:27–8.

[86]   Burton borrows both the term and the praise for "Algebra" from Christopher Clavius's 1608 commentary on Euclid's *Elements*.

connote the torpor induced by wonder or sorrow, as in the common alliterative doublet "stupendious stupiditie."[87] Burton adds "stupend" to his synonyms for the delights of algebra ("so abstruse, and recondite, so bewitching, so miraculous, so ravishing, so easie withal and full of delight") that linguistically echo the algebraic signs by which the infinite may be imagined. Throughout the *Anatomy*, but especially in the third partition, the concept of infinity militates against despair by metonymically invoking God's infinite mercy.[88] In the "Digression of the Ayre," Burton considers Nicholas Hill's hypothesis of an infinite universe populated with other habitable worlds as a testament to God's greatness, which serves as a synonym for grace: "Why should not an infinite cause (As God is) produce infinite effects, as *Nic. Hill Democrit. philos.* disputes?" (2:52). Burton invokes Hill's Epicureanism (along, perhaps, with his dissident Catholicism)[89] as an argument not only for universal grace but for a universe alive with spirit. As Reid Barbour observes, Hill's "atoms are not lifeless but animated ... they are the media through which God's spirit is diffused into an infinite universe." [90] Burton's "stupend" wonder strips the infiniteness of the universe of its providential terror.[91] This is not quite the naturalization of divine wonder that Katherine Park and Lorraine Daston regard as the calling card of the natural philosophers but a fundamentally benign representation of cosmic infinitude and of the spiritual condition induced by its contemplation.[92]

The endless prospect of study consoles the melancholic by providing relief in the recognition that there is, in fact, too much to learn. Much as he argues that the

---

[87] See Daniel Price, *Spirituall Odours* (London, 1618), 7; David Hayward, *Davids Tears* (London, 1623), 97. The *Oxford English Dictionary* lists Burton's use of "stupend" here as its first and last example from the seventeenth century. See s.v. "stupend, adj.," accessed September 22, 2014, http://www.oed.com.libezproxy2.syr.edu/view/Entry/19220 9?rskey=ZR6x0X&result=1&isAdvanced=false. However, the adjective occurs in Robert Heath, *Paradoxicall Assertions and Philosophical Problems Ful of Delight and Recreation for All Ladies* (London, 1659), 40. Thomas Lawrence refers to "stupend rarefactions of air" to describe nitrous explosions (*Mercurius Centralis* [London: 1664], 39).

[88] See Lund on Burton's reading of Niels Hemmingsen and John Chrysostom ("Reading and the Cure of Despair in *The Anatomy of Melancholy*," 545).

[89] See Hugh Trevor-Roper, *Catholics, Anglicans and Puritans: Seventeenth-Century Essays* (Chicago: Chicago University Press, 1987), 1–39.

[90] Reid Barbour, *English Epicures and Stoics: Ancient Legacies in Early Stuart Culture* (Amherst: University of Massachusetts Press, 1998), 60–65.

[91] The association between stupor and wonder in ecclesiastical literature accrues around translations of the Hebrew verb שָׁמֵם, meaning to desolate, appall, or cause horror (Brown, Driver, and Briggs, *The New Brown-Driver-Briggs—Gesenius Hebrew and English Lexicon* [Peabody, MA: Hendrickson Publishers, 1979], 1030b [8074]). The translation of Jeremiah 5:30 *stupor et mirabilia facta* in the Vulgate and its subsequent translation in the Geneva Bible and KJV as "a wonderfull and horrible thing" illustrates the early, semantic association of *mirabilia* with fearsome or terrible wonder.

[92] Lorraine Daston and Katharine Park, *Wonders and the Order of Nature, 1150–1750* (New York: Zone Books, 2001), chap. 8, "The Enlightenment and the Anti-Marvelous."

vast ocean of God's grace drowns even the gravest sins (3:428), the infinite horizon of the Burtonian episteme seeks to relieve a melancholic of despair-inducing pride by trumping the solipsistic desire for mastery. Burton's ecstatic study provokes a wondrous sense of gratitude, much like Browne's "*o altitudo,*" for the bounty of mystery that human reason with all its power could never hope to exhaust. Burton's is clearly not the Aristotelian wonder that "is generated by a difficult problem and … dissipated by a solution to that problem." It finds a closer cousin in Francisco Patrizi's understanding of *maraviglia* and *admiratio,* of wonder that is, as Peter Platt characterizes it, "ongoing and its own end."[93] This sense of wonder belongs to what Platt describes as the "other" mode of Renaissance wonder whose history has been obscured by the predominantly Aristotelian view, of which Bacon is an odd defender.[94] Whereas for Francis Bacon, wonder enslaves by "fixing the mind upon one object of cogitation, whereby it does not spatiate and transcur,"[95] for Burton, wonder releases spirits congealed by melancholic rumination. Bacon regards wonder as potentially idolatrous in the indiscriminate reverence or thrall it induces. Burton regards wonder as releasing religious melancholics (and scholarly divines) from pietistic dread.

Burton's theological commitments remain stubbornly opaque despite the seeming transparency of his institutional affiliations and the until-recently prevailing argument that dissident soteriology would have been impossible at Oxford in his time.[96] The royal proclamations of 1626 and subsequent addenda prohibiting disputation of predestination remind us that Burton would have had good reason to be subtle on the subject,[97] and yet where he speaks directly about election he is, as David Renaker and Lund have shown, considerably more liberal

---

[93]   Peter G. Platt, *Reason Diminished: Shakespeare and the Marvelous* (Lincoln: University of Nebraska Press, 1997), 15. For Platt's fuller argument, see "'Not Before Either Known or Dreamt of': Francesco Patrizi and the Power of Wonder in Renaissance Poetics," *Review of English Studies* 43 (1992): 387–94.

[94]   "For it is better to make a beginning of a thing which has a chance of an end, than to get caught up in things which have no end, in perpetual struggle and exertion" (Francis Bacon, *The New Organon,* ed. Lisa Jardine and Michael Silverthorne [Cambridge: Cambridge University Press, 2000], 3).

[95]   Francis Bacon, "Sylva Sylvarum," in *The Works of Francis Bacon,* ed. James Spedding, Leslie Ellis, and Douglas Heath (London: Longman, 1857), 2:570.

[96]   Peter Lake has shown that it was possible for prominent theologians to criticize Calvinism and rise in the ranks of the Stuart church, even if such remarks were guarded from public dissemination. See Peter Lake, "Calvinism and the English Church," *Past and Present* 114 (1987): 32–76. For the opposing view, see Peter White's articles, to which Lake is responding, especially "The Rise of Arminianism Reconsidered," *Past and Present* 101 (1983): 34–54.

[97]   See Gowland, *The Worlds of Renaissance Melancholy,* 143–51. Gowland suggests that the medical framework of the section on religious melancholy serves to "conceal (and so permit) the author's participation in theological and ecclesiological controversy" (ibid., 140).

than recognized by previous scholars. Renaker notes that Burton's declared faith in the supralapsarianism of the English Church is not only contradicted by the immediately preceding assurance that "all are saved" but undermined by this entirely false characterization of the Caroline Church of England.[98] More recently, Lund has challenged Burton's presumed orthodoxy by examining his subtle but significant misquotations of William Perkins and Robert Bolton, who both become considerably more flexible in his representation.[99] Burton's doctrinal unorthodoxy is perhaps most striking, however, in his compassionate treatment of suicide, a threat that looms large over his book. He impersonates the siren call of every ledge, bridge, and cliff for the suffering melancholic: "Dost thou see that steepe place, that river, that pit, that tree, there's liberty at hand" (1:435). Against the impressive list of writers and civilizations (both Pagan and Christian) that have defended suicides, Burton's capitulation that "these are false and Pagan propositions, prophane Stoicall Paradoxes" (1:437) seems suspiciously weak. He further undermines the reprobation of suicides by urging the reader to be merciful toward those who "free themselves from misery," suggesting that such compassion is in better keeping with the character of a merciful, Christian God.[100]

Burton's extended *ethopoeia* on suicide serves as a cautionary reminder that it is by the "worme of conscience" that the devil persecutes us (3:411). The many assurances that appear in the "Cure for Despaire" do not provide an antidote to this "Divels bath" of melancholic doubt. Like the "Cure of Jealousy" and "Cure of Lovesickness" that precede it in the final partition, the "Cure for Despaire" exposes the very limitations of direct persuasion. Burton's arguments against despair are resolutely affirmative, but they dramatize the purely instrumental character of rational assurance. He ends the book by urging the reader to "speedily remove the cause," avert his thoughts from such scrupulous matters altogether, and "by all opposite meanes, art, and industry ... refresh and recreate his distressed soule" (3:445). For the antidote to despair we are sent back to his prescription and demonstration of a study cure in "Exercise Rectified of Body and Mind,"

---

[98]   David Renaker, "Robert Burton's Palinodes," *Studies in Philology* 76, no. 2 (1979): 178. Burton's revision of this declared faith in "predestination" in the 1624 edition to "supralapsarianism" in 1628 indicates what Renaker calls the "noose around the neck" of any university man who dared discuss this topic, which had been outlawed by the Articles of Religion published the same year (176).

[99]   Lund considers Burton's debt to the controversial Hemmingsen but stops short of suggesting that he shared Hemmingsen's Arminianism ("Reading and the Cure for Despair"). See also John Stachniewski's reading of Burton against the grain of Nicholas Tyacke's representation of Calvinist orthodoxy, *The Persecutory Imagination: English Puritanism and the Literature of Religious Despair* (Oxford: Clarendon Press, 1991), chap. 5.

[100]   "God alone can tell, his mercy may come *inter pontem, & fontem, inter gladium & jugulum*, betwixt the bridge and the brooke, the knife and the throte." Finally, he argues, we ought not judge lest we be tried as well: "Who knows how he may be tempted? It is his case, it may be thine?" (1:438).

and to the "ample fields of ayre" that signify more than simply the atmospheric element whose properties affect humoral well-being. The "Ayre Rectified" in the "Digression of the Ayre" is the air of discourse, the pneumatic medium of scholarly debate, and thought itself. The flight of the hawk "whistled off the fist," following a particularly tedious discussion of melancholy and venery, evokes the audible shock of air suddenly admitted into close quarters. The cosmological romp by which Burton "freely expatiate[s] and exercise[s]" himself rectifies an air grown stale with melancholy doctrine (2:33). It is this gravitas that his study cure opposes. The *roving* humor, as he calls it (1:4), requires a roving cure to refresh, recreate, and revive the spirits. Far from circumscribing the permissible realms of knowledge to the simple, trifling, or inconsequential, Burton's advice that we temper *"serious studies and businesse"* with *"jests and conceits, playes and toyes"*[101] should be read as a positive course of *exhilaration* for the malady that *"begines with sorrow"* and *"must be expelled with hilarity"* (2:122–3).

---

[101]   Attributed by Burton to Prospero Calano, who gave this advice to the "melancholy Cardinall *Caesius*" who was his patient (2:122).

Chapter 4
"Exonerating" Melancholy

With its dizzying, airborne survey of the mysteries of the natural world, the "Digression of the Ayre" would appear to be the paramount example of the study cure examined in the previous chapter, but the objects of its inquiry are rather less eclectic than those Burton recommends for the exercise of the mind and spirits. They pursue a pneumatic theme that is both explicit and at the same time so subtle as to have gone almost unremarked. Why the topic of "air" would serve as the provocation for what Burton describes as his exceptional speculative freedom in the Digression is a question that has scarcely been asked.[1] The ostensible logic of the subsection in which the Digression appears is its treatment of air as one of the six non-natural principles of hygiene that may be "rectified" in order to treat, prevent, or "cure" melancholy. However, the hygienic consideration of air is put off for the vast majority of the subsection, which instead begins with a digression whose relation to the prescribed theme Burton analogizes in the following way:

> As a long-winged Hawke when hee is first whistled off the fist, mounts aloft, and for his pleasure fetcheth many a circuit in the Ayre, still soaring higher and higher, till hee bee come to his full pitch; and in the end when the game is sprung, comes downe amaine, and stoopes upon a sudden: so will I, having now come at last to these ample fields of Ayre, wherein I may freely expatiate and exercise my selfe, for my recreation a while rove, wander round about the world, mount aloft to those aethereall orbes and celestiall spheres, and so descend to my former elements againe.[2]

The epic simile that begins the Digression foregrounds the analogy between the "ample fields of ayre" in which the hawk delights and the pneumatic medium of thought and scholarly discourse in which Burton "expatiates" and

---

[1]   The symbolic value of air *vis-à-vis* Burton's therapeutic and philosophical purposes is briefly hinted at in an unpublished paper by Steven Connor: "The extraordinary, crazy, infirm variability of Burton's own habit of mind and writing, which for him was the cure for his vaporous melancholy, takes its image from the air itself. Air as change, digression, instability is the redemption of air distorted into formula and *idée fixe*" ("The Vapours," accessed September 4, 2014, http://www.stevenconnor.com/vapours/).

[2]   Robert Burton, *The Anatomy of Melancholy*, ed. Thomas C. Faulkner, Nicolas K. Kiessling, and Rhonda Blair, Introduction and Commentary by J.B. Bamborough and Martin Dodsworth, 6 vols. (Oxford: Clarendon Press, 1989), 2:33. Unless otherwise indicated, all references to the *Anatomy* are to this edition, hereafter cited parenthetically in text by volume and page number.

"exercises" himself. Burton's arrival at the topic of air serves as the occasion for a "flight" of fancy whose escalating pitch is not to be regarded as a distraction from the hunt but the very means by which he is able to "stoope" and seize his prey or "game." This choice of words reminds us of the surreptitious mode of argument that the ludic *cento* cleverly disguises. But the game of citation and miscitation we have marked elsewhere is not the sport we are witnessing here. Burton's preface to the Digression hints at the purposiveness of its circumambulatory meditations and to a kind of logic in the mounting gyres of its speculative flight that this chapter will attempt to trace.

Burton investigates matters cosmographical, hydrographical, astronomical, and geological in the Digression, seeming to fly every which way the wind blows. The critical consensus that the Digression's wanderings amount to a random survey of cosmological opinions that Burton held no particular stake in has been challenged by Richard Barlow, who argues that the Digression follows the itinerary of a more or less Lucianic cosmic journey and that Burton ends up as a proponent of the theory of infinite worlds, even if earlier editions and sections of the *Anatomy* suggest that he initially believed otherwise.[3] There is, however, a further logic to the Digression that we may observe when we compare the objects and questions that arrest Burton mid-flight. In what follows, I will attempt to show how the relation of these objects to one another constitutes a pneumatic and hydraulic theme that prepares the way for the Digression's profound Epicurean consolation. The first task of this chapter will be to track this theme in the images of wind, spirit, and breath that Burton uses to represent the processes of earthly mutability and cataclysm that he suggestively characterizes as "exonerations." In the second part of the chapter, I will argue that these meditations offer consolation for melancholy in the Lucretian, Ovidian, and Longinian traditions of translating apocalyptic terror into wonder and, in Burton's Christianized Epicureanism, converting despair at the mutability and vicissitudes of the earth and cosmos into hope for regenerative, indeed, salvific, transformation. The third part of the chapter explores the relationship between the logic of "exoneration" that underwrites his consolatory program and his analysis of the social and economic causes of melancholy. I conclude by returning to the theme of the breath that we will trace below in a coda that considers Burton's representation of humanist writing and citing as a pneumatic exchange of spirit and a more generous and salubrious alternative to melancholy-inducing jealousy and retentive greed.

---

[3]   Richard G. Barlow, "Infinite Worlds: Robert Burton's Cosmic Voyage," *Journal of the History of Ideas* 34, no. 2 (1973): 291–302. Barlow responds to the characterizations of the Digression's intellectual and stylistic aimlessness by Lawrence Babb, *Sanity in Bedlam: A Study of Robert Burton's "Anatomy of Melancholy"* (East Lansing: Michigan State University Press, 1959), and Robert M. Browne, "Robert Burton and the New Cosmology," *Modern Language Quarterly* 13 (1952): 131. Both Babb and Browne note that the near doubling in size of the subsection between the first and fifth edition reflects both the keenness and currency of Burton's reading on the topics surveyed in the Digression.

I. Sublime Vicissitudes: From Torpidity to Apocalypse

Burton's imaginary flight begins with a meditation on lodestones and magnets at the poles of the earth but, as if drawn by ocean currents themselves, quickly pursues a hydraulic theme with a series of questions about the navigability of distant bodies of water and the broader questions of earthly vicissitude to which these lead.[4] He starts at the Arctic, Hudson's "new-found Ocean," then, moving west, he wonders whether California is a cape or an island and how the western winds make possible that strange reputed phenomenon whereby the "Nepe tides equall ... the Spring."[5] He travels farther west, wondering whether "there be any probability to passe by the Straights of *Anian* to *China* by the Promontory of *Tabin*."[6] If so, he says, he would investigate the stories of Marco Polo, "of that great Citty of *Quinsay* and *Cambalu*," or those of the Jesuit Matteo Ricci regarding the magnitude of these lands.[7] He would discover whether the legendary, lost kingdom of Prester John was in Asia or Africa, whether *"Guinea"* (New Guinea) is an island or part of "that hungry Spaniards discovery of *Terra Australis Incognita*, or *Magellanica*," and whether these recently published reports "be as true as that of *Mercurius Britannicus*, or his of *Utopia*, or his of *Lucinia*," which is to say, as "true" as Joseph Hall's and Thomas More's fictional worlds. "And yet," he asks, why wouldn't such marvelous stories of lost, ancient civilizations be true if they have proven so in the Americas? Their unlikelihood, he suggests, is a problem of perception that inheres in the gap between the pace of human and geological time: "for without all question it [Australia] being extended from the Tropicke of *Capricorne* to the circle *Antartick*, and lying as it doth in the temperate *Zone*,

---

[4]   For a brief overview of the state of Renaissance hydraulic engineering in relation to developments in navigation and cartography, see Richard S. Westfall, "Science and Technology during the Scientific Revolution: An Empirical Approach," in *Renaissance and Revolution: Humanists, Scholars, Craftsmen and Natural Philosophers in Early Modern Europe*, ed. Judith Veronica Field and Frank A.J.L. James (Cambridge: Cambridge University Press, 1997), 67–70. For the argument that the state of Renaissance hydraulics was more advanced than has been recognized and has failed to command due scholarly attention, see Martin Schmid, "The Environmental History of Rivers in the Early Modern Period," in *An Environmental History of the Early Modern Period: Experiments and Perspectives*, ed. Martin Knoll and Reinhold Reith (Zurich: Lit Verlag Münster, 2014).

[5]   Neap and spring tides are when high tide reaches its lowest and highest levels respectively. For an overview of Renaissance debates concerning the difference between neap and spring tides leading up to Newton's equilibrium theory in the *Principia*, see David Edgar Cartwright, *Tides: A Scientific History* (Cambridge: Cambridge University Press, 2000), chaps. 4 and 5.

[6]   The Clarendon commentators point out that Baffin's disappointed hopes for a northwest passage in 1615 and 1616 were revived by 1631 with Luke Fox's voyage (5:110), which Burton mentions in the fifth edition.

[7]   *De Christiana expeditione apud Sinas suscepta ab Societate Jesu* (Augsburg, Germany, 1615), published shortly after Ricci's death, was based on journals he kept during his 27-year mission in China.

cannot chuse but yield in time, some flourishing kingdomes to succeeding ages, as *America* did unto the *Spaniards*" (2:34). The theme of geological change will be invoked throughout the Digression to console melancholy fears of the apocalypse, but here it sounds out a faint but audible warning about the vicissitudes of empire wrought by greed.

Having got rather close to what feels like a "mark" in the last remark, Burton swiftly pulls back, the swooping gyres of his flight echoing the rise and fall of empire and the cyclicality of time. And off he goes, searching out "more convenient passage to *Mare Pacificum*" with our "moderne *Argonautes*," describing the mysteries and marvels he would seek out on this hypothetical journey, collapsing authorities past and present and objects empirical and mythical:

> As I goe by *Madagascar* I would see that great bird *Rucke* that can carry a man and horse, or an Elephant, with that *Arabian Phoenix* described by *Adricomius*; see the Pellicanes of *Aegypt*, those *Scythian* Gryphes in *Asia*: And afterwards in *Africk* examine the fountaines of *Nilus*, whether *Herodotus, Seneca, Plin. lib. 5. cap 9. Strabo lib. 5* give a true cause of his annual flowing, *Pagaphetta* discourse rightly of it, or of *Niger* and *Senega*, examine *Cardan, Scaligers* reasons, and the rest. (2:34–5)

The seemingly haphazard relationship between birds, myths, and hydraulics begins to take shape as Burton goes on, from the elusive source of the Nile, to contemplate the mysterious current of the Atlantic and the fabled, swift winds off the Indian Ocean. Then, still very much in the subjunctive mood of Burton's study cure, Burton tells us that he "would examine the *Caspian* Sea, and see where and how it exonerates it selfe." By "exonerate," Burton means to empty or disburden, a characterization of hydraulic pressure whose various implications we will consider throughout this chapter. [8] His synonyms for this process, "ventilation" and "exhalation," make clear that he is thinking of exoneration in pneumatic terms, as a kind of breathing of bodies of water into one another: "What vent the *Mexican* lake hath, the *Titicacan* in *Peru*, or that circular poole in the vale of *Terapeia* … the Spring of which boils up in the middle twenty foot square, and hath no vent but exhalation."

Burton's meditations on the mysterious sources, movements, and eruptions of bodies of water seem to hint allegorically at the power of divine spirit that is both unfathomable and irrepressible and is analogous to the animating *pneuma* or spirit that resides in the breath. The same zeugma in which Burton says, "I would examine the *Caspian* Sea, and see where and how it exonerates itself," continues as follows:

---

[8]   "Exoneration," which here ostensibly means physical disburdening, acquires greater religious and psychological significance when considered in the context of its increasingly spiritual resonance in seventeenth-century English writing. See *Oxford English Dictionary Online*, s.v. "exonerate, n. 1," accessed May 8, 2014, http://www.oed.com.libezproxy2.syr.edu/view/Entry/66330?redirectedFrom=exoneration#eid.

> And if I could, [I would] observe what becomes of Swallowes, Storkes, Cranes,
> Cuckowes, Nightingales, Redstarts, and many other kinde of singing birds,
> water-fowles, Hawkes, &c. some of them are only seene in Sommer, some in
> Winter, some are observed in the snowe, and at no other times, each have their
> seasons. (2:36)

Suddenly, the forward momentum of the zeugma stalls and Burton reverses its
direction. The front-loaded or prozeugmatic "And if I could" is replaced with the
hypozeugmatic "How comes it to passe?" (2:36). He shifts from heaping congeries
to a partial end-stop, drawing the reader close in anticipation of something grand at
the end of the sentence—and grand it is. Syntactical suspense imitates the mystery
of the "breath" that we suddenly realize has been the object of this dizzying pursuit:

> In winter not a bird is in *Muscovy* to bee found, but at the spring in an instant
> the woods and hedges are full of them, saith *Herbastein*. How comes it to passe?
> Doe they sleepe in winter, like *Gesners* Alpine mice, or doe they ly hid (as *Olaus*
> affirmes) *in the bottome of lakes and rivers*, spiritum continentes? *often so found
> by Fishermen in Poland & Scandia, two together, mouth to mouth, wing to wing,
> & when the spring comes they revive againe, or if they be brought into a stove,
> or to the fire side.* (2:36–7)

Burton's flight pauses at its rhetorical apex to admire this remarkable *totentanz*
of hibernating waterfowl; his breathless prose stops to admire the marvel of the
breath suspended between seemingly inanimate birds. The image of two birds
entwined in a hibernatory kiss, torpid but living at the bottom of frozen waters,
provides a sublime, Longinian counterpoint to the narrative arc of his imaginary
hawk's flight. Indeed, capturing the sense of both height and depth in Longinus'
"*altitudo*," Burton's prose reaches its loftiest register as it peers into depths made
surveyable only from the imagined heights of the hawk's lofty "circuit."

The wonderful conceit of frozen birds sustained by the exchange of spirit
provides Burton with an almost emblematic figure for the experience of melancholic
torpor and reanimation. However, before he proceeds to consider human torpidity,
Burton pauses to examine the bibliography on this ancient mystery concerning
the disappearance of birds in winter.[9] He cites Peter Martyr, who "manifestly
convicts" that he "saw swallowes, Spanish kites, and many such other *European*
birds, in December and January" when he served as ambassador in Egypt. But this
explanation seems not to satisfy Burton, who is, of course, personifying a bird
in these meditations about birds. It disappoints precisely for its failure to capture
the suggestiveness of the question as it pertains to melancholy. That is, it fails to

---

[9]   It was not until the middle of the twentieth century that stories similar to those
Burton cites became cause for serious reassessment proving that some waterfowl do
indeed enter torpid states. See Robert C. Lasiewski and Henry J. Thompson, "Field
Observation of Torpidity in the Violet-Green Swallow," *The Condor* 68, no. 1 (1966):
102–3; W.L. McAtee, "Torpidity in Birds," *American Midland Naturalist* 38, no. 1 (1947):
191–206; George T. Austin and W. Glen Bradley, "Additional Responses of the Poor-Will
to Low Temperatures," *The Auk* 86, no. 4 (1969): 717–25.

capture the affective experience of melancholic withdrawal that the mystery seems to analogize. Melancholic people do not remove to sunny climes; they withdraw to dark, forgotten, dangerous places, like the "caves, rockes and hollow trees" where "most thinke" they lie hid in winter, or the "deepe *Tinne mines or Seacliffes*" that Carew and Olaus suggest.[10] Burton insists on treating the matter as a mystery, and one no less elusive than the whereabouts of the monstrous storks who terrorize Indian pygmies in Munster's *Cosmographia*: "I conclude of them all, for my part as *Munster* doth of Cranes and Storkes: whence they come, whither they goe, *incompertum adhuc*, as yet we know not … . *Their comming and going is sure in the night, in the plaines of Asia* (saith he) *the storkes meet on such a set day, hee that comes last is torne in peeces, and so they get them gone*" (2:37).

As if recoiling at the image of Munster's carnivorous birds, or perhaps at the symbolic ravaging of melancholy's "winter" on those whom it afflicts, Burton pulls back to fetch another circuit over "*Isthmi, Euripi, Chersonesi*, creekes, havens, promontories, straights, lakes, bathes, rockes, mountaines, places and fields," places "where citties have bin ruined or swallowed, battles fought." But these melancholy thoughts dissolve with the wonders that come into view from a loftier vantage and Burton returns to the wondrous possibility of the "*spiritum continentes*," a sublime suspension of the breath.[11] He circles back to the question of human hibernation, offering, by way of obscure anecdote, another remarkable analogy for melancholic recovery, here as a spring reawakening from death-like sleep:

> Many rare creatures and novelties each part of the world affords: amongst the rest, I would know for a certaine, whether there be any such men, as *Leo Suavius* in his comment on *Paracelsus de sanit. tuend.* and *Gaguinus* records in his description of *Muscovy*, that in Lucomoria, a province in Russia, lye fast asleepe as dead all winter, from the 27th of November, like froggs and swallowes, benum'd with cold, but about the 24 of Aprill in the spring, they revive againe, and goe about their businesse. (2:37–8)

The anecdote in this retelling is as much about recovery from melancholy as recovery of the literary and textual kind. Burton's named source is Alessandro Guagnini, who reports in his *Description of Sarmatian Europe* that an elaborate

---

10   The image of the birds "mouth to mouth, wing to wing" is in Olaus Magnus, *Historia de gentibus Septentrionalibus* (Rome, 1555), 19:29. Carew expands in his *History of Cornwall* (1602) upon Olaus's account of the "lurking places" where wintering birds have been discovered, adding the language of resurrection: these birds "fall downe into certaine great lakes or pooles amongst the C[r]anes, from whence at the next Spring, they receiue a new resurrection." See Richard Carew, *Survey of Cornwall* (London, 1602), f25 v; Peter Foote, ed., *Olaus Magnus: A Description of the Northern Peoples, 1555, vol. 1*, trans. Peter Fisher and Humphrey Higgens (London: Hakluyt Society, 1996), 980–81.

11   The Clarendon commentators note that while Burton is drawing mainly from Olaus, the phrase "spiritum continentes" and marginal note, "*Immergunt se fluminibus, lacubusque per hiemem totam, &c.*," are taken from Julius Bellius, *Hermes Politicus sive: De peregrinatio prudentia libri tres* (Frankfurt, 1608) (5:117).

trade ritual is enacted annually in Lucomoria (which we might translate as the "retiring" or "dying" place)[12] before the people "die" in winter.[13] According to Guagnini, the Lucomorians leave goods for one another whose worthiness becomes the subject of heated debate when they wake in the spring and either find their exchanged goods equitable or squabble over the difference. Sigismond von Herberstein tells a similar story in his *Rerum Moscoviticarum Comentarii* (1549), retold by Hakluyt in the *Principall Navigations*. The Jesuit demonologist Martin del Rio comments upon Guagnini's report and refers to Herberstein in response to the question of whether a devil can make a man rise from the dead. Kepler, citing del Rio, wonders about the souls of the undead Lucomorians in his posthumously published astronomical fantasy, the *Somnium*. Guagnini called the story an "incredible tale." Herberstein called it a fable.[14] Burton's stake on the truth of the matter might seem pointed when he says he "would know for certaine" whether such men exist or not, but as the complex chain of transmission attests, the story circulated as a matter of legendary speculation that is strengthened, like the wind, by the power of its circulation.

Burton's desire to "know for certain" is a tag that runs throughout the Digression, ironically underscoring its hypothetical quality and subjunctive mood. His inquisition into the true and exact character of natural phenomena is, in fact, far from demystifying and can hardly be called empirical. That said, the historiographical opposition between a wonder-filled premodern mode of inquiry associated with natural history and a modern experimental science that subdues wonder in the name of objectivity and reproducibility has proven inept for understanding—much less classifying—Burton and his unwieldy book. This artificial dichotomy fails to account for the expression in the *Anatomy* of a desire for an exact and true scientific knowledge that takes epic, myth, and anecdote as its guides. Burton says he would know the precise heights of "*Athos, Pelion, Olympus, Ossa, Caucasus, Atlas,*" and learn whether they "be so high as *Pliny, Solinus, Mela* relate, above Clouds, Meteors ... 1250 paces high, according to that measure of *Dicearchus*, or 78 miles perpendicularly high, as *Jacobus Mazonius sec. 3. & 4. ...* or rather 32. stadiums as the most received opinion is, or 4. Miles ... . The pike of *Teneriffe* how high it is? 70 miles or 52, as *Patritius* holds, or 9. as *Snellius* demonstrates in his *Eratosthenes* ... " (2:35–6).[15] He seems to be suggesting that

---

[12] "*lucus*," grove; "*mora*," delay, pause. By the nineteenth century, the term made its way into the medical lexicon as a diagnosis for "morbid sleep persisting for several days." See entry for "Lucumorianus," in Robley Dunglison, *A Dictionary of Medical Science* (Philadelphia: Lea Brothers & Co., 1895), 650.

[13] Alessandro Guagnini, or "Alexander Guagnin," Italian enlistee and eventual commander in the Polish army. This story appears in his "Description of Muscovy," in *Sarmatiae Europeae descriptio* (Cracow, 1578).

[14] See Appendix M in Johannes Kepler, *Kepler's Somnium: The Dream, or Posthumous Work on Lunar Astronomy* (Madison: University of Wisconsin Press, 1967), 136–7.

[15] As the Clarendon commentators note, Patritius sets the height of the pike at 72 not 52 miles, and Snellius does not specify a height but rather a range (greater than 43 stadia but not more than 76 and 2/3) (5:116).

the desire for exact and certain knowledge of the physical dimensions of such wonders misses the point. According to the legends by which Burton knows these mountains, they are the mythic transfigurations or *metamorphoses* of erstwhile gods. Burton might have misremembered his sources or not checked them carefully enough, as David Renaker has argued of other instances of Burton's inaccuracies.[16] It seems likelier that the number game is ironic, a parody of the neo-Scholastic tendencies of the new experimental science in a bid for the therapeutic value of speculative rather than empirical inquiry and the transformative power of myth. Burton's quantitative questions repeatedly yield over to qualitative concerns. We see him lose interest in the precise height of the Teneriffe, chasing instead after the wondrous sight of "that strange *Cirknickzerksey* lake in *Carniola*, whose waters gush so fast out of the ground, that they will overtake a swift horseman, and by and by with as incredible celerity are supped up, which *Lazius* and *Warnerus* make an argument of the *Argonautes* sayling under ground" (2:36). These waters, like the fabled mountains, are more interesting for their mythological significance, their symbolism, and their capacity to induce salubrious wonder than their physical proportions.

Burton turns from the anecdote of the hibernating Lucomorians to a series of apocalyptic speculations, also expressed as desire for wonderfully elusive knowledge: He *would know* which is likelier to overwhelm or "overflow" the other: the earth or the sea? He *would search* the depths for "that variety of Sea monsters and fishes, Mare-maides, Sea men, Horses, &c. which it affords" (2:38). The fantastic flight would take him off in search of Solomon's Ophir and other famed cities of gold, a journey motivated equally by the desire to correct misperceptions of these distant places as to discover new ones. He says he "would censure" the lies of Pliny, Olaus (his source on torpid, kissing birds), Solinus, Strabo, Mandeville, and Marco Polo. He would "correct," "reforme," and "rectifie" errors in navigation, cosmographical charts, and longitudes, "if it were possible; not by the compasse, as some dreame, with *Marke Ridley* in his treatise of magneticall bodies," but "observe some better means to find them out" (2:38). The subjunctive mood of his epistemological fantasy is again underscored by a sense of patent impossibility, which in turn underscores that we are in the province of myth, allegory, and analogy, even as we pursue matters of "science."

Burton's "better means" of discovery would have him find "a convenient place to goe downe with *Orpheus, Ulysses, Hercules, Lucians Menippus*, at St. *Patricks* Purgatory, at *Trophonius* denne, *Hecla* in Island [Iceland], *Aetna* in *Sicily*; to descend and see what is done in the bowels of the earth." He ostensibly toes the empiricist line, saying he rejects the observations of others, preferring to discover for himself what lies in the bowels of the earth. However, he would take poets and mythic heroes for his guides and companions to find "certain" answers to geological conundrums he knows only from legend, for example, of a ship discovered "50. fathome deepe" inside an Alpine mountain, or of the presence of

---

16   David Renaker, "Robert Burton's Tricks of Memory," *PMLA* 87, no. 3 (1972): 391–6.

trees buried in hills and marshes, or the discovery of "fish bones, shelles, beames, iron-workes, many fathomes under ground, & anchors in mountaines far remote from all seas" (2:38). Burton attributes this report to Simmler and Ortelius.[17] The story had, however, more recently appeared in Hakluyt's 1601 publication of António Galvão's *Discoveries of the World*.[18] The Clarendon editors suggest that Burton borrows it from Fracastoro and other neoteric sources (5:120).[19] I will suggest, in the second part of this chapter, that Burton is drawing from the story's more ancient appearances and purposes in the consolatory visions of earthly vicissitude offered by Lucretius and Ovid.

Burton dismisses explanations that these bones, shells, and anchors are the remnants of earthquakes, or that they came "from *Noahs* flood, as Christians suppose" in order to dilate more broadly on the "vicissitude of Sea and Land," the mutability of a world in constant renovation:

> as *Anaximenes* held of old, the mountaines of *Thessaly* would become Seas, and Seas againe Mountaines? The whole world belike should be new moulded, when it seemed good to those all-commanding Powers, and turned inside out, as we doe hay-cocks in Harvest, toppe to bottome, or bottome to top: or as we turne apples to the fire, move the world upon his Center; that which is under the *Poles* now, should be translated to the *Aequinoctiall*, and that which is under the torrid Zone to the Circle *Artique* and *Antartique* another while, and so be reciprocally warmed by the Sunne. (2:39)

Burton bandies about the prospect of a world "turned inside out" and "toppe to bottome" in the evocative language of hearth and harvest. He invites us to meditate on cosmic upheaval not with a terror of Christian apocalypse but with the conjured scent of freshly turned hay and roasting apples as we imagine new, potentially infinite worlds born out of such cosmic mutability: "or if the worlds be infinite, and every fixed starre a Sunne, with his compassing Planets ... cast three or foure Worlds into one; or else of one old world make three or four new, as it shall seeme to them best" (2:39).

Burton elaborates this theme of plural worlds a few pages later: "We may likewise insert with *Campanella* and *Brunus*, that which *Pythagoras, Aristarchus Samius, Heraclitus, Epicurus, Melissus, Democritus, Leucippus* maintained in their ages, there be *infinite Worlds*, and infinite Earths or systemes, *in infinito aethere*." He all but declares himself an Epicurean on the subject, twice quoting

---

[17] Josias Simmler, *De Helvetiorum republica* (1577); Abraham Ortelius, *Theatrum orbis terrarum* (1584).

[18] See Sir Edward Burnett Tylor, *Researches into the Early History of Mankind and the Development of Civilization* (Henry Holt, 1878), 329; António Galvão and Richard Hakluyt, *The Discoveries of the World: From Their First Original unto the Year of Our Lord 1555*, ed. Charles Ramsay Drinkwater Bethune (London: Hakluyt Society, 1862), 26.

[19] Girolamo Fracastoro, *De sympathia*; Georgius Merula, *Memorabilia*; Julius Bellius, *Hermes politicus*.

Nicholas Hill as a brave proponent of a theory that, he laments, "some sticke not still to maintaine and publikely defend":

> If our world be small in respect, why may we not suppose a plurality of worlds, those infinite starres visible in the Firmament to be so many Sunnes, with particular fixt Centers; to have likewise their subordinate planets, as the Sunne hath his dancing still round him? ... . Why should not an infinite cause (as God is) produce infinite effects, as *Nic. Hill Democrit. philos.* disputes? (2:52)

Burton finds Kepler's apparent ambivalence on the plurality of worlds to be something of a smokescreen, hiding convictions that must be discerned "betwixt jest & earnest" (2:53)—a strategy he is quick to detect, it would seem, on account of his own expertise. He condemns "moderne Divines" for being "too severe and rigid against Mathematitians, ignorant and peevish, in not admitting their true demonstrations and certaine observations, that they tyrannize over arte, science, and all philosophy, in suppressing their labours ... forbidding them to write, to speake a truth, all to maintaine their superstition" (2:53).[20] But he holds in worse contempt those who mangle their findings to appease theological authorities: "the World is tossed in a blanket amongst them, they hoyse the earth up and downe like a ball, make it stand and goe at their pleasures" to such a point that "it is to be feared, the Sunne and Moone will hide themselves, and be as much offended as shee [the moon] was with those [philosophers in Lucian] and send another message to *Jupiter*, by some new-fangled *Icaromenippus*, to make an end of all those curious Controversies, and scatter them abroad" (2:55).

The allusion to Lucian's poetic representation of divine fury disguises the profundity of the questions that follow under a veneer of levity and disdain: "The Jewish Thalmudists take upon them to determine how God spends his whole time, sometimes playing with Leviathan, sometimes overseeing the world ... like *Lucian's Jupiter*, that spent much of the yeare in painting butterflies wings and seeing who offered sacrifice" (2:56). The Pagans "mangle [God] after a thousand fashions; our Hereticks, Schismaticks, and some Schoolemen, come not farre behind," as they would know

> why good and bad are punished together, war, fires, plagues, infest all alike, why wicked men flourish good are poore, in prison, sicke, and ill at ease? Why doth he suffer so much mischiefe & evill to be done, if he be able to helpe? Why doth he not assist good, or resist bad, reforme our wills, if he be not the author of sinne, and let such enormities be committed, unworthy of his knowledge, wisdome, government, mercy, and providence, why lets hee all things be done by fortune & chance? (2:56)

Burton spirals these questions into a *reductio ad absurdum* from which he pantomimes a fainting fit:

---

[20] Burton is notably careful here to credit this particular complaint about censorship to Pomponazzi.

Some againe curious phantasticks, will know more then this, and enquire with *Epicurus* what God did before the World was made? was he idle? Where did he bide? What did hee make the world of? why did he then make it and not before? ... . If God be infinitely and only good, why should he alter or destroy the world? if he confound that which is good, how shall himselfe continue good? If hee pull it down because evill, how shall he be free from the evill that made it evill? &c. with many such absurd and brainsicke questions, intricacies, froth of humane wit and excrements of curiosity, & c. which, as our Saviour told his inquisitive disciples, are not fit for them to know. But hoo? I am now gone quite out of sight, I am almost giddy with roving about. (2:57)

He recovers by deferring such inquiries to those with "stronger wits ... better ability" and, suggestively, "happier leisure to wade into such Philosophicall mysteries" (2:57). Burton concludes with Samuel Daniel that *"God in his providence to checke our presumptuous inquisition, wraps things in uncertainty, barres us from long antiquity, and bounds our search within the compasse of some few ages."*[21] But the questions have been asked and remain in the air, so to speak, despite their disavowal, and they do so all the more potently by their swift and equally theatrical abandonment. Now no longer a hawk but a melancholy spaniel, Burton descends to chase the game he says he's been after all along: "my melancholy spaniels quest, my game is sprung, and I must suddenly come downe and follow" (2:58). He proceeds, for the rest of the Digression, to describe the kinds and qualities of air that aggravate and ameliorate melancholy. However, this shift into the mode of the medical *practica* for the remaining eight pages of the Digression does little to attenuate the power of the meditations on "exoneration" and vicissitude to which we have been privy in the preceding 26 and whose philosophical, rhetorical, and political resonance we shall now consider in greater detail.

II. Epicurean Consolations

Burton claims that the Digression is modeled after Lucian's *Icaromenippus*, and, indeed, there are obvious parallels between his and Lucian's cosmic flights (not least of which are the satirical investments shared by both writers), but the marks and tones of Mennipean satire found elsewhere in the *Anatomy* are strikingly absent from the Digression, which owes far greater debts to Lucretius and Ovid, and these debts have gone largely unremarked.[22] Burton's Epicureanism, where it has been treated, has been interpreted, especially in more recent criticism, as an expression of Stoic moral psychology.[23] However, the consolatory purposes

---

[21] From *The first part of the Historie of England* (London, 1612), 3.

[22] Rosalie Colie, *Paradoxia Epidemica: The Renaissance Tradition of Paradox* (Princeton, NJ: Princeton University Press, 1966), 307.

[23] Angus Gowland, *The Worlds of Renaissance Melancholy: Robert Burton in Context* (Cambridge and New York: Cambridge University Press, 2006), 12–16; Jeremy Schmidt, "Melancholy and the Therapeutic Language of Moral Philosophy in Seventeenth-Century Thought," *Journal of the History of Ideas* 65, no. 4 (2004): 583–601. Reid Barbour

to which both Ovid and Lucretius deploy Epicurean physics and theories of mutability find striking parallels in the themes of the Digression and in Burton's broader interest in and understanding of the creative and curative powers of transformation. One of the principal aims of the *Anatomy*, as of *De rerum natura*, is to dispel irrational fears of divine punishment. Burton cites Lucretius more than two dozen times, mostly in the third partition, giving rather damning testimony of religious inducements to despair. These references appear mainly in Burton's discussion of atheism, under the heading "Religious melancholy in defect."[24] Here Burton makes a wry distinction between the ancient philosophers who scorned "superstition" and "simple" atheists who call Christian doctrine superstitious, offering a covert bid for the latter by defending the former. Indeed, he notes the thankless work of those who have prosecuted the Epicurean cause, chief among them, Lucretius:

> there be those that Apologise for *Epicurus*, but all in vaine: *Lucian* scoffes at all, *Epicurus* he denies all, & *Lucretius* his scholler defends him in it,
>> *Humana ante oculos foedè cum vita jaceret,*
>> *In terris oppressa gravi sub religione,*
>> *Quae caput à coeli regionibus ostendebat,*
>> *Horribili super aspectu mortalibus instans, &c.*
>> When humane kinde was drench't in supersitition,
>> With gastly lookes aloft which frighted mortall men, &c.[25]
> He alone, as another *Hercules*, did vindicate the world from that monster. (3:404)

Burton lauds Lucretius as "another Hercules" for having rid the world of a suggestively plastic monster of superstition, horrible both for the groundless fears it inspires and the ravages it wreaks in war, which he counts as a further symptom (and cause) of religious melancholy. On this point, a few pages earlier, he also quotes Lucretius: "*Tantum religio potuit suadere malorum.*[26] Not there onely, but all over *Europe*, we read of bloody battels, rackes and wheeles, seditions, factions, oppositions ..." (3:367).

Burton's cosmic meditations in the Digression resemble the sixth book of *De rerum* in their attempts to dissuade the reader from the belief that natural

---

regards Burton's Epicureanism as a "model for both the calculus of pleasure and the proper endurance of pain," but foregrounds the place of this ethic within a politics of liberation from the "fear-inducing strictures of the state" (*English Epicures and Stoics: Ancient Legacies in Early Stuart Culture* [Amherst: University of Massachusetts Press, 1998], 65–6). I am making a similar point in this chapter about the importance of freedom from religious terror that Burton is drawing from the Epicurean tradition.

[24]   Full title of the subsection: "Religious Melancholy in Defect, Parties affected, Epicures, Atheists, Hypocrites, Worldly Secure, Carnalists, all Impious Persons, Impenitent Sinners, &c."

[25]   Burton is quoting from *De rerum natura*, 1:62–5.

[26]   "So much of evil could religion prompt" (Titus Lucretius Carus, *The Nature of Things*, trans. Frank O. Copley (New York: W.W. Norton & Company, 1977), 1.101.

calamities are divinely ordained.[27] Lucretius complains that "men see in heaven and here on earth / things happen, that often fills their minds with fear, / and humble their hearts with terror of the gods."[28] Burton likewise emphasizes the natural causes of cosmic and geological upheaval (2:38–9) and, like Lucretius and Ovid, he routinely borrows from myth and legend in so doing. Lucretius' use of myth has long vexed scholars who view it as a contradiction of the poem's didactic purposes.[29] But in Burton's spiritual therapeutics we see the same terms of consolation work in tandem with myth in two ways: first as a means of inducing a therapeutic sense of wonder and delight, and second as a means of rendering providential analyses of natural cataclysm into myths themselves.

Burton's revisions and additions to the *Anatomy* reveal a systematic effort to dispel fears promoted by millennial doomsayers. As Robert Hallwachs noted, Burton made repeated addition of the word "secure" to the second edition.[30] He changed the original text of this sentence in the subsection on "Perturbations of the Mind Rectified" from "Many are fully cured when they ... enjoy their desires or be satisfied in their minds" to "Many are fully cured when they ... enjoy their desires, *or be secured* and satisfied in their minds."[31] "Secure" here qualifies "satisfaction," implying that there can be no real comforting or abatement of melancholy without the removal of cause, and that cause is fear. "Feare," Burton warns, "dissolves the spirits, infects the heart, attenuates the soule: and for these causes all passions and perturbations must to the uttermost of our power, and most seriously be removed" (2:100). He emphasizes the point that the removal of fear is no easy task. As we have already seen in Chapter 2, Burton compares the relationship between the melancholic and fear to the body and its shadow, saying that you "may as well bid him that is sicke of an ague, not to bee adry; or him that is wounded, not to feele paine" as try to dispell irrational fear through reason (1:420). He is hard pressed then in the second partition to explain how one goes about removing fears that so infect the heart and soul: "Yea but you will here infer, that this is excellent food indeed if it could be done, but how shall it be effected,

---

27   Reject such thoughts! Far from your mind remove them,
     Unworthy of gods and alien to their peace!
     Else power divine, belittled by you, will often
     Harm you—not that gods' power can be so damaged
     That anger would drive them panting for fierce revenge,
     But that you'll picture these placid, peaceful, harmless
     Creatures aboil with billows of rolling wrath,
     And then won't enter their temples with peace at heart. (Ibid., 6.68–75)

28   Ibid., 6.50–52.

29   See Monica R. Gale, *Myth and Poetry in Lucretius* (Cambridge: Cambridge University Press, 1994).

30   Robert G. Hallwachs, "Additions and Revisions in the Second Edition of Burton's *Anatomy of Melancholy*: A Study of Burton's Chief Interests and of his Style as Shown in his Revisions" (PhD diss., Princeton University, 1942), 81.

31   Robert Burton, *The Anatomy of Melancholy* (Oxford, 1624), 239; italics mine.

by whom, what art, what meanes?" (2:100). Burton suggests various checks and restraints to *"false, frivolous Imaginations, absurd conceits, fained feares and sorrowes"* (2:101). He prescribes busyness ("If it be idlenesse hath caused this infirmity"), and company (if "he perceave himselfe given to solitarinesse"), and all manner of pleasant recreations (2:102). But his chief advice, as the full title of the subsection makes plain, is that the melancholic disburden himself by "confessing his griefe to a friend" (2:99). When judgment and self-moderation fail, and he intimates that they inevitably do, "The best way for ease is to impart our misery to some friend, not to smother it up in our owne breast" (2:104). This disburdening, which he characterizes as exoneration, is an even greater balm than the friend's consolation: "good words are cheerefull and powerfull of themselves," but "the simple narration many times easeth our distressed minde, and in the midst of greatest extremities, so diverse have beene relieved, by exonerating themselves to a faithfull friend" (2:105).

This therapeutic disburdening is quite different from the confessional absolution of sin. Burton is reworking the idea of exoneration as the removal of irrational fears of one's reprobation. The increased emphasis on spiritual consolation in the second and subsequent editions of the *Anatomy* suggests that Burton had come to regard despair not only as the more prevalent but also the more preventable variety of melancholy. Whereas "simple" or "physical" melancholy presents as "irrational" fear or sadness—that is, sadness without objective cause—spiritual melancholy, says Burton, is largely the result of fears imposed from without and, therefore, as the Epicurean poets demonstrate, may be allayed, abated, and avoided through means of external persuasion.

If Burton's cosmological meditations in the Digression echo Lucretius in their explanatory and consolatory purposes, they recall Pythagoras' Epicurean oration in the fifteenth book of Ovid's *Metamorphoses* even more precisely. Burton invokes (without naming) Pythagoras' theory of benign, cosmic, and geological mutability in the Digression when he tells us he "would descend and see what is done in the bowels of the earth," asking an extraordinary list of questions that directly echo Ovid: "doe stones and mettles grow there still? how come firre trees to be digged out from tops of hills, as in our mosses, and marshes all over *Europe*? How come they to digge up fish bones, shelles, beames, iron works, many fathomes under ground, & anchors in mountaines far remote from all seas?" (2:38). Golding's Pythagoras illustrates his lesson on impermanence with the very same examples:

> Euen so the ages of the world from gold too Iron past.
> Euen so haue places oftentymes exchaunged theyr estate.
> For I haue séene it sea which was substanciall ground alate,
> Ageine where sea was, I haue séene the same become dry lond,
> And shelles and scales of Seafish farre haue lyen from any strond.
> And in the toppes of mountaynes hygh old Anchors haue béene found.[32]

---

[32]   Ovid, *The XV Bookes of P. Ouidius Naso, Entytuled Metamorphosis*, trans. Arthur Golding (London, 1567), 190r.

This lesson is not a *memento mori* so much as a consolatory discourse on the immutability and immortality of the soul that passes between all living things, man to beast and vice versa, and it famously serves as the foundation for Pythagoras' argument for vegetarianism. His lecture on metempsychosis ties the theme of the mutability and translation of the soul to the movement and transformation of the earth's elements—fire thickening into air, water becoming earth—pointing at the endurance and translatability of all matter despite formal alteration:

> The earth resoluing leysurely dooth melt too water shéere.
> The water fyned turnes too aire. The aire éeke purged cléere
> From grossenesse, spyreth vp aloft, and there becommeth fyre.
> From thence in order contrary they backe ageine retyre.
> Fyre thickening passeth intoo Aire, and Ayër wexing grosse,
> Returnes too water: Water éeke congealing intoo drosse,
> Becommeth earth. No kind of thing kéepes ay his shape and hew.
> For nature louing euer chaunge repayres one shape a new
> Uppon another neyther dooth there perrish aught (trust mée)
> In all the world, but altring takes new shape.[33]

In support of this point that it is only the shape of things that changes, Ovid lists the same aforementioned curiosities (anchors in mountaintops and fish found far from water) that Burton cites to describe the radical changes of the earth over time. Golding's Pythagoras elaborates this theme of natural vicissitude through examples of hydraulic transformation: hills worn down "by force of gulling" into the sea, gravel where marshes lay previously, and lakes in places that "Erst did suffer drowght." The *Oxford English Dictionary* specifically offers Golding's translation in its definition of "gulling" as a hydraulic transformation—a "wearing away or hollowing out effected by the action of running water or other means."[34] Ovid's inventory of lakes and rivers that have changed direction and shape and of mainlands turned islands or drowned completely brings us back to the hydraulic theme of Burton's meditations in the early part of the Digression. Considering their place in Pythagoras' lecture on metempsychosis allows their consolatory purpose in the *Anatomy* to come into sharper view.

The hydraulic transformation of the earth serves Ovid, as it does Burton, as a powerful analogy for the perseverance of immortal spirit as a kind of world soul. This, of course, is a crucial difference from Lucretius' Epicureanism, which insists on the mortality of the soul and is therefore less easily assimilated into the Christian Epicureanism of the late sixteenth and early seventeenth centuries.[35]

---

[33] Ibid.

[34] *Oxford English Dictionary Online*, s.v. "gulling, n. 2," accessed March 4, 2014, http://www.oed.com.libezproxy2.syr.edu/view/Entry/82471.

[35] On Ovid's rewriting of Lucretius, see Philip Hardie, "The Speech of Pythagoras in Ovid Metamorphoses 15: Empedoclean Epos," *The Classical Quarterly* 45, no. 1 (1995): 204–14. The revival and influence of Epicureanism before Gassendi's Christian Epicureanism has been a focus of the recent swell of scholarship on Lucretius that

Especially in Golding's translation, Pythagorean metempsychosis is the process by which this world soul not only survives but also compels transformation, ensuring its continuity through metamorphosis:

> Al things doo chauge. But nothing sure dooth perrish. This same spright
> Dooth fléete, and fisking héere and there dooth swiftly take his flyght
> From one place too another place, and entreth euery wyght,
> Remouing out of man too beast, and out of beast too man.
> But yit it neuer perrisheth nor neuer perrish can ...
> The soule is ay the selfsame thing it was and yit astray
> It fléeteth intoo sundry shapes.[36]

Cosmic upheaval and earthly decay become the very harbingers of renewal according to Pythagoras' teaching. Living things are born of death: hornets are bred from the carcass of a horse, scorpions from crab mold, butterflies from caterpillars, snakes from human spines in the grave, the phoenix risen from its own corpse in a nest of fragrant spices.

With the phoenix and hyena, Ovid shifts from the theme of postmortem transformation to transformations *in vivo*. The laughing hyena changes sex from female to male and back again. The chameleon changes its hue by imitating its surroundings: "All colours that it leaneth too doth counterfeit by kind." The urine of a spotted lynx turns to stone as sea coral hardens when it touches air. Ovid's *mirabilia naturae*, both locally in Pythagoras' oration and thematically in the stories of transformation told in the rest of the *Metamorphoses*, provide a key stylistic and substantive model for Burton's meditations on mimetic transformation. Despite the excruciations of Ovid's transfigured subjects and of melancholic suffering as experienced in the myriad forms studied by Burton, mutability functions as a sign of regenerative *copia* in both the *Metamorphoses* and the *Anatomy*. As Pythagoras says, coming to the end of his lecture by way of Burton's favorite device of the *occupatio*: "The day would end, / And *Phebus* panting stéedes should in the *Ocean* déepe descend, / Before all alterations I in woordes could comprehend."[37] For Ovid and Burton alike, the rhetorical gesture of insufficiency to relate such numberless examples is the ultimate sign of hope in plenitude. At the very least, these examples argue against providential readings of cosmic upheaval and calamity. At best, they offer hope for recovery (and in Burton's Christianized Epicureanism, redemption)

---

includes Stephen Greenblatt, *The Swerve: How the World Became Modern* (New York: W.W. Norton, 2011); Gerard Paul Passannante, *The Lucretian Renaissance: Philology and the Afterlife of Tradition* (Chicago: University of Chicago Press, 2011); Philip R. Hardie, *Lucretian Receptions: History, the Sublime, Knowledge* (Cambridge: Cambridge University Press, 2009); Stuart Gillespie, "Lucretius in the English Renaissance," in *The Cambridge Companion to Lucretius*, ed. Philip Hardie and Stuart Gillespie (Cambridge: Cambridge University Press, 2007), 242–53; Alison Brown, *The Return of Lucretius to Renaissance Florence* (Cambridge, MA: Harvard University Press, 2010).

[36]   Ovid, *The XV Bookes of P. Ouidius Naso, Entytuled Metamorphosis*, 189r.
[37]   Ibid., 193v.

with the inevitable changes that come with the passing of time and the hydraulic force or "gulling" of grace.

Burton's benign representation of cosmic mutability had company among contemporary French and English writers who looked to Lucretius to counter the argument that the world had been deteriorating since the Fall.[38] The Digression's vision of mutability echoes Louis le Roy's repudiation of theories of universal decay in *De la vicissitude* (1575) and anticipates similar arguments made by George Hakewill in his *Apologie* (1627).[39] For Le Roy, mutability in the natural world serves as an analogy for the perpetual flux of human experience. Nations, governments, and philosophies rise and fall, he says, but these fluctuations portend no general demise for humanity. Quite the contrary—new technological and geographic discoveries prove the vitality of human wit and ingenuity. In Le Roy's view, knowledge at the turn of the seventeenth century was positively advancing, not proliferating in vain.[40] Hakewill adapted Le Roy's argument to refute Godfrey Goodman's doomsday prophesying in the millenarian *The Fall of Man* (1616), offering evidence of what he called history's "circular progresse."[41] He suggests that even the greatest tumults and catastrophes are but momentary interruptions of a process whereby things "have their *birth*, their *growth*, their *flourishing*, their *failing*, their *fading*, and within a while after their *resurrection* and *reflourishing* againe."[42] While Burton is less interested in championing progress than Le Roy or Hakewill, he is undeniably enthusiastic about the momentum of scientific

---

[38] On the themes of benevolent mutability and transformation in Renaissance art and humanism, see Michel Jeanneret, *Perpetual Motion: Transforming Shapes in the Renaissance from Da Vinci to Montaigne*, trans. Nidra Poller (Baltimore: Johns Hopkins University Press, 2000). On the relationship between the arguments concerning the decay of man and the decay of the world, see Victor Harris, *All Coherence Gone* (Chicago: University of Chicago Press, 1949); Richard F. Jones, *The Seventeenth Century: Studies in the History of English Thought and Literature from Bacon to Pope* (Stanford: Stanford University Press, 1951), 10–15; Meredith Jane Donaldson, "Moveable Text: Mutability, Monumentality, and the Representation of Motion in British Renaissance Literature" (PhD diss., McGill University, 2011), chap. 5.

[39] The Digression and the Preface were the two most expanded sections of the second edition of the *Anatomy*, but it was not until the third edition in 1636, after Hakewill's controversial treatise was published, that Burton added the most poetic and Pythagorean flourishes to his meditations on cosmic vicissitude, such as this one: "*Josephus Blancanus* ... foolishly feares, and in a just tract proves ... that in time the Sea will wast away the land, and all the globe of the earth shall be covered with waters, *risum teneatis amici*? what the sea takes away in one place it addes in another ..." (2:38). Another key addition is the comparison of worlds turned inside out to the turning of "apples to the fire" (2:39) discussed above.

[40] See Jeanneret, *Perpetual Motion*, chap. 7.

[41] See Godfrey Goodman, *The Fall of Man, or the Corruption of Nature, Proued by the Light of Our Naturall Reason* (London, 1616).

[42] George Hakewill, *An Apologie of the Power and Providence of God in the Government of the World* (Oxford, 1635), 259.

discovery and the vitality of late Renaissance natural philosophy. Whereas early twentieth-century critics such as Williamson tied the mutability theme in seventeenth-century literature to the obfuscating and disorienting discoveries of the new "science," this confusion is a source of exuberance in the *Anatomy*, and in the Digression in particular.[43] Burton delights in the bounty of unresolved scientific controversies much as he delights in the anatomizing of melancholy and its innumerable expositors' conflicting views. The hawk that "fetcheth many a circuit" is content to hover amongst the constellations of opinion enumerated by his widening gyres. Such irresolution is the signal feature of Burton's centonic style and a key component of its cure; the *Anatomy*'s "confusion" of bibliographical voices has special therapeutic value for melancholy caused by a desire to fix opinion and discover "with certainty" what experience shows to be partial, provisional, and contingent. In other words, a survey of the "vicissitudes" of the un/knowable world is the very thing Burton offers the readers of his generation who might have been sent reeling by the very same.

Longinian Vicissitudes

The therapeutic substitution of awe and wonder for fear and terror that we see both in the Digression and the traditions of Epicurean consolation to which it is indebted is further illuminated by Longinian rhetorical theory. It is plain to see that Burton's imaginary hawk tours the heights and depths in a way that evokes the double meaning of *altus* in Longinus' treatise on the sublime. I would, however, emphasize some of the more subtle ways in which the Digression (and, by extension, the digressive mode of the *Anatomy*) borrows from the *techne* of the Longinian sublime in order to both represent and respond to the psychological experience of his melancholy readers. Longinus defined the sublime as an effect of the twinned representation of cosmic and psychological cataclysm, typically expressed through literary synesthesia and a poetics of psychic interruption. He points to Sappho for his definitive example:[44]

> Speechless I gaze: the flame within
> Runs swift o'er all my quivering skin;

---

[43]   George Williamson, "Mutability, Decay, and Seventeenth-Century Melancholy," *ELH* 2, no. 2 (1935): 121–50.

[44]   As with the baroque, the category of the sublime in seventeenth-century literature has been examined mainly in respect to French texts. Recent examples include Emma Gilby, *Sublime Words: Early Modern French Literature* (London: Legenda, 2006); and John D. Lyons, "Sublime Accidents," in *Chance, Literature, and Culture in Early Modern France*, ed. John D. Lyons and Kathleen Wine (Burlington, VT: Ashgate, 2009), 95–110. Some exceptions include chapters in Joshua Scodel, *Excess and the Mean in Early Modern English Literature* (Princeton, NJ: Princeton University Press, 2002); and *Translations of the Sublime: The Early Modern Reception and Dissemination of Longinus' Peri Hupsous in Rhetoric, the Visual Arts, Architecture and the Theatre*, ed. Caroline van Eck (Leiden: Brill, 2012).

My eyeballs swim; with dizzy din
   My brain reels round;
And cold drops fall; and tremblings frail
Seize every limb; and grassy pale
I grow; and then—together fail
   Both sight and sound.[45]

Longinus compares the chaos of erotic desire here to Homer's depiction of the Battle of the Gods, "when earth is torn up from its foundations, and Tartarus itself laid bare, and the Universe suffers overthrow and dissolution."[46] He remarks Sappho's uncanny ability to "gather soul and body into one," praising her "power of first selecting and then closely combining those [emotions] which are conspicuous and intense."[47] The sublime, exemplified by Sapphic longing, is synesthetic not only in its combining of the lover's individual senses but in its concentration of the symptoms "found severally in lovers" in the poet's single expression of longing.[48] It transports the solitary reader into an imagined community that collectively shares the disordered passions of the lyricist.[49]

The resonance of Longinus' psychological insights with Burton's ethical and therapeutic project becomes more apparent when we consider that the success of the Longinian sublime depends upon the simultaneous articulation and disarticulation of the private experience of psychic disturbance.[50] Sublime ecstasy (*ekstasis*) is a transport of and from one's individual subject position. One hears one's thoughts and feelings echoed by another and is thereby simultaneously humbled (literally broken down and disabused of the fiction of one's uniqueness) and, at the same time, hoisted up to share the poet's vantage of universal suffering. Burton's oft-repeated description of the melancholic as "*fracti animis*,"[51] or broken in spirit, suggests the sublime discontinuity of melancholic experience. Rather than signaling the failure of the melancholic subject to cohere as a constant self, the fractured spirit is one that may be fortunately transformed. Its very discontinuity allows for the possibility of positive transformation.

---

[45]   Longinus, *On the Sublime*, trans. A.O. Prickard (Oxford: Clarendon, 1906), 23.

[46]   Ibid., 17.

[47]   Ibid., 23.

[48]   "All the symptoms are found severally in lovers; to the choice of those which are conspicuous, and to their concentration into one, is due, the pre-eminent merit here. So it is, I think, with the Poet and his storms ..." (ibid., 24).

[49]   Suzanne Guerlac describes this transportation or *hypsous* as a flight in two phases, "first a sense of being 'scattered,'" then of being "uplifted with a sense of proud possession ... as if we had ourselves produced the very thing we heard" ("Longinus and the Subject of the Sublime," *New Literary History* 16, no. 2 [1985]: 275).

[50]   Guerlac describes this destabilizing effect of the sublime in terms of iteration and reception, enunciation and enunciator: "The transport of the sublime ... includes a slippage among the positions of enunciation, as the *destinateur* gets 'transported' into the message and the *destinataire* achieves a fictive identification with the speaker" (ibid.).

[51]   For example, 1:331; 2:83; 2:101.

Burton's rhetorical techniques in the Digression and, indeed, throughout the *Anatomy* evoke what we might refer to as a melancholic sublime. The power of his use of asyndeton especially is illuminated by Longinus' remarks on the liberating discontinuity of sublime rhetoric. Longinus admires the propulsive force of the asyndeton and the freedom of a syntax unshackled by coordinating conjunctions. He compares the effects of a highly restrictive syntax to the binding of a runner's limbs. The writer's passions, like the runner's limbs, "chafe" against the resistance of these "connecting links and other appendages" that impede their course, which otherwise would advance "as though from an engine of war."[52] By this analogy, the sublime is animated by an emotional power whose vehemence is represented as brute force.[53] The pleasure of rhetoric becomes, in Longinus' description, a masochistic pleasure in the attack upon the auditor's resistance to the powers of oratory. The rhetorician's tools are likened to modes of physical assault: a blow to the face that stirs and makes men "frantic." Such erotic battery destabilizes the subject, making a different kind of order out of the disorderliness of the broken mind and spirit.[54] This paradoxical "disorderly order" furthermore reduplicates the striven quality of the sublime as the effect of a disturbed syntax that imitates emotional disturbance, giving us a sense of the highly mimetic aesthetic tradition upon which Burton is drawing.[55] The sublime does simply lend itself to mimetic reproduction. Its description requires the aesthetic sympathy of sublime language. To invoke the sublime is, therefore, to enact the sublime or, to echo Suzanne Guerlac, the sublime is brought into being by force of its articulation. It is always citational, always *artificial*, even as it is felicitated by the discontinuity of lived experience.[56]

III. Earthly and Spiritual Exonerations

With these philosophical and rhetorical contexts in mind we are better able to evaluate the purposes to which Burton puts the themes of the Digression to use in his comments on the religious, economic, and sociopolitical provocations to melancholy. To assess the religious implications of Burton's Epicurean meditations, we must return to the Digression's images of regenerative eversion, or the outward movement of the earth's center to its periphery: "The whole world belike should be new moulded ... and turned inside out, as we doe hay-cocks in Harvest, toppe to bottome, or bottome to top" (2:39). This image leads Burton

---

[52]   Longinus, *On the Sublime*, 23.

[53]   He refers to the speaker as the "striker," elaborating as follows on the violence of his gesture, presence, and physical engagement with the audience: "There are many things which the striker may do," he says, quoting from Demosthenes, "by gesture, by look, by voice" (ibid., 44).

[54]   Ibid.

[55]   See Chapter 2.

[56]   Guerlac, "Longinus and the Subject of the Sublime," 287.

to announce the possibility of infinite worlds that he goes on to elaborate, as we have seen above, but before doing so he digresses to plumb the earth's center, describing the "underworld" with a natural historian's sense of eclectic wonder about its natural properties and mythical character alike:

> What is the center of the Earth, is it pure element only, as *Aristotle* decrees, inhabited (as *Paracelsus* thinks) with creatures, whose Chaos is Earth: or with *Fayries*, as the woods and waters (according to him) are with *Nymphes*; or the Aire with spirits? *Dionisiodorus* ... that sent a letter *ad superos*, after he was dead, from the Center of the earth, to signifie what distance the same center was from the *superficies* of the same, *viz. 4200 stadiums*, might have done well to have satisfied all these doubts. (2:39)

The story of Dionysiodorus is borrowed from Pliny's *Natural History*,[57] and in Pliny's same style of mythical reportage, Burton goes on to examine the reputed characteristics of the Pagan underworld and Christian hell: "Or is it the place of Hell, as Virgill in his *Aeneides, Plato, Lucian, Dantes*, and others poetically describe it, and as many of our Divines thinke?" (2:39). He rejects stories of reputed hell-mouths as "fables and illusions," like "that poeticall Infernus, where *Homers* soule was seene hanging on a tree ... to which they ferried over in *Charons* boat" (2:40). The charge of improbability carries suggestively over to Burton's handling of the nature of a Christian hell: "*Better doubt of thing concealed, then to contend about uncertainties*," he concludes, quoting Augustine.

Burton dismisses all Scholastic inquiries as to hell's dimensions (how many damned souls it will hold and in what manner of torment, etc.), turning his attention instead to the "spiritous" energy at the center of the earth, where all things become fluid. The earth's ores are a "fountaine of mettles" and the heated air springs up in the form of water to "moisten the Earthes superficies" by way of secret passages or, literally, the "bowels of the earth" (2:41). The belly of the world is rendered as the earth's nutritive core, a vital and propulsive engine of benevolent transformation rather than the pit of hell.[58] "Exoneration" here suggests

---

[57] "*Dionysodorus* in another kind would be beleeved: (for I will not beguile you of the greatest example of Grecian vanitie.) This man was a Melian, famous for his skill in Geometrie ... his neere kinswomen ... solemnized his funerals, & accompanied him to his grave. These women (as they came some fewe dayes after to his sepulchre for to perfourme some solemne obsequies thereto belonging) by report, found in his monument an Epistle ... written in his owne name To them above, that is to say, To the Living: and to this effect, namely, That hee had made a step from his sepulchre to the bottome and centre of the earth ..." (Pliny, the Elder, *The Historie of the World*, trans. Philemon Holland (London, 1601), 49.

[58] We might also read this nutritive and expulsive core as the Galenic heart, giving Burton's emphasis here on "exoneration" a more obviously spiritual hue. On the "heart's expulsive power" in Crooke's Galenic physiology, see Ann Blair, *The Theater of Nature* (Princeton, NJ: Princeton University Press, 1997), 21; Robert A. Erickson, *The Language of the Heart: 1600–1750* (Philadelphia: University of Pennsylvania Press, 1997), 15.

the necessity of physical disburdening and release, both of the earth's elements and the humoral body to which it is analogous.[59] Burton's geohumoral exonerations echo his nearly Arminian insistence on the power of a universally available grace.[60] As we have seen, Burton recommends disburdening oneself to a friend as the most effective means of healing distressed spirits,[61] but there is a further sense in which the efficacy of psychic disburdening as "exoneration" is yoked to a mechanic of grace whose forceful abundance inheres in the very structure and physics of the universe. In the third partition, Burton counsels his readers to yield the pride that underscores religious despair over to the plenum of God's mercy, which he calls an "Alexipharmicum" and characterizes in pronouncedly hydraulic terms: "As a drop of water is to the Sea, so are thy misdeeds to his mercy, nay there is no such proportion to bee given, for the Sea though great, may yet be measured, but God's mercy cannot be circumscribed" (3:437).

The analogy between grace and hydraulics resides in the suggestion that the power of grace, like the great wonders of geology surveyed in the Digression, may be witnessed in the passages wrought by the force of "spirit" in what would otherwise appear to be impregnable impasses and remote deeps. Landlocked waters and unfathomable depths stand in for the imperviousness of the desperate to the workings of grace and the bottomlessness of their sense of sin. Burton ties the theme of recovery from despair to the images of birds and men revived from the seeming grave of winter slumbers. Upon mention of these marvelous reanimations, Burton raises and dismisses the possibility that the earth will either be drowned by the sea or "dry up the vast Ocean with sand and ashes," suggestively pointing the reader to the wonders of the deep and its evidence of regeneration: "Search the depth, and see that variety of Sea monsters and fishes, Mare-maides, Sea men, Horses, c. which it affords" and "see what is done in the bowels of the earth ... doe stones and mettles grow there still?" (2:38). He goes on from here to survey Ovid's examples of geological inversion and eversion in his apocalyptic reverie that, informed by Pythagorean metempsychosis, argues for the triumph of life despite the apparent death of all things.

The recourse to wonder is, of course, the very spirit of Lucretian consolation elaborated in Ovid's poetic theme of metamorphosis. For Burton, it implies that the cure for melancholy lies in awe or wonder, which activates the healing powers of the imagination and renders the recalcitrant or hardened spirit amenable to grace. This is the very substance of Burtonian "repentance," which he later characterizes as "an attractive loadstone" that "draw[s] Gods mercy and graces unto us" (3:428), "effect[s] prodigious cures" and "make[s] a stupend metamorphosis" (3:429).

---

[59]   To "exonerate" could refer to the disburdening of the bowels as well as the soul (*Oxford English Dictionary Online*, s.v. "exonerate," accessed September 7, 2014, http://www.oed.com.libezproxy2.syr.edu/view/Entry/66328).

[60]   See Mary Ann Lund, *Melancholy, Medicine and Religion in Early Modern England: Reading "The Anatomy of Melancholy"* (New York: Cambridge University Press, 2010), chap. 2.

[61]   See Chapter 3 and Michael O'Connell, *Robert Burton* (Boston: Twayne, 1986), chap. 4.

God's love draws human love through an irresistible force of attraction that draws like to like. It is the engine, so to speak, of Burton's hydraulic account of grace, but it borrows from more ancient and occult understandings of the power of eros as a generator of sympathetic magic.[62] It is a force seen everywhere in nature: "This love is manifest, I say, in inanimate creatures, how comes a load-stone to draw iron to it? Jet? chaffe? The ground to covet shores, but for love? No creature, S. *Hierom* concludes, is to be found, *quod non aliquid amat*, no stock, no stone, that hath not some feeling of love" (3:13–14). Burton goes on to show how these feelings are evident in the "great Sympathy" between certain plants (trees especially, as we shall see in the coda to this chapter) and in the "Sensible love ... of brute beasts" and the "pleasure they take in the Act of Generation" (3:14). The "golden chaine" of love that "reacheth downe from Heaven to Earth ... " is less a hierarchy from base to best than a chain of mimetic transference that inclines humanity toward God through loving and charitable acts: "as the Sunne in the Firmament, (I say) so is love in the world ... *The love of God begets the love of man, and by this love of our neighbor, the love of God is nourished and increased*" (3:31–2).

Burton stresses throughout the *Anatomy* that love is the antidote to melancholy: love of others, love of God and of men. He quotes Bernard on Corinthians 13:13, saying that love "*inflames our soules with a divine heat, and being so inflamed purgeth, and so purged, elevates to God, makes an attonement and reconciles us unto him.*" This transformation of the soul by love's fiery purgation invites comparison to the ways in which earlier commentators understood melancholy to be transformed through heat. The classical authorities typically regarded adust (heated, burnt, or combusted) melancholy as an especially dangerous, manic form of the disease, characterized by frenzy.[63] This understanding shaped the views of Renaissance physicians such as Jacques Ferrand on the deleterious effects of eros and the passions on the melancholically inclined.[64] Ficino, on the other hand, argued that such frenzy in the moderately adust melancholic is a state of inspiration and a hallmark of melancholic genius.[65] In the *Anatomy*, the "heat" of love transforms melancholy from a cold and dark humor into one that facilitates empathy and charity, the absence of which is repeatedly made out to be the root cause of melancholic suffering in the world. In what follows, I outline some of the ways in which Burton analogously extends the Digression's exonerative theme to argue for the necessity of more equitable distributions of wealth and resources, including the resources of faith or "credit" between men and women.

---

[62]   See Ioan P. Culianu, *Eros and Magic in the Renaissance* (Chicago: University of Chicago Press, 1987).

[63]   See Galen, *On the Affected Parts*, trans. Rudolph E. Siegel (New York: Karger, 1976), 88–90.

[64]   Jacques Ferrand, *A Treatise on Lovesickness*, ed. and trans. Donald A. Beecher and Massimo Ciavolella (Syracuse, NY: Syracuse University Press, 1994), 115.

[65]   Noel L. Brann, *The Debate Over the Origin of Genius During the Italian Renaissance: The Theories of Supernatural Frenzy and Natural Melancholy in Accord and in Conflict on the Treshold of the Scientific* (Leiden: Brill, 2002), 285.

Exonerations of the Body Politic

Burton's study of the exonerative movements and ventilations of waters, spirits, and metals of the earth finds an important parallel in his discussion of economic circulation and its malignant obstruction. As has been noted throughout this study, Burton's writing is itself "ventilated" by citation. His citations are, moreover, scored or punctured by other citations, miscitations, and theatrical interruptions to such a point as to make it notoriously difficult to detect Burton's own views. However, if we can measure his skepticism by the degree of mischief to which he subjects his sources, we might cautiously detect his earnestness where he subdues or interrupts long stretches of centonic ventriloquism and offers what appears to be more direct critique.[66] Several such instances occur in places where Burton offers arguments for the salutary disburdening of obstructed social systems, and this is perhaps most strikingly the case in the political and economic critique offered by way of his satirical utopia in the Preface. Burton blames England's economic insularism for a variety of social and political ills. He repeatedly ties economic congestion to the preponderance of melancholic disease in England. By contrast, he praises the Dutch for their salutary use of channels and waterways, which allow for healthy ingress and egress of goods and commodities. Burton argues that if the English similarly transformed their marshes and fens, they would procure more favorable balances of trade and advance their position among competing mercantile nations.[67] In this way, Burton folds the logic and language of humoral and spiritual exoneration into an argument for the greater circulation of wealth and political power. This is an idea that finds parallels if not in Harvey's own explanation of the circulation of the blood (*De Motu Cordis*, 1628) then in the interpretation of this discovery and fear of its political ramifications as elaborated by Harvey's detractors.[68]

Burton condemns primogeniture as a systematic obstruction of English health as well as wealth, as it concentrates riches in the same deleterious way that it

---

[66]   Mary Ann Lund similarly observes that when "fifty wise precepts are quoted together" in the *Anatomy*, "they appear to be comically meaningless. By contrast, when simple instructions are interspersed with complex pieces of advice ... their effectiveness as serious advice can instead be heightened" (*Melancholy, Medicine and Religion in Early Modern England*, 193).

[67]   As William Mueller noted, Burton's economic critique of English dependence upon precious metals reflects the unprecedented devaluation of gold and silver during the sixteenth and seventeenth centuries (*The Anatomy of Robert Burton's England* [Berkeley: University of California Press, 1952], 41). The inflation of rents and commodities that ensued dwarfed raises in wages, and land values were further inflated by scarcity brought on by enclosure, a system Burton describes in the same terms as Thomas More as one wherein "Sheepe demolish Townes, devoure men" (1:55).

[68]   William Harvey's controversial "discovery" of the circulation of the blood was rejected by many for its deemed threat to the political and social hierarchy, despite Harvey's own affinity to the king. See Christopher Hill, *Intellectual Origins of the English Revolution: Revisited* (Oxford: Oxford University Press, 1997), 344–5.

corrupts and degrades English bloodlines.[69] He reminds us several times that he is writing his book as a "second son," restricted in his choice of occupation and prevented from marrying by birth order. Primogeniture is therefore presented not only as a cause of his scholarly melancholy, having compelled him to a scholarly life, but also a cause of his sensitivity to the plight of the oppressed. He cites the accident of his birth order as the reason for his particular sympathy toward those who are melancholy for want of love, means, and liberty.[70] His identification with the landless and dispossessed therefore makes his colonial "solution" to the problem of English overpopulation all the more suspicious. He proposes that "if people overabound" in his "little utopia," they "shall be eased by Colonies" (1:95). The simplicity of this solution echoes the arguments of many of Burton's contemporaries, not least of them William Vaughan, whose allegorical poem *The Golden Fleece* argues that "all of the spiritual and material defects of the English commonwealth may be remedied by the planting and fishing of Newfoundland."[71] In the same spirit, the colonial propagandist Robert Johnson compared England to an overgrown garden in need of weeding. Several decades earlier, Richard Hakluyt had famously suggested that England sweep the prisons for able-bodied recruits to populate the colonies.[72]

We cannot say with certainty whether Burton's indictment of English inheritance law carries over to this handy solution for England's population crisis. His tone in the Preface and its utopia is prone to sudden shifts that destabilize our sense of its earnestness and prescriptive force. However, it is difficult not to take Burton's colonial solution as at least partly parodic of the alternately naïve and apocalyptic devices that early modern utopias such as More's, Campanella's, Bacon's, and Hall's routinely use to establish the convenient fictions for

---

[69] See his account of the improved health of the English as its blood was transfused with each successive historical invasion. This commonplace representation of English history appears in a variety of contemporary writings, including Lucy Hutchinson's autobiographical memoir of her husband's life. See Lucy Apsley Hutchinson, *Memoirs of the Life of Colonel Hutchinson, Governor of Nottingham Castle and Town* (London: G. Bell & Sons, 1908), 4–5.

[70] Unmarried men were imagined to suffer complications from the retention of seed just as women were thought to suffer green-sickness for the same reason, although with very different symptomatic expressions. On the poisonous retention of semen, see Pseudo-Albertus Magnus, *Women's Secrets: A Translation of Pseudo-Albertus Magnus's De Secretis Mulierum*, trans. Helen Rodnite Lemay (Albany: State University of New York Press, 1992), 48; Ferrand, *A Treatise on Lovesickness*, 61.

[71] Sandra Djwa, "Early Explorations: New Founde Landys (1496–1729)," *Studies in Canadian Literature/Études En Littérature Canadienne* 4, no. 2 (1979), http://journals.hil. unb.ca/index.php/SCL/article/view/7918.

[72] Robert Johnson, *Noua Britannia Offring Most Excellent Fruites by Planting in Virginia*, 1609; Hakluyt, "Preface to *Divers Voyages*," reprinted in Richard Hakluyt, *The Original Writings & Correspondence of the Two Richard Hakluyts* (London: Hakluyt Society, 1935).

their possibility. The evidence for this satirical reading inheres in the hydraulic reasoning he deploys to substantiate this solution, which directly follows the elaboration of marriage laws in his "poeticall commonwealth." Poverty, he says, "shall hinder no man from marriage" (1:94–5). There will be no dowry for the rich, great dowries for the foul, none or very little for the fair (1:94). The colonies provide a quick and tidy answer to the likely outcome of so much wedding and bedding, and so his solution mimics the humoral analogy in Robert Gray's analogy for the colonial solution to overpopulation as a purgative "exoneration" of the blood for the avoidance of corruption: "euen as bloud though it be the best humour in the body, yet if it abound in greater quantitie then the state of the body will beare, doth indanger the bodie, & oftentimes destroyes it."[73]

Freedom in Burton's utopia cannily hinges on the possibility of unlimited space *elsewhere*, as space in Burton's utopia is completely utilized: "no bogs, fens, marshes, vast woods, deserts, heaths, commons, but all inclosed, for that which is common, and every man's is no man's." No waste and no wasted space. This perfect utility is balanced, as in More's *Utopia*, with prescribed time for leisure. In Burton's imagined commonwealth, people will be permitted "once a weeke to sing or dance, (though not all at once) or doe whatsoever he shall please" (1:93–4). The parenthetically anti-Puritan jeer further hints that Burton's utopia has slid into parody, but if that were not enough of a clue to the satirical play at hand, he interrupts his utopian reverie just as he arrives at the topic of war and taxes: "*Manum de tabella*, I have beene over tedious in this subject, I could have here willingly ranged, but these straits wherein I am included, will not permit" (1:97). His alibi for abandoning the utopian project in *medias res* is, notably, a lack of space. The "straits" or conventions of the utopian form, and of the realpolitik eventually demanded by the imagining of an ideal society are, he laments, too narrow for his purposes. In this playfully acerbic way, Burton postpones his more explicit political and economic critique for his discussions of melancholy caused by poverty and loss of liberty and of the misery of scholars later in the first and second partitions. But the hydraulic analogy and its ethical resonance resurfaces in the critique that underlies Burton's discussions of jealousy in the third partition. Here he takes up the theme of failed economic circulation more subtly but arguably much more profoundly in the distinctions he draws between love as a hydraulic force characterized by generosity and jealousy as its pathological obstruction.

Exonerating Jealousy

Among the various affective disorders listed in Burton's extensive discussion of love melancholy, the most common are those that result from obstructed desire. After giving dozens of ribald, even scatological, suggestions for turning lovers "off" of their beloved, Burton famously advises that the last (and best) cure is to let lovers have their way (3:242). There is, however, no such simple solution for unrequited love. Burton reproduces long tracts of classical arguments used

---

[73]   Robert Gray, *A Good Speed to Virginia* (London, 1609), B3v.

to dissuade lovers from pursuing the uninterested or unavailable. He cites well-known antifeminist disparagements of marriage and female beauty that advise the lover to consider every one of his beloved's flaws: to doubt, fear, and distrust her. The "friend" of the afflicted is advised to "Tell him but how he was scoffed at behinde his back ... that his love is false, and entertaines another, rejectes him, cares not for him, or that she is a foole." If this fails, the beloved should be called "a nasty queane, a slut, a fixen [sic], a scold, a divell" (2:14). As the hyperbole of Burton's asyndeton becomes more lurid, the desire that motivates this aversion therapy becomes more desperate. The friend's effort to induce revulsion becomes as absurd as the antifeminist arguments to which these cures are imputed:

> Tell him ... that hee or shee hath some loathsome filthy disease, gout, stone, strangury, falling sicknesse, and that they are hereditary, not to bee avoided, he is subject to a consumption, hath the Poxe, that hee hath three or foure incurable tetters, issues: that she is bald, her breath stinkes, she is mad by inheritance, and so are all the kindred, a hair-braine, with many other secret infirmities, which I will not so much as name, belonging to women. That he is a Hermaphrodite, an Eunuch, imperfect, impotent, a spendthrift, a gamester, a foole, a gull, a beggar, a whoremaster, farre in debt, and not able to maintaine her, a common drunkard, his mother was a witch, his father hanged, that he hath a wolfe in his bosome, a sore leg, he is a leper, hath some incurable disease, that he will surely beat her, he cannot hold his water, that he cries out or walkes in the night, will stab his bedfellow, tell all his secrets in his sleepe, and that nobody dare lye with him, his house is haunted with spirits, with such fearfull and tragicall things, able to avert and terrifie any man or woman living. (3:214)

Note how the pronoun conspicuously switches from feminine to masculine throughout the passage, suggesting that the gender of the beloved (and, indeed, of the lover) is beside the point. The implied irrelevance of gender underscores the point that desire makes its object (and its diversion) inconsequential and that cures by dissuasion are doomed to fail.

The most infamous part of this subsection is borrowed from the French medieval physician Bernardus Gordonius and is reproduced in the *Anatomy* in the original Latin (as is the case with the majority of Burton's more salacious quotations). As the passage has been widely cited in English as evidence of Burton's supposed antifeminism, I too will give the English version, which has become somewhat overly familiar not only in Burton criticism but in the more general scholarship on early modern melancholy, gender, and desire:[74]

> Let some old woman of the vilest appearance, in dirty and disgusting clothes, be prepared: and let her carry a sanitary towel under her apron, and let her say

---

[74]   See, for instance, Lesel Dawson, *Lovesickness and Gender in Early Modern English Literature* (Oxford: Oxford University Press, 2008), 197; Carol Thomas Neely, *Distracted Subjects: Madness and Gender in Shakespeare and Early Modern Culture* (Ithaca, NY: Cornell University Press, 2004), 102–3; Mark Breitenberg, *Anxious Masculinity in Early Modern England* (Cambridge: Cambridge University Press, 1996), 48.

that her friend is drunken, and that she pisses her bed, and that she is epileptic and unchaste and that on her body there are enormous growths, that her breath stinks, and other monstrous things, in which old women are knowledgeable: if he will not be persuaded by these arguments, let her suddenly produce the sanitary towel, and brandish it before his face, crying "This is what your loved one is like!," and if he doesn't give up at this, he is not a man but a devil incarnate.[75]

If Gordonius's suggestion fails, Chrysostom offers yet another rhetorical cure that Burton supplies, this time in English:

> Take her skinne from her face, and thou shalt see all loathsomenesse under it, that beauty is a superficiall skinne and bones, nerves, sinewes: suppose her sicke ... hoarie-headed, hollow cheeked, old; within she is full of filthy fleame, stinking, putride, excrementall stuffe: snot and snevill in her nostrils, spittle in her mouth, water in her eyes, what filth in her braines, &c. (3:226)

Burton adds his own *occupatio* to the recommended scripts above: "I will say nothing of the vices of their mindes, their pride, envy, inconstancy, weaknesse, malice, selfewill, lightnesse, insatiable lust, jealousie" (3:228). He then slips into a highly conventional and patently comic routine on marriage, making sport of its clichéd antifeminisms. He underscores the conventionality of the routine, insinuating that it is older than time by beginning with the ancient Sirach and Solomon: "*Ecclus. 25.14. No malice to a womans: no bitterness like to hers, Eccles. 7. 28. And as the same author urgeth Prov 31.10. Who shall finde a virtuous woman?*" Terence gets a word in on female incorrigibility: "*They know neither equities, good nor bad, bee it better or worse* (as the Comicall poet hath it) *beneficiall or hurtfull, they will doe what they list*" (3:228).[76] We hear Hesiod call women a scourge and punishment, Diogenes dismiss the entire female sex, and Chaucer recycle the misogyny of the *Romaunt of the Rose*:

> Every each of them hath some vice
> If one be of Villany,
> Another hath a liquorish eye,
> If one be full of wantonnesse,
> Another is a Chideresse. (3:228–9)

---

[75]   The Latin quotation, taken from Bernard de Gordon (Gordonius), *Opus lilium medicinae inscriptum, de morborum prope omnium curatione* (Lyons, 1574), is as follows: "*& portet subtus gremium pannum menstrualem, & dicat quod amica sua sit ebriosa, & quòd mingat in lecto, & quòd est epileptica & impudica;& quòd in corpore suo sunt excrescentiae enormes, cum faetore anhelitus, & aliae enormitates, quibus vetulae sunt edoctae: si nolit his persuaderi, subitò extrahat pannum menstrualem, coram facie portando, exclamando, talis est amica tua; & si ex his non demiserit, non est homo, sed diabolus incarnatus*" (3:214–15). The English translation cited above is from the commentary to the Clarendon *Anatomy* (6:139). Unless otherwise specified, translations below are taken from this commentary and will be referred to by volume and page number.

[76]   From *Heauton Timorumenos*, or *Self Tormentor*.

Burton puts this rhetoric of blame into comic relief with exaggerated misogynistic zeal, claiming that Hero's lantern remained tragically unlit because no man could be found who had good success in love, which he speciously declares "can refer to nought, but the inconstancy and lightnesse of women."

Burton concludes his routine with Ariosto, who tells us that *"in a thousand, good there is not one, / All be so proud, unthankfull and unkinde"* but suggestively adds: *"But more herein to speake I am forbidden, / Sometime for speaking truth one may be chidden."* The echo of Chaucer's "chideresse" in Ariosto's self-censoring fear of being "chidden" recalls countless instances in the *Anatomy* where Burton strikes a similar defensively mute pose. Moreover, the gendered association with chiding points to the self-consciously ambivalent sense of his own gendering as a critic. What distinguishes the barking satirist from the "chideresse" or, for that matter, the Democritean remonstration from the nagging of a hag?[77] Burton alerts us to the ironic resemblance between the two, turning suddenly to say he is "not willing ... to prosecute the cause" against women:

> therefore take heed you mistake me not, *matronam nullam ego tango*, I honour the sex, with all good men ... and such women haters bare the blame, if ought bee said amisse, I have not writ a tenth of that which might bee urged out of them and others ... And that which I have said (to speake truth) no more concerned them then men, though women be more frequently named in this tract (to Apologise once for all) I am neither partiall against them, or therefore bitter: what is said of the one, *mutato nomine*, may most part be understood of the other. (3:229)

Not quite the proto-feminism of the humanist apologias,[78] Burton's professed equanimity reveals his ventriloquized misogyny to be a variety of and indeed a mask for the more general misanthropy subtending the antimatrimonial tradition: "If women in general be so bad (and men worse then they) what a hazard is it to marry, where shall a man finde a good wife, or a woman a good husband?" (3:229–30). Burton cites Scaliger and Lipsius, Plautus and Seneca, whose good authority he begs us accept: "I pray you learne of them that have experience, for I have none, παῖδας ἐγὼ λόγους ἐγενησάμην, libri mentis liberi" (3:230). The Greek verse, which Burton Latinizes for the reader, is Synesius' and its meaning is "I have begotten books as my children; books are the children of the mind."[79]

---

[77] See Chapter 1.

[78] For example, those written by Equicola and Capra. See "Agrippa and the Feminist Tradition," in Henricus Cornelius Agrippa, *Declamation on the Nobility and Preeminence of the Female Sex*, ed. and trans. Albert Rabil Jr. (Chicago: University of Chicago Press, 1996). On this tradition see Constance Jordan, "Feminism and the Humanists: The Case for Sir Thomas Elyot's Defense of Good Women," in *Rewriting the Renaissance: The Discourses of Sexual Difference in Early Modern Europe*, ed. Margaret W. Ferguson and Maureen Quilligan (Chicago: University of Chicago Press, 1986); Sarah Apetrei, *Women, Feminism and Religion in Early Enlightenment England* (Cambridge: Cambridge University Press, 2010), chap. 1.

[79] 6:148.

The substitution of literary production for genetic offspring, while comedic, has teeth: both in Burton's repeated lament at not having had a family of his own and in its intimation of the erotic and procreative qualities of humanist writing and citing, to which we will soon return.

Burton gives the conspicuous lie to his elective bachelorhood when he says that he will "dissemble" with Lipsius:

> *Este procul nymphae, fallax genus este puellae,*
> *Vita jugata meo non facit ingenio:*
> *Me juvat, &c.* (3:230)[80]

The original quote, as it appears in Lipsius's *Lectiones Antiquae*, in fact shoos away the young nymphs out of conjugal commitment. Lipsius's speaker rejects the *single*, not marital life.[81] However, Burton has substituted "*vita jugata*" (the married life) for "*via soluta*" (the solitary way), perhaps accidentally, perhaps by design, perhaps even to declare other and unnamed desires and preferences. In any case, the miscited lines underscore the speciousness of authority on the subject of marriage claimed on the basis not of experience but *inexperience*. This rhetorical gesture ("I wouldn't know but hear it's awful") undermines the misogyny of the subsection with something like Antonio's bachelor machismo in Webster's *Duchess of Malfi*:

> Say a man never marry, nor have children,
> What takes that from him? Only the bare name
> Of being a father, or the weak delight
> To see the little wanton ride a-cock horse
> Upon a painted stick, or hear him chatter
> Like a taught starling. (1.1.389–394)[82]

We might read Burton's protested disinterest in marriage similarly as a kind of conspicuously false stoicism, especially as in the succeeding pages the misogynist arguments become more plainly visible as misanthropy, indicting the derider rather than the object of derision and insinuating that the misanthropy of the *auctoritas* points to a more hateful melancholy than the kind suffered by those sick with love.

Burton follows his long section on cures "*By Counsell and Perswasion, Fouleness of the Fact, Mens, Women Faults, Miseries of Marriage, Events of Lust, &c*" with a short discussion of potions and other "*Philters, Magicall and Poeticall Cures.*" These "unlawefull means" (to which those unremedied by

---

[80]   "Stay away from me, ye nymphs, deceitful tribe! Stay away, ye girls! Married life is not for me: I like, &c." (6:148–9).

[81]   Justus Lipsius, *Antiquarum lectionum commentarius* (Antwerp, 1575), 126.

[82]   John Webster, *The Duchess of Malfi and Other Plays*, ed. René Weis (Oxford: Oxford University Press, 2009), 1.1.384–6. The Duchess observes Antonio's suddenly red eyes as he speaks these lines and offers him her wedding ring as a "cure."

"perswasions" are desperately driven) include the highly symbolic "pissing through a ring" and other "absurd remedies" such as ingesting the beloved's blood or placing the beloved's excrement under the lover's pillow. Burton's tone in this brief section barely pretends at solemnity. He notes, for instance, that the most famous "remedy" for lovesickness is suicide, naming one particularly well-known jumping-spot, "*Leucata Petra*, that renowned rocke in *Greece*, of which *Strabo* writes ... . From which rocke if any Lover flung himself downe headlong, he was instantly cured." Burton wryly jokes in the margin that the moral of the story is that "vehement Feare expels Love." The joke, of course, reverses the *Anatomy*'s insistent counsel throughout and especially in the third partition that love expels fear.

Several further examples of magical cures for love melancholy follow from myth and poetry, underscoring their improbability and, indeed, the impossibility of dispelling desire by revulsion or repression. Noting such, Burton declares that "where none of all these remedies will take place ... all Lovers must make an head, and rebell ... and crucifie *Cupid* till hee grant their request, or satisfie their desires." All the arguments against love, women, and marriage in the preceding 23 pages are finally rendered as absurd as erotic desire itself. They are offered in unabashed excess of their supposed function of dissuasion, suggesting nothing if not the insufficiency of convention, artifice, or language itself to stave it off. The comic routine stages nothing, in other words, if not the argument that desire will "have its way." And so, as Burton advises in the title of the following subsection, "*The last and best Cure of Love Melancholy, is, to let them have their Desire*" (3:242). Burton proposes venery as a cure for venery, or to put it in hydraulic and hygienic terms, he proposes venereal release as a cure for the insufficient release of venereal desire and its excess stores of humor and bodily spirits. He cites examples of maids cured of madness by marriage and virgins cured of amenorrhea after rowdy sexual escapades. "*Many mad-men, melancholy, and labouring of the falling sicknesse, have been cured by this alone*," he says, citing Montaltus, who "will have it drive away sorrow, and all illusions of the braine, to purge the heart and braine from ill smoakes and vapours that offend them" (2:30). Burton momentarily equivocates on this advice, giving Aristotle's evidence, witnessed in sparrows, who are "short lived because of their salacity," in order to suggest that "extremes being both bad, the medium is to be kept" with regard to venery (2:32). But lest we take his bid for temperance too stringently, Burton follows up with a line borrowed from Kaspar Barth's quick-tongued prostitute, Celestina: "*occidi vero paucas per ventrem vidisti*"[83] (leaving out Sempronio's reply: "Occidi nullas, confodi multas").[84] It is with this witty quip that Burton concludes his discussion of love melancholy and proceeds from the theme of cure by venereal release directly to the hydraulic meditations of the "Digression of Ayre."

---

[83] "You have seen few killed through the belly" (5:107).

[84] "None killed, many ruined" (ibid.). Kaspar Barth, *Pornoboscodidascalus Latinus* (Frankfurt, 1624), 24.

'Tis All One: Windy Substitutions

Scott Blanchard insists that Burton's "venereal cure" is offered merely to debunk the authority of humanist and classical learning.[85] According to Blanchard, the scatological focus of Burton's cited authorities is reproduced in the *Anatomy* in order to indicate the degree to which these authors are implicated by their own critiques, taking voyeuristic pleasure in the abjectness of their studied objects.[86] We may detect a curious pattern in modern Burton criticism here, whereby Burton's citations are taken earnestly when they condemn pleasure but skeptically when they marshal arguments in its favor. Blanchard argues that Burton hopes to convert his readers by holding up a mirror to their sins. At the same time, he recognizes Burton's habit of turning "deadpan discussions" into "copious piece[s] of nonsense punctuated by accumulating formulae" as a strategy for incriminating the "hopelessly bankrupt epistemology" of humanism and the meaninglessness of a world in which melancholy is everything.[87]

Burton's explorations of the universality of melancholy register as a kind of tautology in this way for Blanchard and other late twentieth-century readers of the *Anatomy* who interpret Burton's perennial tag, "'tis all one," as a statement of universal nihilism.[88] I propose a different reading of this oft-repeated phrase—one that foregrounds the association Burton makes between a melancholic inclination toward analogy, literary copia, and abundance. "'Tis all one" does not imply that all is nought, or "waste" as Grant Williams, for instance, has suggested.[89] It is a propaedeutic dictum tending toward euphoria, not despair. Instead of a melancholic "waste of the same," Burton offers a plenum of infinite variation. His asyndetic, amplificatory sentences delight in variety (even while they spiral to infinity) much as Erasmus delights in the myriad ways one may choose to write, "your letter gives me pleasure."[90] However, whereas the animating principle of Erasmian copia is the generation of a variety of substitutable forms, Burton's copia is somewhat cannier. He buries the heterotopic under the illusion of homogeneity. The reader's task is to discern better from worse arguments among the endless array of cited opinions.

---

[85]   He interprets Burton's "praise of nymphomania," as he does Burton's praise of poverty, as a mock-encomiastic instance of Menippean satire. W. Scott Blanchard, *Scholars' Bedlam: Menippean Satire in the Renaissance* (Lewisburg, PA: Bucknell University Press, 1995), 139.

[86]   Ibid., 152.

[87]   Ibid., 149.

[88]   Ibid., 135–6.

[89]   Robert Grant Williams, "Heterological Rhetoric: Textual Waste in *The Anatomy of Melancholy*" (London, ON: University of Western Ontario, 1995).

[90]   Desiderius Erasmus, "Foundations of the Abundant Style (*De duplici copia verborum ac rerum commentarii duo*)," in *Collected Works of Erasmus*, ed. and trans. Betty Knott, vol. 24 (Toronto, ON: University of Toronto Press, 1978), 348–54.

The "'tis all one" refrain in the *Anatomy* sends up the Christian critique of "vanity" by calling attention to the theatricality of the dismissive wave of the hand over a protested morass of the "same." Burton alerts us to this ironic gesture early in the Preface with his conspicuously elided citation of Ecclesiastes:

> That men are so mis-affected, melancholy, mad giddy-headed, heare the testimony of *Solomon, Eccl.2.12. And I turned to behold wisdome, madnesse and folly, &c.* And *Ver.23. All his daies are sorrow, his travell griefe, and his heart taketh no rest in the night.* So that take Melancholy in what sense you will, properly or improperly, in disposition or habit, for pleasure or for paine, dotage, discontent, feare, sorrow, madnesse, for part, or all, truly, or metaphorically, 'tis all one. (1:25)

Conspicuous in its absence is the twenty-fourth verse of Ecclesiastes 1, in which the speaker turns abruptly from his critique of *vanitas* to declare that "there is nothing better for a man, than that he should eat and drink, and that he should make his soul enjoy good in his labor." This resonant affirmation of the ethical value of pleasure underwrites Burton's therapeutic approach throughout the *Anatomy*. Its elision here is therefore all the more striking and seems to parody the Christian Neostoic cultivation of imperturbability in the face of the unpredictable. The indiscriminate swerve of the atom that renders us vulnerable to the vicissitude of things in Lucretian Epicureanism is, by contrast, what makes us free. This seemingly paradoxical freedom *in* vulnerability is the heart of Democritus Junior's melancholic laughter and the very soul of his wit and wisdom. Burton's "'tis all one" pantomimes the Stoic dismissal of the uniqueness of individual suffering even while it lists and lists, serving up variety under the disguise of sameness. Read this way, the so-called excessiveness of Burton's copious style, sometimes referred to as "mannerist" or "baroque," becomes more clearly a sign of affirmation and generation than of cynicism and decay.[91] To use the vocabulary of Ecclesiastes, it is in recognition of the vanity of life that life comes to signify *despite* death and that Burtonian copia spites its own vanity.[92]

Burton's Epicureanism makes a wonderfully clever "windy" substitution of folly as pneumatic medicine for the maligned Ecclesiastical "striving after wind." Foolish speech is in one sense "insubstantial" speech, or it aims to pass, however facetiously, as such. The English noun "folly" corresponds to the Latin *follies*, which means bellows, but was used in late popular Latin to suggest a

---

[91]   On the generative mode of the baroque, see Terence Cave, *The Cornucopian Text: Problems of Writing in the French Renaissance* (Oxford: Clarendon Press, 1979); José Antonio Maravall, *Culture of the Baroque: Analysis of a Historical Structure* (Manchester: Manchester University Press, 1986); Giancarlo Maiorino, *The Cornucopian Mind and the Baroque Unity of the Arts* (University Park: Pennsylvania State University Press, 1990).

[92]   As we saw in Chapter 1, Burton further rectifies the Stoic interpretation of Epicurean mutability by emphasizing the vanity and illusoriness of proprietary notions of authorship and selfhood, especially as endorsed by Christian Neostoics and spiritual physicians who drew on these principles in their prescriptions for moral hygiene.

"windbag, empty-headed person, fool."[93] In this way, "windiness" conveys the substancelessness of foolish speech, but considered in the ways we are invited to by Burton in his meditations on air and hypochondria, windiness also conveys cosmic and pneumatic spirit. The game of foolery in the *Anatomy* resides in the play between the apparent insubstantiality of foolish airs and the early modern understanding of air itself as full of matter. Like Erasmus's Dame Folly, Democritus Junior's playing medium is the air and wind of learned discourse. As we saw in Chapter 1, Burton plays the fool or ingénue by claiming he is merely citing authorities who are in fact parodied by their hyperbolic parroting. We might say that Burton hyperventilates his authorities through his own windiness. What I have tried to show in the discussion above is how his hyperventilation or "airing out" of the authorities draws on a logic of salubrious ventilation that underwrites his ethical and physiological prescriptions. This reasoning is more recognizable still in the critiques of jealousy that symbolically bridge the discussions of love and religious melancholy.

Cognate to Burton's "'tis all one" refrain is another of his catchphrases, which is also the epigraph to his first edition of the *Anatomy*: "*omne meum, nihil meum*" (it is all mine and nothing mine). With this rejoinder, Burton both proclaims and disclaims responsibility for the potential offense of his parodic citing throughout the *Anatomy*. "'Tis all one" functions similarly to reinforce the comic *mise-en-abyme* whereby Burton signals his distance from his cited authorities. We see an illuminating instance of this in his apology for unwittingly offending the female sex by his recited obloquies on the subject of marriage. Burton ironically compares his depiction of the sexes to "Passus'" picture in Lucian's *Encomium Demosthenis*. He explains that "Passus," or Pauson as he is generally referred to in classical literature, was commissioned to depict a horse with "heeles upward, tumbling on his backe." The painter, however, depicted him "passant," he says, using the heraldic term for an animal standing with three feet on the ground and forefoot lifted in a trot.[94] Burton tells us that when the buyer came to retrieve the painting, he "was very angry, and said, it was quite opposite to his minde; but *Passus* instantly turned the Picture upside downe, shewed him the horse at that site which he requested, and so gave him satisfaction" (3:229). The rhyming assimilation of "Pauson" to "Passus," who depicted the horse "passant" draws attention to Burton's conspicuously alliterated misnomer. Pauson was immortalized by Aristotle as the painter who represented his subjects in the worst possible light. Aristotle tells us in the *Poetics* that men may be depicted as better, worse, or just as they are in life and names examples of artists who exemplified each approach: "Polygnotus

---

[93]   Wind and foolery are connected linguistically in the origins of the word "buffoon," which derives from Italian, *buffare*, to "puff" as in to puff out the cheeks in comic gesture (*Oxford English Dictionary Online*, s.v. "buffoon, n.," accessed September 7, 2014, http://www.oed.com.libezproxy2.syr.edu/view/Entry/24337).

[94]   *Oxford English Dictionary Online*, s.v. "passant, adj. 3," accessed February 21, 2013, http://www.oed.com.libezproxy2.syr.edu/view/Entry/138448?redirectedFrom= passant#eid.

depicted men as nobler than they are, Pauson as less noble, Dionysius drew them true to life."[95] Comparing himself to the painter remembered for his skepticism and translating the name of the painter from "Pauson" to "Passus," Burton styles himself as the artist who suffers (*passus*) for his satire, showing things not only as they are, or *passant* (the more common early modern use of the term being similar to the French) but as we need to see them if we are to be reformed.[96] Burton glosses the "Passus" anecdote as follows: "If any man take exception at my words, let him alter the name, reade him for her, and 'tis all one in effect" (3:229). If we don't like what we read, in other words, we may simply turn the picture—or book—upside down, just as Burton does shortly thereafter.

Near the end of his lengthy discussion of jealously, Burton turns the misogynistic catalogue of melancholic complaints against the incontinence of female sexuality on its head. Continence, or rather the lover's fixation upon his beloved's sexual incontinence, is made out to be the hollow conceit of the jealous lover's melancholic imagination. Burton tells the husband who is convinced his wife has made him a cuckold that he had better hope the child he suspects to be another's is indeed not his own. Better a bastard than the product of so miserable a man: "Even this which thou so much abhorrest, it may be for thy progenies good, better be any mans son then thine ... for thou thy selfe hast peradventure more diseases than an horse, more infirmities of body and minde, a cankered soule, crabbed conditions ..." (3:310). Burton's remonstrance makes a joke of the jealous husband and a hero of the credulous cuckold. He delights in examples of husbandly generosity trumping "solicitousness" and champions "willing credulity" over niggardly suspicion. He recounts the following anecdote to illustrate: "*A good fellow, when his wife was brought to bed before her time, bought halfe a dozen of Cradles before hand for so many children, as if his wife should continue to beare children at every two months*" (3:314). In Burton's deft retelling, the story of a man who happily invests in the fecundity of a wife who promises to gestate "every two months" becomes a generous and salubrious alternative to the asphyxiate economy of marital jealousy upon which the cuckold joke is based.

Burton accounts for jealousy in physiological terms as a constriction of the heart and diminishment of the vital spirit that makes one quite literally pusillanimous or small-spirited. It has an insidious power of corruption about it: the dark, unsympathetic power of the melancholic imagination that is the inverse of the hypochondriac's magnanimous sensitivity. Burton calls jealousy a "bastard-branch" of melancholy, remarking that none are so badly affected by this disease as jealous husbands. Such men drive their wives to infidelity by depriving them of their due good faith: "He was jealous, and she made him a cuckold for keeping her up: suspition without a cause, hard usage, is able of it selfe to make a woman

---

[95]   Aristotle, *The Poetics of Aristotle*, ed. and trans. S.H. Butcher (London: Macmillan, 1902), II, 1448a.

[96]   *Oxford English Dictionary Online*, s.v. "passant, adj. 1," accessed February 21, 2013, http://www.oed.com.libezproxy2.syr.edu/view/Entry/138448?redirectedFrom= passant#eid.

fly out, that was otherwise honest" (3:284). A man, says Burton, is duty bound to trust his wife. He goes so far as to equate a deficit of trust with a lack of sexual ability or failure of sexual obligation, remarking that a husband who neglects this duty is "negligent in his businesse, *quando lecto danda opera*" (3:287).[97] Having neglected this conjugal responsibility, and thereby being "slack" in his bed-labors, the jealous husband courts his own cuckolding. He has, as Burton point out, already betrayed her by cheating her of her due credit. Therefore, he asks: "Who will pitty them … or bee much offended with such wives … if they deceave those that cosened them first?" (3:287)

At the end of this subsection, Burton teases the reader with the promise of a remedy for jealousy that he says he cannot divulge—not because he himself is "jealous" of it, he assures, but for other suggestively nameless reasons: "One other soveraigne remedy I could repeat, an especiall Antidote against Jealousie, an excellent cure, but I am not now disposed to tell it, not that like a covetous Empiricke, I conceale it for any gaine, but some other reasons, I am not willing to publish it; if you be very desirous to know it, when I meet you next, I will peradventure tell you what it is in your eare" (3:329). With nearly 22,000 words spent on the causes, kinds, and cures for jealousy, Burton's withholding of a final cure for melancholy is exquisitely ironic. His analogy pokes fun at the jealous "Empiricke" whose covetous watch over his experiments resembles the cuckold's paranoia over his wife's honor.[98] But the last joke is on the reader who has read thus far in hopes of coming away with an easy cure. Burton plays a continuous game of disclosure and occlusion with the reader, emblazoning learned opinion in a vast, encyclopedic array that obfuscates the writer's own position—a position withheld, he playfully suggests, because it can only be transpired, mouth to ear, when next the reader and writer meet.

Coda: The Cure Transpired

We have throughout this study considered the rhetorical dimensions of Burton's cure and attended, in this chapter, to the aesthetic, philosophical, economic, and ethical registers of Burton's pneumatic and hydraulic themes and imagery. I will end by considering the way in which Burton represents his own reading and writing as a pneumatic encounter between distant minds and bodies. Burton's joke about the unrepeatable cure for jealousy suggestively postpones the delivery of this secret remedy to an *in vivo* encounter between author and reader rendered as a pneumatic rather than corporeal exchange.[99] The author promises a whispered intimacy rather

---

[97]   "When there was business to be done in bed" (6:181). Burton is quoting from a letter describing a lawsuit brought against one lawyer by his neglected wife in Aristaenetus, *Epistolae Amatoria*, trans. Josias Mercer (Paris, 1595), bk. 2, letter 3.

[98]   Middleton and Rowley make a similar association in *The Changeling*, wherein the jealous husband keeps a closet full of potions used for the discernment of female chastity.

[99]   Cicero offers an analogous image of the breath as the transmission of the author's spirit in *Tusculan Disputations* 1.xv.34, when he quotes Ennius' epitaph: "Let no one

than a press, so to speak, of the flesh. However, the joke is not on the reader who mistakes the airy substitute for the thing itself but the reader who misses the point that the book is itself a living whisper; its exchanges with living and dead authors, readers past and present, are real, substantial, and intimate and—as shall be made clearer by the following illustration—even erotic encounters in their own right.

In the subsection titled "Love's Power and Extent," Burton renders testimony as a kind of literary kissing to which he compares the reputed phenomenon of "Love amongst the Vegetalls," a much beloved theme in classical and neoteric natural history.[100] He remarks that there are "many pregnant proofes and familiar examples ... especially of palme trees, which are both he and she, & expresse not a sympathy but a love passion" (3:42). Burton cites Claudian's description of the temple of Venus:

> *Vivunt in venerem frondes, omnisque vicissim*
> *Foelix arbor amat, nutant ad mutua palmae*
> *Foedere, populeo suspirat populus ictu,*
> *Et platano platanus, alnoque assibilat alnus.* (3:42)[101]

Burton continues with the report, attributed to Florentius by the seventh-century compilers of the agricultural history, the *Geōponika*, "of a Palme tree that lov'd most fervently, *and would not be comforted untill such time her love applied himselfe unto her, you might see the two trees bend, and of their owne accords stretch out their boughes to embrace and kisse each other*" (3:42).[102] Citing the Roman historian Ammianus Marcellinus, he further reports that palme trees "marry one another, and fall in love if they grow in sight, and when the wind brings the smell to them, they are marvelously affected" (3:42).[103] Burton notes that Philostratus observes as much, as does Galen, whom he quotes, quoting Constantine saying

---

honour me with tears or on my ashes weep. / For why? From lips to lips of men I pass and living keep" (*Tusculan Disputations*, trans. J.E. King, vol. 8, Loeb Classical Library 141 [London: Heinemann, 1927], 41).

[100]   See Lynn Thorndike, *A History of Magic and Experimental Science*, vol. 1 (New York: Macmillan, 1923), 85.

[101]   Claudius Claudianus, *Epithalamium de nuptiis Honorii Augusti*, 65–8. "The very leaves live for love and in his season every happy tree experiences love's power: palm bends down to mate with palm, poplar sighs its passion for poplar, plane whispers to plane, alder to alder" (*Claudian*, ed. and trans. Maurice Platnauer, vol.1 [New York: Heinemann, 1922], 247).

[102]   Cassianus Bassus, *Geōponika: Agricultural Pursuits*, trans. T. Owen, vol. 2 (London, 1805), 7. For a suggestive association between this logic of sympathy, antipathy, and Epicurean mutability, see Book XV in which Bassus connects the doctrine of the similitudes to a discussion of spontaneous generation.

[103]   Ammianus interrupts his account of the Emperor Julian's war with the Persians to describe the landscape and lovingly digresses on the topic of love amongst palm trees; *Rerum Gestarum*, 24.3. See Ammianus Marcellinus, *Ammianus Marcellinus*, trans. John Rolfe, vol. 2, Loeb (Cambridge: Heinemann, 1935), 429.

that trees "will be sicke for love, ready to dye and pine away, which the husband men perceiving ... *stroke many Palmes that grow together, and so stroking again the Palme that is enamored they carry kisses from the one to the other*" (3:42–3).

Burton's juxtaposition of "pine" and "Palme" evokes the metamorphosis of Attis in Ovid's catalogue of the trees that uproot themselves and gather to shelter Orpheus when he sings of his beloved Eurydice's death.[104] Last in this list is the pine tree that was once the shepherd Attis. In the *Fasti*, Ovid explains that Attis pledged his chastity to the goddess Cybele, but broke his vow and in his anguish at having done so castrated himself.[105] In the *Metamorphoses*, Ovid ambiguously suggests that Attis is transformed into the hard and bristly pine tree, possibly as punishment, possibly for his own preservation, because he was beloved by Cybele. Golding's translation pauses on the line with a question: "The tree to Cybele, mother of the Goddes, most deere. For why? / Her minion Atys putting off the shape of man, did dye, / And hardened into this same tree." In Golding's translation, Attis' induration is the very inverse of Christ's incarnation. Christ's putting on the soft and suffering flesh makes possible the softening and redemption of man's hard heart. In Burton's meditation on inanimate love, the unbending pine (*arbor infelix* upon which the poet Marsyas was flayed) serves as a homonym for melancholic suffering that symbolically yields to the bowing palm associated with Christ's entry into Jerusalem.

Just as Shakespeare turns the homonymic palm and palm into the "holy palmers' kiss," Burton's meditation on loving palms suggests the metonymic substitution of hand and palm for leaf and page in a kind of loving writer's kiss. Burton thus translates the silvicultural image of tethering or "stroking" lonely trees into a figure for the loving art of citation. The kisses that carry between pining palms echo the lines of transmission whereby one author reads and cites another:

> If any man thinke this which I say to be a tale, let him read that story of two palme trees in *Italy*, the male growing at *Brundusium*, the female at *Otranto* (related by *Jovianus Pontanus* in an excellent Poem, sometimes Tutor to *Alphonsus Junior*, King of *Naples*, his Secretary of State and a great Philosopher) *which were barren and so continued a long time*, till they came to see one another by growing up higher, though many *Stadiums* asunder. *Pierius* in his *Hierogliphicks*, and *Melchior Guilandinus memb. 3. Tract. de papyro*, cites this story of *Pontanus* for a truth. (3:43)

This congeries of testimony on love amongst the palm trees imitates the object of its description, making humanist citing out to be kind of scholarly yearning like that of the palm trees that reach for one another "*by the bending of boughs, and inclination of their bodies*" (3:43). Burton defies the skeptical reader to read the story as it appears in a poem by the Italian humanist Pontano, who is cited by the early symbologist Pierius (Pierio Valeriano) and also by the Prussian botanist

---

[104]   Ovid, *Metamorphoses*, 10.86–105.

[105]   Ovid, *Fasti*, 4.223–44.

Guilandinus (Melchior Wieland) who cites "this story of *Pontanus* for a truth." What would appear to the modern reader to be a suspiciously circuitous string of references is an illustration of the way in which the anecdote accrues a kind of intensification through its repetition. This is no self-consuming artifact of the humanist imagination but a testament to the pneumatic power of discourse. The frozen kiss of torpid birds discovered mouth-to-mouth is remembered here in what we might describe as an emblem for citation as transpiration. The centonic art by which Burton finds comfort and offers us the same is recognizable here as an *ars amatoria*—an artful dilation propelled by the same desire that inclines Burton to his books and us to him.

Epilogue
Loving Burton, or Burton for Amateurs

It is hard to imagine that Samuel Johnson would have sprung out of bed "two hours sooner than he wished" to read *The Anatomy of Melancholy* as it is described by many contemporary scholars.[1] The impassivity that one encounters in modern Burton scholarship is all the more surprising when set against evidence of the *Anatomy*'s early reception. We know that the book sold very well during and after Burton's lifetime, reputedly making his publisher, Henry Cripps, a small fortune. Thomas Fuller described the *Anatomy* as "an excellent Book ... wherein [the author] hath piled up variety of much excellent Learning,"[2] and remarks that "Scarce any Book of *Philology* [which he defines as 'the *Roses* of learning, without the *prickles*'[3]] ... in so short a time passed so many *Impressions*" in England.[4] While it is a more complicated matter to ascertain the ways in which early readers made use of the *Anatomy*, reader marks in surviving copies of seventeenth-century editions provide us with something of a window. Of course, as Mary Ann Lund notes in her survey of many of these volumes, it is notoriously difficult to draw conclusions about reader-reception based on marks and annotations whose makers and motives remain largely unknown to us.[5] That said, there are patterns to be detected both of distribution and kind in the 40-odd seventeenth-century copies I consulted at libraries in the UK, Canada, and the United States.[6] It is true that marks in these copies reflect a diverse set of interests, from the kinds and causes of melancholy[7] to practical advice concerning diet, exercise and habitation[8] and from occult themes to history and industry, often with marks pertaining to all the above in the same volume.[9] But there are, generally speaking, fewer marks

---

[1]   James Boswell, *The Life of Samuel Johnson* (London, 1791), 217.

[2]   Thomas Fuller, *The History of the Worthies of England* (London, 1662), 134.

[3]   Ibid., 26.

[4]   Ibid., 134.

[5]   Mary Ann Lund, *Melancholy, Medicine and Religion in Early Modern England: Reading "The Anatomy of Melancholy"* (New York: Cambridge University Press, 2010), 198.

[6]   I viewed all seventeenth-century copies held at the Bodleian Library, Brasenose College, Lincoln College, Christ Church College, and the English Faculty Library at Oxford University, the British Library, the Wellcome Library, the Houghton Library at Harvard University, and the Osler Medical Library at McGill University. I refer to all annotated copies below by library, shelfmark, and date.

[7]   Bodleian, Gibson 245 (1638), 46–7.

[8]   For example, Brasenose UB SIII 75 (1651); Bodleian, Antiq.d.1638.2.

[9]   As in British Library, 715.i.13 (1652).

on more strictly speaking "medical" topics than spiritual and philosophical ones, and of all sections, the Preface and sections on love and religious melancholy are the most heavily marked. We may observe further patterns in the kinds of material marked even within these sections. A majority of the marked passages are aphoristic or anecdotal. These include witty sayings, incisive comments, jokes, and illustrations that encapsulate the sense or wisdom of much longer, preceding discussions. It is from this store that the canon of the more quotable Burton is largely drawn, and many of the same passages are copied in surviving manuscript collections of notes taken from the *Anatomy*.[10] Readers also regularly marked passages describing strange and marvelous occurrences in nature and human behavior as well as quiddities, curiosities, and particularly memorable stories and examples, suggesting that the *Anatomy*'s modeled technique for rectifying the spirits by vivid engagement of the imagination seems likely to have been effective for many.[11]

In addition to these marks and annotations, we have printed evidence that readers regarded the book as a storehouse of wonderful stories, as the poet Robert Howard saw fit to use them.[12] Numerous seventeenth-century readers and writers recognized the *Anatomy*'s narrative and literary pleasures as evidence of the genius of the "ingenious Robert Burton."[13] The *Anatomy* is the first book that comes to William Leybourn's mind in his inventory of activities recommended "to recreate ingenious spirits, because, as the seventeenth-century historian Thomas Fuller wrote, 'Recreation is a second Creation.'"[14] Moreover, with the notable exception of William Prynne, who cites Burton at face value a number of times in his *Pleasant Purge for a Roman Catholike*,[15] early references to the *Anatomy* seem

---

[10]   Compare, for instance, Lincoln L.3.14 (1628) and Bodleian, Bliss B.406 (1651) with British Library, Sloane MS 2521; Sloane MS 1965; and Sloane MS 1677. The (James) Boswell copy, Houghton, HEW 5.11.7 (1628), includes a penciled index of such phrases.

[11]   See, especially, Wellcome, 7092/B (1621); Bodleian, Bliss B.406 (1651); Bodleian, NN 17 Th (1624); Brasenose UB SIII 75 (1651); English Faculty, YJ 37.1 [Ana] (1638). The story of duke's trick, for instance, discussed in Chapter 3, is marked in Bodleian, Gibson 245; Wellcome, 7092/B (1621); Bodleian, Antiq.d.1638.2.

[12]   Sir Robert Howard, "Statius, his Achilleis, with Annotations," *Poems* (London, 1660), 210–11.

[13]   Gerard Langbaine, *An Account of the English Dramatic Poets* (Oxford, 1691).

[14]   Thomas Fuller, *The Holy State by Thomas Fuller* (London, 1642), 183. Leybourn commences his 1694 study of *Pleasures with Profit* with this defense of recreation: "When *Weariness* hath almost annihilated our *Spirits* ~ It is the *breathing* of the *Soul*, which would otherwise be *stifled* with continual *Business* ... . And this Interval of *Rest* or *Recreation* produceth the same *effects*, as well in *Sensitives* and *Vegitives*, as it doth in *Man*" (*Pleasure with Profit Consisting of Recreations of Divers Kinds, Viz., Numerical, Geometrical, Mechanical, Statical, Astronomical, Horometrical, Cryptographical, Magnetical, Automatical, Chymical, and Historical* ... [London, 1694], 1).

[15]   William Prynne, *A Pleasant Purge for a Roman Catholike to Evacuate His Evill Humours* (London, 1642), 2:155.

to understand that Burton was offering a restorative form of recreation that was as ingenious as it was irreverent.[16] David Lloyd counts Burton among the friends and teachers of the royalist Dudley Digges in his martyrological *Memoires*. He describes the *Anatomy* as being "as full of all variety of learning as [the author] himself, wherein Gentlemen, that have lost time, and are put upon an aftergame of learning, pick many choice things to furnish them for discourse or writing."[17] Lloyd admiringly reports that when the young Burton met the Earl of Dorset, then Chancellor of the University, he had the audacity to address him as "Mr. Dorset" and proceeded "to discourse" with him amiably for "an hour together."[18] The story suggests that Burton liked a risky game in person as much as he did in print and that a significant pleasure for early modern readers of the *Anatomy* lay in the author's unsanctimoniousness. At least one seventeenth-century reader recognized Burton's subversive take on the misogynist *auctoritas*. James Norris calls on Burton as his first modern witness to the cause of defending women against the ancient tropes of antifeminism.[19]

Why the comparatively grave reception then by modern scholars? Earlier in the process of writing this book I came to the hasty conclusion that the reason for Burton's recent (relative) neglect, misreading, and maligning was simply that most scholars who cite the book do not read the *Anatomy* in full or carefully enough to recognize its ironies. The *Anatomy* is a big book, though there are bigger, and a difficult one, though this tends to be said less with respect to the density of its prose, arguments, and references, and more often to indict the personality who speaks through the *Anatomy* as a willfully opaque and obfuscating narrator who refuses to yield to the reader's desire for authorial transparency. To be fair, unprecedented expectations for productivity of a particularly historicist and archival style, combined with a deceptive sense of the comprehensiveness and immediacy of an ever-expanding and "searchable" archive, makes nonfiction prose works such as Burton's particularly vulnerable to decontextualized "consultation" and therefore to the kinds of misreadings or, rather, missed readings that I have marked throughout this study.

Discovering while dissertating on Burton just how few early modernists had read the *Anatomy* in full, I came to the further conclusion that only a graduate fellowship or independent fortune could allow one to read Burton pleasurably. These seemed to me to be the only conditions under which a person might have access both to the arcane volumes out of which Burton's *cento* is composed and

---

[16]   James Granger calls it a "very ingenious" cento (*Biographical History of England*, 1769).

[17]   David Lloyd, *Memoires of the Lives, Actions, Sufferings & Deaths of Those Noble, Reverend and Excellent Personages* (London: S. Speed, 1668), 428.

[18]   Ibid.

[19]   James Norris, *Haec & Hic; or, the Feminine Gender More Worthy than the Masculine. Being a Vindication of that Ingenious and Innocent Sex from the Biting Sarcasms, Bitter Satyrs, and Opprobrious Calumnies, Wherewith they are Daily, tho Undeservedly, Aspers'd by the Virulent Tongues and Pens of Malevolent Men* ... (London, 1683), 89.

the time required to discern his mischief with them. It was around that time that I met a prominent early modernist who asked me what I was working on. When I told him he replied simply by calling the *Anatomy* a "black hole." I presumed he meant it as a caution: that way danger lies. Dissertations on Burton are left to die in a graveyard of monographs never published or, worse, never written. I became increasingly anxious each time I discovered another thesis on the *Anatomy* by an author whose name appeared nowhere else in scholarly print. Was this senior scholar warning me about the fate of lost friends and colleagues who fell prey to this intractably difficult book with so little general appeal as to mean certain publishing doom and academic failure? I later came to sense that this scholar was describing other dangers posed by prolonged exposure to Burton: risks of being lost in the vortex of his pleonasm, his dizzying citations, belligerent opacity, and unwillingness to perform a self-same narratorial identity. I have since come to wonder whether we might account for the Burtonian black hole as a vanishing syndrome of another sort, a Circean lure of rhetorical pleasures that threaten to engulf scholarly objectives and turn them into something else. One might regard the disappearing act of hopeful Burtonists as the result of their porcine feasting upon a kind of excremental literary excess, as some later twentieth-century writers have characterized Burtonian *copia*. Or we might surmise that scholars have disappeared into the *Anatomy* only to be transformed in temperament and spirit (as Burton expressly hopes) into affectively impressionable or "passionate" readers who go now by a different name: amateurs, or fans—to whom I will shortly return.

The attrition of Burton scholars from the academy might only seem more conspicuous given the relative scarcity of titles on the *Anatomy* outside of the dissertations database. But if indeed this attrition is more marked among Burtonists, I suspect that this reveals an elective phenomenon rather than one compelled by failure. It might in fact reflect Burton's successful persuasion of his scholarly readers to avoid the conditions that aggravate melancholy by getting out of academia, out of doors, out of a life he calls "most uncertaine, unrespected, subject to all casualties, and hazards." In his lengthy discussion of scholarly melancholy, Burton remarks that many "a polite and terse Academicke," having too long suffered the injuries of their profession, find they "must turne rusticke, rude, melancholise alone, learne to forget, or else, as many doe become Maultsters, Grasiers, Chapmen, &c. (now banished from the Academy, all commerce of the Muses, and confined to a country village, as *Ovid* was from *Rome* to *Pontus*,) and daily converse with a company of Idiots and Clownes" (1:324). I recite these fulminations not to lament how little has changed but rather to suggest that the earnest complaint underlying Burton's comic railing may shed light on the reason why, recently at least, it seems that those outside the ivory tower have been readier to delight in his raucous prose. However, as we have already seen, this was not always the case. Neither is it the case that privilege alone affords the conditions required for Burton's appreciation.

The *Anatomy* continues to rank highly on popular "best books" and desert island reading lists, recalling the manner in which Paul Jordan-Smith called it

"The Book for a Desert Island."[20] Geoffrey Keynes prefaced his review of Jordan-Smith's book by remarking that "if a vote were taken among the brotherhood of bibliographers as to what single volume afforded them the greatest amount of interest among all the books they knew, it is possible that *The Anatomy of Melancholy* would come out high in the list." Keynes further remarked that he envied Jordan-Smith for "the pleasure he must have derived from the compilation of his [work]."[21] This expression of envy for the pleasure of "compilation" hints at profound tensions in the early academy between a still-emerging professional imperative to distinguish scholarly labor from literary pleasure and to do so by policing sympathetic and mimetic engagement with the objects of one's study in the name of maintaining objectivity and critical distance. Keynes observes the pseudo-Burtonian style in which Jordan-Smith's laudatory preface is written—and the rightness of this, being "well suited to the subject at hand."[22] A noted bibliophile himself, Keynes might have similarly praised Holbrook Jackson's rhapsodic *Anatomy of Bibliomania*, perhaps the best example of modern mimetic meditation upon Burton's bibliophilia.[23] These are books about the love of books and the love of Burton's love of books—a characterization that will, no doubt, make them seem profoundly unscholarly to most modern scholars, but I would ask whether the policing of affective impressionability and mimetic assimilation assists or obstructs in our efforts to better "apprehend" the literatures and cultures of early modernity. Impressionability and imitation are hardly endorsed practices in mainstream contemporary scholarship, but the same was not true for early modern readers, whose rhetorical trainings aimed precisely to move, affect, convert, inspire, and console: to alter and be altered.

Curious to compare modern scholarly and popular responses to Burton, I consulted the Amazon reviews for the 2001 New York Review Books Classics edition of the *Anatomy*. Even when written by ostensibly professional academics, these reviews follow the quintessential pattern of online product recommendations, giving advice as to the utilitarian value of the book: "buy it, don't buy it, it's 'worth' it; it '*works*.'" "If you like good literature," one customer writes, "you'll love this book. If you like psychology, you'll love this book. If you want to seem pretentious, you need this book."[24] Lord Byron, incidentally, said more or less the same thing, calling the book "most useful to a man who wishes to acquire

---

20 Paul Jordan-Smith, *Bibliographia Burtoniana: A Study of Robert Burton's "The Anatomy of Melancholy"* (Stanford: Stanford University Press, 1931), 3.

21 Geoffrey Keynes, "Bibliographia Burtonia," *The Review of English Studies* 35 (1933): 337.

22 Ibid., 338.

23 Holbrook Jackson, *The Anatomy of Bibliomania* (Urbana: University of Illinois Press, 2001 [1950]).

24 A Customer, "Absolutely the Best Book Ever Written … Bar None," Review, *The Anatomy of Melancholy* (New York Review Books Classics), February 24, 2002, http://www.amazon.com/review/R344MS4EB0GOB7/ref=cm_srch_res_rtr_alt_2.

the reputation of being well read, with the least trouble."[25] Amazon fans also appreciate the *omnium gatherum* quality of the *Anatomy*, whose delights may be accessed in a random, haphazard manner, as one might look upon curiosities in an early modern cabinet. Some reviewers offer suggestions for use: "*The Anatomy of Melancholy* wasn't meant to be read from the first page to the last; I have never met anyone who did that and one would have to be more than a little mad to even try."[26] Alfred Newton earlier in the twentieth century said this too, quoting Samuel Johnson, who famously rejected the idea that one has to read a book through to derive its benefits.[27] The same Amazon customer writes: "Just pick up the book. Open it to any page. You may find lists, digressions, bits of 17th century prose, quotes, much Latin. Whatever you find, it is sure to please if you only give it half a chance." In the same vein, another Amazon reviewer cautions that the *Anatomy* is "a reference book and not a novel, and therefore shouldn't be read in a continuous way. It becomes tedious and incomprehensible. Like grandma used to say: 'Take small bites so you don't choke!'"[28] But if this reader sees fit to offer dosing instructions for the *Anatomy*'s consumption, others seem to derive benefits from its surfeit and repetition: "Where to begin discussing this book? How about again and again? For it begs never to be put down, and if finished (as if that's even possible) to be picked up again and pored over. Again. And again. And again … a bricolage (I think) to be devoured ravenously and chewed interminably like an everlasting gobstopper—a joy to exhaust your mind and body by … ."[29]

In an editorial for the *Telegraph* (extracted from his introduction to the handsome Folio Society reissue of the Holbrook Jackson edition) the bestselling fantasy writer Philip Pullman remarks on the therapeutic effects of the *Anatomy*'s interminable energy:

> Those readers who have some experience of the disorder of the mind we now call depression will know that the opposite of that dire state is not happiness but energy; and energy is contagious. We can catch it from others. They cheer us up. Burton's energy is as free and abounding as that of Rabelais, and its effect on the reader is similar: an invigorating of the natural spirits (created in the liver),

---

25 Thomas More, *Life of Lord Byron* (London: Murray, 1851), 48.

26 A Customer, "Absolutely the Best Book Ever Written … Bar None."

27 The early twentieth-century bibliophile Alfred Newton wrote that he read the *Anatomy* with "delight, not cover to cover,—for, as Dr. Johnson once inquired, 'who reads a book through?'—but I have read most of it once, and parts of it several times" (Alfred Edward Newton, *End Papers: Literary Recreations* [Boston: Little, Brown, 1933], 98–9).

28 Scott Schwartz, "Take Small Bites!" Review, *The Anatomy of Melancholy* (New York Review Books Classics) (Paperback), June 16, 2008, http://www.amazon.com/review/R1EF6JHBOLQ98A/ref=cm_srch_res_rtr_alt_1.

29 Nouche "Nouche!" "Vivisect Your Mind," Review, *The Anatomy of Melancholy* (New York Review Books Classics) (Paperback), August 30, 2006, http://www.amazon.com/review/RPORVS8S9BGAM/ref=cm_srch_res_rtr_alt_1.

causing a quickening of the vital spirits (produced in the heart), leading to a stimulation of the animal spirits (formed in the brain). In other words, a tonic.[30]

Pullman ends by inverting Johnson's quip about *Paradise Lost*, suggesting somewhat scandalously that no one "would wish [the *Anatomy*] a sentence shorter, or be without one of [its] thousands of anecdotes and quotations. This is one of the indispensable books; for my money, it is the best of all."[31]

If there's something to be observed in this survey of modern, lay responses to Burton, it is the seeming tautology that one needs to be a fan in order to appreciate him. The pleasure afforded by the *Anatomy* would appear to be a measure of its efficacy as medicine—a potion that delivers both solace and entertainment and, like any good therapy, demands a certain suspension of disbelief and a commitment to the cure. One needs to approach the book with a willingness to be entertained and distracted from ruminating preoccupations, to be busied for seemingly endless stretches of prose and time. It would appear, as much as we might have expected otherwise, that "getting" Burton—both his jokes and the beneficial pleasure of his book—does not necessarily require fluency with the arcane materials with which he plays. Nonacademic readers recognize Burton's satire and theatricality, his bombast and antics, in tone if not in proof. Burton seems to have been eager to ensure that this would be the case, protesting the undoubtedly false complaint that he was forced to write the book in English (1:16).

Scholarly misapprehension of Burton's ludic and therapeutic performance seems to illustrate the inadmissibility of aesthetic feeling in modern scholarly practice. After more than a decade of the so-called return (or "revenge") of aesthetics, the literary humanities may have repatriated formalism but not the wonder, pleasure, and impressionability that frequently precedes critical impulse. The deprivileging of formal reading, especially of early modern prose, goes a long way toward explaining the oversight of the ways the *Anatomy* exhibits what Michael Clark calls the "power to complicate that is also a power to undermine."[32] Antiformalist interests have weighed against the kind of interpretive work that would, among other things, translate Burton's jokes because such work has been regarded as a glossing of surfaces rather than an exposition of historical and cultural practices. Recent historicist revaluations of the *Anatomy*, from John Stachniewski's and Mary Ann Lund's examinations of Burton's spiritual counsel to Angus Gowland's reassessment of Burton's retrograde literary humanism, have prepared the way for the preceding study and will, I hope, foster further study of the *Anatomy*. But such good work on Burton and other neglected nonfiction prose writers of the late Renaissance demands a reader who is unafraid, as Svetlana

---

30   Philip Pullman, "Reasons to Be Cheerful," *Telegraph.co.uk*, April 10, 2005, sec. books, http://www.telegraph.co.uk/culture/books/3640566/Reasons-to-be-cheerful.html.

31   Ibid.

32   Michael Clark, *Revenge of the Aesthetic: The Place of Literature in Theory Today* (Berkeley: University of California Press, 2000), 11.

Alpers suggests, to attend to the *surface* of things and become "passible" readers, to use Timothy Reiss's term, in their own right.[33] For so long as we predicate scholarly research on anaesthetic objectivity and resist stylistic analyses on the grounds of their supposed subjectivity and presentism (while supposing materialist historicism to be immune to such limitations) the worlds not only of early modern melancholy but its many other modes of feeling and being will continue to seem occult, which is to say, hidden from us.

---

[33]   Svetlana Alpers, *The Art of Describing: Dutch Art in the Seventeenth Century* (Chicago: University of Chicago Press, 1983); Timothy J. Reiss, *Mirages of the Selfe: Patterns of Personhood in Ancient and Early Modern Europe* (Stanford: Stanford University Press, 2003), 96.

Works Cited

Manuscript Sources

British Library, Sloane MS 1677.
British Library, Sloane MS 1965.
British Library, Sloane MS 2521.

Printed Primary Sources

Abernethy, John. *A Christian and Heauenly Treatise*. London, 1622.
Agrippa, Henricus Cornelius. *Declamation on the Nobility and Preeminence of the Female Sex*. Edited and translated by Albert Rabil Jr. University of Chicago Press, 1996.
———. *Three Books of Occult Philosophy*. Translated by John French. London, 1651.
Alexander of Tralles. *Oeuvres Médicales d'Alexandre de Tralles, Le Dernier Auteur Classique Des Grands Médicins Grecs de L'antiquité*. Edited by Felix Brunet. Vol. 1. Paris: Geuthner, 1933.
Anon. *Democritus Natu Minimus*. 1647.
Aristaenetus. *Epistolae Amatoriae*. Translated by Josias Mercer. Paris, 1595.
Aristotle. *Generation of Animals*. Translated by Arthur Leslie Peck. Loeb Classical Library. Cambridge, MA: Harvard University Press, 1943.
———. *The Poetics of Aristotle*. Edited and translated by S.H. Butcher. London: Macmillan, 1902.
Ausonius. *Ausonius*. Translated by Hugh G. Evelyn White. Vol. 1. London: Heinemann, 1919.
Bacon, Francis. *Francis Bacon: The New Organon*. Edited by Lisa Jardine and Michael Silverthorne. Cambridge: Cambridge University Press, 2000.
———. "Sylva Sylvarum." In *The Works of Francis Bacon*, edited by James Spedding, Leslie Ellis, and Douglas Heath. Vol. 2. London: Longman, 1857.
———. *Sylva Sylvarum, or, A Naturall Historie in Ten Centuries*. London, 1627.
Bacon, Nathaniel. *A Relation of the Fearefull Estate of Francis Spira in the Yeare, 1548*. London, 1638.
Barth, Kaspar. *Pornoboscodidascalus Latinus*. 1624.
Bassus, Cassianus. *Geōponika: Agricultural Pursuits*. Translated by T. Owen. Vol. 2. London, 1805.
Baxter, Richard. "The Cure of Melancholy and Overmuch-Sorrow by Faith and Physick." In *A Continuation of Morning-Exercise Questions and Cases of Conscience Practically Resolved by Sundry Ministers in October, 1682*, edited by Samuel Annesley, 263–303. London, 1683.

Beard, Thomas. *The Theatre of Gods Iudgements: Or, A Collection of Histories out of Sacred, Ecclesiasticall, and Prophane Authours, Concerning the Admirable Iudgements of God Vpon the Transgressours of His Commandments.* London, 1597.

Bolton, Robert. *A Discourse about the State of True Happinesse.* London, 1611.

———. *Instructions for a Right Comforting of Afflicted Consciences.* London, 1631.

Bright, Timothie. *A Treatise of Melancholie.* London, 1586.

Browne, Thomas. *Pseudodoxia Epidemica, or, Enquiries into very many received tenents and commonly presumed truths.* London, 1646.

Burton, Robert. *The Anatomy of Melancholy.* Oxford, 1621.

———. *The Anatomy of Melancholy.* Oxford, 1624.

———. *The Anatomy of Melancholy.* Edited by Thomas C. Faulkner, Nicolas K. Kiessling, and Rhonda Blair. Introduction and Commentary by J.B. Bamborough and Martin Dodsworth. 6 vols. Oxford: Clarendon Press, 1989–2000.

Cardano, Girolamo. *The Book on Games of Chance (Liber de Ludo Aleae).* New York: Holt, Rinehart and Winston, 1961.

Carew, Richard. *Survey of Cornwall.* London, 1602.

Cassian, John. *John Cassian: The Conferences.* Edited and translated by Boniface Ramsey. New York: The Newman Press, 1997.

Cervantes, Miguel de. *Exemplary Stories.* Translated by Lesley Lipson. Oxford: Oxford University Press, 1998.

———. *Novelas Ejemplares.* Madrid, 1613.

Church of England. *Articles ... accordyng to the Computation of the Churche of England, for Thauoydyng of the Diuersities of Opinions, and for the Stablyshyng of Consent Touchyng True Religion.* London, 1563.

Cicero. *Tusculan Disputations.* Translated by J.E. King. Vol. 8. Loeb Classical Library 141. London: Heinemann, 1927.

Claudianus, Claudius. *Epithalamium de nuptiis Honorii Augustii.* In *Claudian,* edited and translated by Maurice Platnauer. Vol. 1. New York: Heinemann, 1922.

Crooke, Helkiah. *Mikrokosmographia: A Description of the Body of Man.* London, 1615.

Daniel, Samuel. *The first part of the Historie of England.* London, 1612.

Day, Angel. *The English Secretorie.* London, 1595.

du Laurens, André. *A Discourse of the Preservation of the Sight.* Translated by Richard Surphlet. London, 1599.

Du Vair, Guillaume. *A Buckler Against Adversitie: or, A Treatise of Constancie.* Translated by Andrew Court. London, 1622.

Ephesus, Rufus of, and Peter E. Pormann. *On Melancholy.* Tübingen: Mohr Siebeck, 2008.

Erasmus, Desiderius. "Foundations of the Abundant Style (*De duplici copia verborum ac rerum commentarii duo*)." In *Collected Works of Erasmus,* edited and translated by Betty Knott. Vol. 24. Toronto, ON: University of Toronto Press, 1978.

————. "A Short Debate Concerning the Distress, Alarm, and Sorrow of Jesus." In *Collected Works of Erasmus*, edited by J.W. O'Malley. Translated by Michael J. Heath. Vol. 70. Toronto, ON: University of Toronto Press, 1998.

Ferrand, Jacques. *A Treatise on Lovesickness*. Edited and translated by Donald A. Beecher and Massimo Ciavolella. Syracuse, NY: Syracuse University Press, 1994.

Ficino, Marsilio. *The Letters of Marsilio Ficino*. Translated by Members of the Language Dept., School of Economic Science. Vol. 1. London: Shepheard-Walwyn, 1975.

————. *Platonic Theology*. Edited by James Hankins and William R. Bowen. Translated by Michael J.B. Allen and John Warden. Vol. 6. I Tatti Renaissance Library. Cambridge, MA: Harvard University Press, 2001.

————. *Three Books on Life*. Edited and translated by Carol Kaske and John Clark. Binghamton: Center for Medieval and Early Renaissance Studies, State University of New York Press, 1989.

Foote, Peter, ed. *Olaus Magnus: A Description of the Northern Peoples, 1555*. Vol. 1. Translated by Peter Fisher and Humphrey Higgens. London: Hakluyt Society, 1996.

Fuller, Thomas. *The History of the Worthies of England*. London, 1662.

————. *The Holy State by Thomas Fuller ...* . London, 1642.

Galen. *On the Affected Parts*. Translated by Rudolph E. Siegel. New York: Karger, 1976.

Galvão, António, and Richard Hakluyt. *The Discoveries of the World: From Their First Original unto the Year of Our Lord 1555*. Edited by Charles Ramsay Drinkwater Bethune. London: Hakluyt Society, 1862.

Garzoni, Tomaso. *The Hospitall of Incurable Fooles*. London, 1600.

Geiger, Malachias. *Microcosmus hypochondriacus sive de melancholia hypochondriaca tractatus, cum curatione hujus affectus*. Monaco: Straub, 1652.

Gordonius, Bernardus. *Opus lilium medicinae inscriptum, de morborum prope omnium curatione*. Lyons, 1574.

Goulart, Simon. *Admirable and Memorable Histories Containing the Wonders of Our Time*. Translated by Edward Grimeston. London, 1607.

Granger, James. *Biographical History of England*. 1769.

Gray, Robert. *A Good Speed to Virginia*. London, 1609.

Greenham, Richard. *A Most Sweete and Assured Comfort for all those that are Afflicted in Consciscience* [sic], *or Troubled in Minde*. London, 1595.

————. *Paramythion: Two Treatises of the Comforting of an Afflicted Conscience*. London, 1598.

Guagnini, Alessandro. *Sarmatiae Europeae descriptio*. Cracow, 1578.

Hakewill, George. *An Apologie of the Povver and Prouidence of God in the Gouernment of the World*. Oxford, 1635.

Hakluyt, Richard. *The Original Writings & Correspondence of the Two Richard Hakluyts*. London: Hakluyt Society, 1935.

————. *Principal Navigations*. London, 1589.

Hayward, David. *David's Tears*. London, 1623.

Heath, Robert. *Paradoxicall Assertions and Philosophical Problems Ful of Delight and Recreation for All Ladies*. London, 1659.

Helmont, Jan Baptist van. *A Ternary of Paradoxes: The Magnetick Cure of Wounds*. Translated by Walter Charleton. London, 1650.

Hippocrates. *Pseudepigraphic Writings*. Edited and translated by Wesley D. Smith. Studies in Ancient Medicine. Vol. 2. Leiden: E.J. Brill, 1990.

Horace. *Sermones*. N.d.

Howard, Robert. *Poems, Viz. 1. A Panegyrick to the King. 2. Songs and Sonnets. 3. The Blind Lady, a Comedy. 4. The Fourth Book of Virgil. 5. Statius his Achilleis, with Annotations. 6. A Panegyrick to Generall Monck*. London, 1660.

Hutchinson, Lucy Apsley. *Memoirs of the Life of Colonel Hutchinson, Governor of Nottingham Castle and Town*. London: G. Bell & Sons, 1908.

Johnson, Robert. *Noua Britannia Offring Most Excellent Fruites by Planting in Virginia*. 1609.

Kepler, Johannes. *Kepler's Somnium: The Dream, or Posthumous Work on Lunar Astronomy*. Madison: University of Wisconsin Press, 1967.

Langbaine, Gerard. *An Account of the English Dramatic Poets*. Oxford, 1691.

Lawrence, Thomas. *Mercurius Centralis*. London, 1664.

le Roy, Louis. *De la vicissitude ou variété des choses en l'univers*. Paris, 1575.

Lemnius, Levinus. *The Secret Miracles of Nature: In Four Books*. London, 1658.

———. *The Touchstone of Complexions*. Translated by Thomas Newton. London, 1576.

Leybourn, William. *Pleasure with Profit Consisting of Recreations of Divers Kinds, Viz., Numerical, Geometrical, Mechanical, Statical, Astronomical, Horometrical, Cryptographical, Magnetical, Automatical, Chymical, and Historical ...* . London, 1694.

Lipsius, Justus. *Antiquarum lectionum commentarius*. Antwerp, 1575.

———. *Politica: Six Books of Politics or Political Instruction*. Edited and translated by Jan Waszink. Assen, Netherlands: Koninklijke Van Gorcum, 2004.

Lloyd, David. *Memoires of the Lives, Actions, Sufferings & Deaths of Those Noble, Reverend and Excellent Personages*. London, 1668.

Longinus. *On the Sublime*. Translated by A.O. Prickard. Oxford: Clarendon, 1906.

Lucretius, Titus Carus. *The Nature of Things*. Translated by Frank O. Copley. New York: W.W. Norton & Company, 1977.

Magnus, Olaus. *Historia de gentibus Septentrionalibus*. Rome, 1555.

Marcellinus, Ammianus. *Ammianus Marcellinus*. Translated by John Rolfe. Vol. 2. Loeb Classical Library. Cambridge: Heinemann, 1935.

Melville, Herman. *Moby-Dick, or The Whale*. Edited by Harrison Hayford, Hershel Parker, and G. Thomas Tanselle. Evanston and Chicago: Northwestern University Press and the Newberry Library, 1988.

Mexia, Pedro, and Antoine Du Verdier. *The Treasurie of Auncient and Moderne Times*. Edited and translated by Thomas Milles. London, 1613.

Middleton, Thomas. *Five Plays*. Edited by Bryan Loughrey and Neil Taylor. London: Penguin, 1988.

Montaigne, Michel de. *Essayes, or Morall, Politicke and Millitarie Discourses.* Translated by John Florio. London, 1603.

Norris, James. *Haec & Hic; or, the Feminine Gender More Worthy than the Masculine. Being a Vindication of that Ingenious and Innocent Sex from the Biting Sarcasms, Bitter Satyrs, and Opprobrious Calumnies, Wherewith they are Daily, tho Undeservedly, Aspers'd by the Virulent Tongues and Pens of Malevolent Men ... .* London, 1683.

Ovid. *Amores.* N.d.

———. *Fasti.* N.d.

———. *Metamorphoses.* N.d.

———. *The XV Bookes of P. Ouidius Naso, Entytuled Metamorphosis.* Translated by Arthur Golding. London, 1567.

Perkins, William. *A Golden Chaine, or the Description of Theologie Containing the Order of the Causes of Saluation and Damnation.* London, 1591.

———. *M. Perkins, His Exhortation to Repentance ... with Two Treatises of the Duties and Dignitie of the Ministrie.* London, 1605.

———, Richard Rogers, Richard Greenham, and George Webb. *A Garden of Spirituall Flowers.* London, 1610.

Pico della Mirandola, Giovanni Francesco. *On the Imagination.* Translated by Harry Caplan. New Haven, CT: Yale University Press, 1930.

Platter, Felix. *Praxeos seu de cognoscendis praedicendis, praecauendis, curandisque, affectibus homini incommodantibus.* Basel, 1602.

Pliny, the Elder. *The Historie of the World.* Translated by Philemon Holland. London, 1601.

Price, Daniel. *Spirituall Odours.* London, 1618.

Prynne, William. *A Pleasant Purge for a Roman Catholike to Evacuate His Evill Humours.* London, 1642.

Pseudo-Albertus Magnus, St. *De Secretis Mulierum.* Translated by Helen Rodnite Lemay. Albany: State University of New York Press, 1992.

Puttenham, George. *The Arte of English Poesie.* London, 1589.

Quintilian. *Institutes of Oratory.* Translated by John Watson. London: Bell, 1907.

Rabelais, François. *Five Books of the Lives, Heroic Deeds and Sayings of Gargantua and His Son Pantagruel.* Translated by Thomas Urquhart and Peter Motteux. London: A.H. Bullen, 1904.

Rainolds, John. *Oxford Lectures on Aristotle's Rhetoric.* Edited and translated by Lawrence D. Green. Cranbury, NJ: Associated University Press, 1986.

Rogers, Richard. *Seven Treatises.* London, 1603.

Sprat, Thomas. *History of the Royal Society.* London, 1667.

Synesius. *The Essays and Hymns of Synesius of Cyrene.* Translated by Augustine Fitzgerald. Oxford: Oxford University Press, 1930.

Terence. *Eunuch.* N.d.

"Tractate Sabbath." Edited by Isidore Epstein. Translated by H. Freedman. In *The Babylonian Talmud: Seder Moed.* Vol. 1. London: Soncino Press, 1938.

Walkington, Thomas. *The Optick Glasse of Humors.* London, 1607.

Wilson, Thomas. *The Rule of Reason, Conteinying the Arte of Logique.* Edited by
  Richard Sprague. Northridge, CA: San Fernando Valley State College, 1972.
Withals, John. *A Shorte Dictionarie for Yonge Beginners.* London, 1566.

Secondary Sources

A Customer. "Absolutely the Best Book Ever Written ... Bar None." Review of *The
  Anatomy of Melancholy*, by Robert Burton. New York Review Books Classics,
  February 24, 2002. http://www.amazon.com/review/R344MS4EB0GOB7/
  ref=cm_srch_res_rtr_alt_2.
Agamben, Giorgio. *Stanzas: Word and Phantasm in Western Culture.* Minneapolis:
  University of Minnesota Press, 1993.
Allderidge, Patricia. "Management and Mismanagement at Bedlam, 1547–1633."
  In *Health, Medicine and Mortality in the Sixteenth Century*, edited by Charles
  Webster, 141–64. Cambridge: Cambridge University Press, 1979.
Alpers, Svetlana. *The Art of Describing: Dutch Art in the Seventeenth Century.*
  Chicago: University of Chicago Press, 1983.
Anglin, Emily. "'The Glass, the School, the Book': The *Anatomy of Melancholy*
  and the Early Stuart University of Oxford." *ESC: English Studies in Canada*
  35, no. 2 (2009): 55–76.
Apetrei, Sarah. *Women, Feminism and Religion in Early Enlightenment England.*
  Cambridge: Cambridge University Press, 2010.
Ashworth, William B. "Natural History and the Emblematic World View." In
  Reappraisals of the Scientific Revolution, edited by David C. Lindberg and
  Robert S. Westman. Cambridge: Cambridge University Press, 1990.
Auski, Peter. *Christian Plain Style: The Evolution of a Spiritual Ideal.* Montreal:
  McGill-Queen's Press, 1995.
Austin, George T., and W. Glen Bradley. "Additional Responses of the Poor-Will
  to Low Temperatures." *The Auk* 86, no. 4 (1969): 717–25.
Babb, Lawrence. *Sanity in Bedlam: A Study of Robert Burton's "Anatomy of
  Melancholy."* East Lansing: Michigan State University Press, 1959.
Bakhtin, Mikhail Mikhaïlovich, and Michael Holquist. *The Dialogic Imagination:
  Four Essays.* Austin: University of Texas Press, 1981.
Barbour, Reid. *English Epicures and Stoics: Ancient Legacies in Early Stuart
  Culture.* Amherst: University of Massachusetts Press, 1998.
Barczyk-Barakonska, Liliana. "'Never to Go Forth of the Limits': Space and
  Melancholy in Robert Burton's Library Project." *Journal of European Studies*
  33, no. 3–4 (2003): 212–26.
Barlow, Richard G. "Infinite Worlds: Robert Burton's Cosmic Voyage." *Journal of
  the History of Ideas* 34, no. 2 (1973): 291–302.
Baur, Susan. *Hypochondria: Woeful Imaginings.* Berkeley: University of
  California Press, 1989.
Benthien, Claudia. *Skin: On the Cultural Border Between Self and the World.* New
  York and Chichester: Columbia University Press, 2004.
Blair, Ann. *The Theater of Nature.* Princeton, NJ: Princeton University Press, 1997.

Blanchard, W. Scott. *Scholars' Bedlam: Menippean Satire in the Renaissance.* Lewisburg, PA: Bucknell University Press, 1995.

Bonansea, Bernardino M. *Tommaso Campanella: Renaissance Pioneer of Modern Thought.* Washington, DC: Catholic University of America Press, 1969.

Bono, James. "Medical Spirits and the Medieval Language of Life." *Traditio* 40 (1984): 91–130.

Bos, A.P. *The Soul and Its Instrumental Body: A Reinterpretation of Aristotle's Philosophy of Living Nature.* Leiden: Brill, 2003.

Bouwsma, William J. "The Two Faces of Humanism: Stoicism and Augustinianism in Renaissance Thought." In *Itinerarium Italicum: The Profile of the Italian Renaissance in the Mirror of Its European Transformations: Dedicated to Paul Oskar Kristeller on the Occasion of His 70th Birthday*, edited by Thomas Allan Brady and Heiko Augustinus Oberman. Leiden: Brill, 1975.

Bozeman, Theodore Dwight. *The Precisianist Strain: Disciplinary Religion and Antinomian Backlash in Puritanism to 1638.* Chapel Hill: University of North Carolina Press, 2004.

Brann, Noel L. *The Debate Over the Origin of Genius During the Italian Renaissance: The Theories of Supernatural Frenzy and Natural Melancholy in Accord and in Conflict on the Threshold of the Scientific.* Leiden: Brill, 2002.

Bregman, Jay. *Synesius of Cyrene: Philosopher-Bishop.* Berkeley: University of California Press, 1982.

Breitenberg, Mark. *Anxious Masculinity in Early Modern England.* Cambridge: Cambridge University Press, 1996.

Brennan, Teresa. *The Transmission of Affect.* Ithaca, NY: Cornell University Press, 2004.

Brooke, Christopher. *Philosophic Pride: Stoicism and Political Thought from Lipsius to Rousseau.* Princeton, NJ: Princeton University Press, 2012.

Brown, Alison. *The Return of Lucretius to Renaissance Florence.* Cambridge, MA: Harvard University Press, 2010.

Browne, Robert M. "Robert Burton and the New Cosmology." *Modern Language Quarterly* 13 (1952): 131–48.

Burchell, David. "Hobbes, Science and Rhetoric Revisited." In *Science, Literature and Rhetoric in Early Modern England*, edited by Juliet Cummins and David Burchell. Aldershot, UK: Ashgate, 2007.

Butler, Judith. *Bodies That Matter: On the Discursive Limits of "Sex."* New York: Routledge, 1993.

Butler, Todd Wayne. *Imagination and Politics in Seventeenth-Century England.* Burlington, VT: Ashgate, 2008.

Caciola, Nancy. *Discerning Spirits: Divine and Demonic Possession in the Middle Ages.* Ithaca, NY: Cornell University Press, 2003.

Campbell, Mary Baine. *Wonder and Science: Imagining Worlds in Early Modern Europe.* Ithaca, NY: Cornell University Press, 2004.

Cartwright, David Edgar. *Tides: A Scientific History.* Cambridge: Cambridge University Press, 2000.

Cave, Terence. *The Cornucopian Text: Problems of Writing in the French Renaissance*. Oxford: Clarendon Press, 1979.

Cefalu, Paul. *Moral Identity in Early Modern English Literature*. Cambridge: Cambridge University Press, 2004.

Chartier, Roger. "Leisure and Sociability: Reading Aloud in Early Modern Europe." In *Urban Life in the Renaissance*, edited by Susan Zimmerman, 103–20. Cranbury, NJ: Associated University Press, 1989.

Clark, Albert C. *Prose Rhythm in English*. Oxford: Oxford University Press, 1913.

Clark, Michael. *Revenge of the Aesthetic: The Place of Literature in Theory Today*. Berkeley: University of California Press, 2000.

Clark, Stuart. *Vanities of the Eye: Vision in Early Modern European Culture*. Oxford: Oxford University Press, 2007.

Colie, Rosalie. *Paradoxia Epidemica: The Renaissance Tradition of Paradox*. Princeton, NJ: Princeton University Press, 1966.

Colish, Marcia L. *The Stoic Tradition from Antiquity to the Early Middle Ages*. 2 vols. Leiden: Brill, 1985–1990.

Connor, Steven. *The Book of Skin*. Ithaca, NY: Cornell University Press, 2004.

———. *The Matter of Air*. London: Reaktion, 2010.

———. "The Vapours." Accessed September 4, 2014. http://www.stevenconnor.com/vapours/.

Coudert, Allison, and Jeffrey S. Shoulson, eds. *Hebraica Veritas? Christian Hebraists and the Study of Judaism in Early Modern Europe*. Philadelphia: University of Pennsylvania Press, 2004.

Covino, William. *Magic, Rhetoric, and Literacy: An Eccentric History of the Composing Imagination*. Albany: State University of New York Press, 1994.

Craik, Katharine. *Reading Sensations in Early Modern England*. Basingstoke, UK: Palgrave Macmillan, 2007.

Croll, Morris William. "'Attic Prose' in the Seventeenth Century." *Studies in Philology* 18, no. 2 (1921): 79–128.

———. "The Baroque Style in Prose." In *"Attic" and Baroque Prose Style: The Anti-Ciceronian Movement*, edited by J. Max Patrick and Robert O. Evans. Princeton, NJ: Princeton University Press, 1969.

———. "The Cadence of English Oratorical Prose." *Studies in Philology* 16, no. 1 (1919): 1–56.

Culianu, Ioan P. *Eros and Magic in the Renaissance*. Chicago: University of Chicago Press, 1987.

Daniel, Drew. *The Melancholy Assemblage: Affect and Epistemology in the English Renaissance*. New York: Fordham University Press, 2013.

Daston, Lorraine, and Katharine Park. *Wonders and the Order of Nature, 1150–1750*. New York: Zone Books, 2001.

Dawson, Lesel. *Lovesickness and Gender in Early Modern English Literature*. Oxford: Oxford University Press, 2008.

Debus, Allen G. *The English Paracelsians*. London: Oldburne, 1965.

Diethelm, Oskar, and Thomas F. Heffernan. "Felix Platter and Psychiatry." *Journal of the History of the Behavioral Sciences* 1, no. 1 (1965): 10–23.

Djwa, Sandra. "Early Explorations: New Founde Landys (1496–1729)." *Studies in Canadian Literature/Études En Littérature Canadienne* 4, no. 2 (June 6, 1979). http://journals.hil.unb.ca/index.php/SCL/article/view/7918.

Donaldson, Meredith Jane. "Moveable Text: Mutability, Monumentality, and the Representation of Motion in British Renaissance Literature." PhD dissertation, McGill University, 2011.

Dunglison, Robley. *A Dictionary of Medical Science*. Philadelphia: Lea Brothers & Co., 1895.

Edwards, Karen L. "Thomas Browne and the Absurdities of Melancholy." In *"A Man Very Well Studyed": New Contexts for Thomas Browne*, edited by Kathryn Murphy and Richard Todd, 211–26. Leiden: Brill, 2008.

Erickson, Robert A. *The Language of the Heart: 1600–1750*. Philadelphia: University of Pennsylvania Press, 1997.

Ernst, Germana. *Tommaso Campanella: The Book and the Body of Nature*. Dordrecht: Springer, 2010.

Evans, Bergen, and George Joseph Mohr. *The Psychiatry of Robert Burton*. New York: Columbia University Press, 1944.

Fanego, Teresa. "English in Transition 1500–1700: On Variation in Second Person Singular Pronoun Usage." In *Sederi vii: Articles and Essays Presented in the 7th Conference of the Society Held at the University of Coruña, Spain, in March 1996*, edited by S.G. Fernández Corugedo, 5–15. La Coruna: Universidad de Coruña, 1996.

Feingold, Mordechai. "Oriental Studies." In *The History of the University of Oxford*, edited by Nicholas Tyacke. Vol. 4. Oxford: Oxford University Press, 1997.

Findlen, Paula. *Possessing Nature: Museums, Collecting, and Scientific Culture in Early Modern Italy*. Berkeley: University of California Press, 1994.

Fish, Stanley Eugene. *Self-Consuming Artifacts: The Experience of Seventeenth-Century Literature*. Berkeley: University of California Press, 1972.

Flashar, Hellmut, ed. *Problemata Physica*. Berlin: Akademie Verlag, 1962.

Floyd-Wilson, Mary. *English Ethnicity and Race in Early Modern Drama*. Cambridge: Cambridge University Press, 2003.

———. *Occult Knowledge, Science and Gender on the Shakespearean Stage*. Cambridge: Cambridge University Press, 2013.

Foucault, Michel. *The Order of Things: An Archaeology of the Human Sciences*. New York: Vintage, 1973.

———. *Power/knowledge: Selected Interviews and Other Writings, 1972–1977*. Edited and translated by Colin Gordon. New York: Pantheon Books, 1980.

Fox, Ruth A. *The Tangled Chain: The Structure of Disorder in "The Anatomy of Melancholy."* Berkeley: University of California Press, 1976.

Frazer, James George. *The Golden Bough: A Study in Magic and Religion*. 3rd ed. London: Macmillan, 1911.

Freud, Sigmund. "On Narcissism: An Introduction." In *The Standard Edition of the Complete Psychological Works of Sigmund Freud*, edited and translated by James Strachey. Vol. 14. London: Hogarth Press, 1961.

Frye, Northrop. *Anatomy of Criticism: Four Essays*. Princeton, NJ: Princeton University Press, 1957.

Gage, Frances. "Exercise for Mind and Body: Giulio Mancini, Collecting, and the Beholding of Landscape Painting in the Seventeenth Century." *Renaissance Quarterly* 61, no. 4 (2008): 1167–207.

Gale, Monica R. *Myth and Poetry in Lucretius*. Cambridge: Cambridge University Press, 1994.

Garber, Marjorie. "Shakespeare in Slow Motion." *Profession* 2010, no. 1 (2010): 151–64.

Gilby, Emma. *Sublime Words: Early Modern French Literature*. London: Legenda, 2006.

Gillespie, Stuart. "Lucretius in the English Renaissance." In *The Cambridge Companion to Lucretius*, edited by Philip Hardie and Stuart Gillespie, 242–53. Cambridge: Cambridge University Press, 2007.

Goldstein, Leonard. "Science and Literary Style in Robert Burton's 'Cento out of Divers Writers.'" *Journal of the Rutgers University Library* 21 (1958): 55–68.

Göttler, Christine, and Wolfgang Neuber. *Spirits Unseen: The Representation of Subtle Bodies in Early Modern European Culture*. Leiden: Brill, 2008.

Gouk, Penelope. *Music, Science, and Natural Magic in Seventeenth-Century England*. New Haven, CT: Yale University Press, 1999.

Gowland, Angus. "Consolations for Melancholy in Renaissance Humanism." *Societate Și Politică* 6, no. 11 (2012): 10–38.

———. "Rhetorical Structure and Function in *The Anatomy of Melancholy*." *Rhetorica: A Journal of the History of Rhetoric* 19, no. 1 (2001): 1–48.

———. *The Worlds of Renaissance Melancholy: Robert Burton in Context*. Cambridge and New York: Cambridge University Press, 2006.

Graham, Kenneth John Emerson. *The Performance of Conviction: Plainness and Rhetoric in the Early English Renaissance*. Ithaca, NY: Cornell University Press, 1994.

Green, Lawrence. "Aristotle's Rhetoric and Renaissance Conceptions of the Soul." In *La Rhétorique d'Aristote: Traditions et Commentaires de l'Antiquité au XVIIe siècle*, edited by Gilbert Dahan and Irène Rosier-Catach, 283–98. Paris: Vrin, 1998.

Greenblatt, Stephen. *The Swerve: How the World Became Modern*. New York: W.W. Norton, 2011.

Grell, Ole Peter. *Paracelsus: The Man and His Reputation, His Ideas and Their Transformation*. Leiden: Brill, 1998.

Grosz, E.A. *Volatile Bodies: Toward a Corporeal Feminism*. Bloomington: Indiana University Press, 1994.

Guerlac, Suzanne. "Longinus and the Subject of the Sublime." *New Literary History* 16, no. 2 (1985): 275–89.

Hackel, Heidi Brayman. *Reading Material in Early Modern England: Print, Gender, and Literacy*. Cambridge: Cambridge University Press, 2005.

Hadas, Moses. "Horace, *Sermones* 1.4.10." *The Classical Weekly* 21, no. 15 (1928): 114.

Hadzsits, George Depue. *Lucretius And His Influence*. New York: Longmans, Green and Co., 1935.

Hall, Anne Drury. "Epistle, Meditation, and Sir Thomas Browne's Religio Medici." *PMLA* 94, no. 2 (1979): 234–46.

Hallwachs, Robert G. "Additions and Revisions in the Second Edition of Burton's *Anatomy of Melancholy*: A Study of Burton's Chief Interests and of his Style as Shown in his Revisions." PhD dissertation, Princeton University, 1942.

Hanegraaff, Wouter J. *Esotericism and the Academy: Rejected Knowledge in Western Culture*. Cambridge: Cambridge University Press, 2012.

Hardie, Philip R. *Lucretian Receptions: History, the Sublime, Knowledge*. Cambridge: Cambridge University Press, 2009.

———. "The Speech of Pythagoras in Ovid Metamorphoses 15: Empedoclean Epos." *The Classical Quarterly* 45, no. 1 (1995): 204–14.

Harris, Victor. *All Coherence Gone*. Chicago: University of Chicago Press, 1949.

Haskell, Yasmin. "The Anatomy of Hypochondria: Malachias Geiger's Microcosmus Hypochondriacus (Munich 1652)." In *Diseases of the Imagination and Imaginary Disease in the Early Modern Period*, edited by Yasmin Haskell, 275–300. Turnhout: Brepols, 2011.

Havenstein, Daniela. *Democratizing Sir Thomas Browne: Religio Medici and Its Imitations*. Oxford: Clarendon Press, 1999.

Heusser, Martin. *The Gilded Pill: A Study of the Reader-Writer Relationship in Robert Burton's "Anatomy of Melancholy."* Tübingen: Stauffenburg, 1987.

Hill, Christopher. *Intellectual Origins of the English Revolution: Revisited*. Oxford: Oxford University Press, 1997.

Hurt, Ellen Louise. "The Prose Style of Robert Burton: The Fruits of Knowledge." PhD dissertation, University of Oregon, 1966.

Hutchison, Keith. "What Happened to Occult Qualities in the Scientific Revolution?" *Isis* 73, no. 2 (1982): 233–53.

J.H.M. "Experto Crede Roberto." *Notes and Queries* 6, no. 144 (1852): 107.

Jackson, Holbrook. *The Anatomy of Bibliomania*. Urbana: University of Illinois Press, 2001.

Jackson, Stanley. *Care of the Psyche: A History of Psychological Healing*. New Haven, CT: Yale University Press, 1999.

———. *Melancholia and Depression: From Hippocratic Times to Modern Times*. New Haven, CT: Yale University Press, 1986.

Jarcho, Saul. "Galen's Six Non-Naturals: A Bibliographic Note and Translation." *Bulletin of the History of Medicine* 44, no. 4 (1970): 372–7.

Jardine, N., J.A. Secord, and E.C. Spary. *Cultures of Natural History*. Cambridge: Cambridge University Press, 1996.

Jeanneret, Michel. *A Feast of Words: Banquets and Table Talk in the Renaissance*. Chicago: University of Chicago Press, 1991.

————. *Perpetual Motion: Transforming Shapes in the Renaissance from Da Vinci to Montaigne*. Translated by Nidra Poller. Baltimore: Johns Hopkins University Press, 2000.

Johns, Adrian. *The Nature of the Book: Print and Knowledge in the Making*. Chicago: University of Chicago Press, 1998.

Jones, Richard F. *The Seventeenth Century: Studies in the History of English Thought and Literature from Bacon to Pope*. Stanford: Stanford University Press, 1951.

Jordan, Constance. "Feminism and the Humanists: The Case for Sir Thomas Elyot's Defense of Good Women." In *Rewriting the Renaissance: The Discourses of Sexual Difference in Early Modern Europe*, edited by Margaret W. Ferguson and Maureen Quilligan. Chicago: University of Chicago Press, 1986.

Jordan-Smith, Paul. *Bibliographia Burtoniana: A Study of Robert Burton's "The Anatomy of Melancholy."* Stanford: Stanford University Press, 1931.

Kenney, E.J. *Latin Literature*. Cambridge: Cambridge University Press, 1982.

Keynes, Geoffrey. "Bibliographia Burtonia." *The Review of English Studies* 35 (1933): 337–9.

Kiessling, Nicolas K. *The Library of Robert Burton*. Oxford: Oxford Bibliographical Society, 1988.

Kitzes, Adam. *The Politics of Melancholy from Spenser to Milton*. New York: Routledge, 2006.

Klibansky, Raymond, Erwin Panofsky, and Fritz Saxl. *Saturn and Melancholy: Studies in the History of Natural Philosophy, Religion, and Art*. New York: Basic Books, 1964.

Knapp, Charles. "Notes on Horace's Sermones." *The American Journal of Philology* 44, no. 1 (1923): 62–6.

Kraye, Jill. "Ἀπάθεια and Προπάθειαι in Early Modern Discussions of the Passions: Stoicism, Christianity and Natural History." *Early Science and Medicine*, 17 (2012): 230–53.

————. "Moral Philosophy." In *The Cambridge History of Renaissance Philosophy*, edited by C.B. Schmitt and Quentin Skinner, 301–86. Cambridge: Cambridge University Press, 1988.

————. "Stoicism in the Renaissance from Petrarch to Lipsius." *Grotiana* 22, no. 1 (2001): 21–45.

Kuriyama, Shigehisa. *The Expressiveness of the Body and the Divergence of Greek and Chinese Medicine*. New York: Zone, 2002.

Lake, Peter. "Calvinism and the English Church." *Past and Present* 114 (1987): 32–76.

Lasiewski, Robert C., and Henry J. Thompson. "Field Observation of Torpidity in the Violet-Green Swallow." *The Condor* 68, no. 1 (1966): 102–3.

Lievsay, John. "Robert Burton's De Consolatione." *South Atlantic Quarterly* 55 (1956): 329–36.

Lund, Mary Ann. *Melancholy, Medicine and Religion in Early Modern England: Reading "The Anatomy of Melancholy."* New York: Cambridge University Press, 2010.

————. "Reading and the Cure of Despair in *The Anatomy of Melancholy.*" *Studies in Philology* 105, no. 4 (Fall 2008): 533–58.

Lüthy, Christoph. "The Fourfold Democritus on the Stage of Early Modern Science." *Isis* 91, no. 3 (January 2000): 443.

Lyons, Bridget Gellert. *Voices of Melancholy: Studies in Literary Treatments of Melancholy in Renaissance England.* London: Routledge & Kegan Paul, 1971.

Lyons, John D. "Sublime Accidents." In *Chance, Literature, and Culture in Early Modern France*, edited by John D. Lyons and Kathleen Wine, 95–110. Burlington, VT: Ashgate, 2009.

MacDonald, Michael. *Mystical Bedlam: Madness, Anxiety and Healing in Seventeenth-Century England.* Cambridge: Cambridge University Press, 1983.

Maclean, Ian. "Foucault's Renaissance Episteme Reassessed: An Aristotelian Counterblast." *Journal of the History of Ideas* 59, no. 1 (1998): 149–66.

Maiorino, Giancarlo. *The Cornucopian Mind and the Baroque Unity of the Arts.* University Park: Pennsylvania State University Press, 1990.

Maravall, José Antonio. *Culture of the Baroque: Analysis of a Historical Structure.* Manchester: Manchester University Press, 1986.

Marcus, Leah S. *The Politics of Mirth: Jonson, Herrick, Milton, Marvell, and the Defense of Old Holiday Pastimes.* Chicago: University of Chicago Press, 1989.

Marshall, Ed. "Experto Crede Roberto." *Notes and Queries* 7, no. 107 (1877): 408.

Mauss, Marcel. *A General Theory of Magic.* London: Routledge, 2005.

Mazzio, Carla. "The History of Air: Hamlet and the Trouble with Instruments." *South Central Review* 26, no. 1 (2009): 153–96.

McAtee, W.L. "Torpidity in Birds." *American Midland Naturalist* 38, no. 1 (1947): 191–206.

McConica, James, ed. *The Collegiate University.* Vol. 3, *The History of the University of Oxford.* Oxford: Clarendon Press, 1986.

McGill, Scott. *Virgil Recomposed: The Mythological and Secular Centos in Antiquity.* New York: Oxford University Press, 2005.

McLean, H.V. "Review of *The Psychiatry of Robert Burton*, by Bergen Evans in Consultation with George J. Mohr, M.D." *Psychoanalytic Quarterly* 15 (1946): 245–8.

Milbank, John. *Being Reconciled: Ontology and Pardon.* New York: Routledge, 2003.

Monsarrat, Gilles D. *Light from the Porch: Stoicism and English Renaissance Literature.* Paris: Didier-Érudition, 1984.

Mueller, William Randolph. *The Anatomy of Robert Burton's England.* Berkeley: University of California Press, 1952.

Muldrew, Craig. *The Economy of Obligation: The Culture of Credit and Social Relations in Early Modern England.* New York: St. Martin's Press, 1998.

Murphy, Kathryn. "Robert Burton and the Problems of Polymathy." *Renaissance Studies* 28, no. 2 (2014): 279–97.

Nardo, Anna K. *The Ludic Self in Seventeenth-Century English Literature.* Albany: State University of New York Press, 1991.

Neely, Carol Thomas. *Distracted Subjects: Madness and Gender in Shakespeare and Early Modern Culture.* Ithaca, NY: Cornell University Press, 2004.

Newton, Alfred Edward. *End Papers: Literary Recreations.* Boston: Little, Brown, 1933.

Nochimson, Richard Leonard. "Robert Burton: A Study of the Man, His Work, and His Critics." PhD dissertation, Columbia University, 1967.

Nouche "Nouche!" "Vivisect Your Mind." Review of *The Anatomy of Melancholy* (New York Review Books Classics). August 30, 2006. http://www.amazon. com/Anatomy-Melancholy-Review-Books-Classics/product-reviews/094032 2668?pageNumber=2.

O'Connell, Michael. *Robert Burton.* Boston: Twayne, 1986.

Olson, Glending. *Literature as Recreation in the Later Middle Ages.* Ithaca, NY: Cornell University Press, 1982.

Osler, Sir William. *Selected Writings of Sir William Osler, 12 July 1849 to 29 December 1919.* London: Oxford University Press, 1951.

Pagel, Walter. *Joan Baptista van Helmont: Reformer of Science and Medicine.* Cambridge: Cambridge University Press, 1982.

———. *Paracelsus: An Introduction to Philosophical Medicine in the Era of the Renaissance.* Basel: Karger, 1982.

Parker, Patricia A. *Literary Fat Ladies: Rhetoric, Gender, Property.* London and New York: Methuen, 1987.

Passannante, Gerard Paul. *The Lucretian Renaissance: Philology and the Afterlife of Tradition.* Chicago: University of Chicago Press, 2011.

Paster, Gail Kern. *The Body Embarrassed: Drama and the Disciplines of Shame in Early Modern England.* Ithaca, NY: Cornell University Press, 1993.

———. *Humoring the Body: Emotions and the Shakespearean Stage.* Chicago: University of Chicago Press, 2010.

Platt, Peter G. "'Not Before Either Known or Dreamt of': Francesco Patrizi and the Power of Wonder in Renaissance Poetics." *Review of English Studies* 43 (1992): 387–94.

———. *Reason Diminished: Shakespeare and the Marvelous.* Lincoln: University of Nebraska Press, 1997.

Pullman, Philip. "Reasons to Be Cheerful." *Telegraph.co.uk*, April 10, 2005, sec. books. http://www.telegraph.co.uk/culture/books/3640566/Reasons-to-be-cheerful.html.

Pumfrey, Stephen. "The Spagyric Art; Or, The Impossible Work of Separating Pure from Impure Paracelsianism: Historiographical Analysis." In *Paracelsus: The Man and His Reputation, His Ideas and Their Transformation*, edited by Ole Peter Grell, 21–52. Leiden: Brill, 1998.

Radden, Jennifer. *The Nature of Melancholy: From Aristotle to Kristeva.* Oxford: Oxford University Press, 2002.

Rebhorn, Wayne A. *The Emperor of Men's Minds: Literature and the Renaissance Discourse of Rhetoric.* Ithaca, NY: Cornell University Press, 1995.

Reid, Edith Gittings, and Sir William Osler. *The Great Physician: A Short Life of Sir William Osler.* London and New York: Oxford University Press, 1931.

Reif, Stefan C., ed. *Hebrew Manuscripts at Cambridge University Library: A Description and Introduction.* Cambridge: Cambridge University Press, 1997.

Reiss, Timothy J. *Against Autonomy: Global Dialectics of Cultural Exchange.* Stanford: Stanford University Press, 2002.

———. *Mirages of the Selfe: Patterns of Personhood in Ancient and Early Modern Europe.* Stanford: Stanford University Press, 2003.

Renaker, David. "Robert Burton and Ramist Method." *Renaissance Quarterly* 24, no. 2 (1971): 210–20.

———. "Robert Burton's Palinodes." *Studies in Philology* 76, no. 2 (1979): 162–81.

———. "Robert Burton's Tricks of Memory." *PMLA* 87, no. 3 (1972): 391–6.

Rener, Frederick M. "Robert Burton's Tricks of Memory." *PMLA* 88, no. 1 (1973): 142–4.

Rosenblatt, Jason P. *Renaissance England's Chief Rabbi: John Selden.* Oxford: Oxford University Press, 2008.

Roth, Cecil. "Sir Thomas Bodley, Hebraist." *Bodleian Library Record* 7 (1966): 242–51.

Rouse, Mary A., and Richard H. Rouse. *Authentic Witnesses: Approaches to Medieval Texts and Manuscripts.* Notre Dame: University of Notre Dame Press, 1991.

Rouse, W.H.D. *Burton the Anatomist: Being Extracts from the "Anatomy of Melancholy" Chosen to Interest the Psychologist in Every Man.* Edited by G.C.F. Mead and Rupert Clift. London: Methuen, 1925.

Saintsbury, George. *Specimens of English Prose Style from Malory to Macaulay.* London: Kegan Paul, 1885.

Sale, Carolyn. "Eating Air, Feeling Smells: Hamlet's Theory of Performance." *Renaissance Drama* 35 (2006): 145–68.

Sawday, Jonathan. "Shapeless Elegance." In *English Renaissance Prose: History, Language, and Politics*, edited by Neil Rhodes. Tempe, AZ: Medieval & Renaissance Texts & Studies, 1997.

Schleiner, Winfried. *Melancholy, Genius, and Utopia in the Renaissance.* Wiesbaden: Otto Harrassowitz, 1991.

Schmelzer, Mary Murphy. *'Tis All One: "The Anatomy of Melancholy" as Belated Copious Discourse.* New York: Peter Lang, 1999.

Schmid, Martin. "The Environmental History of Rivers in the Early Modern Period." In *An Environmental History of the Early Modern Period: Experiments and Perspectives*, edited by Martin Knoll and Reinhold Reith. Zurich: Lit Verlag Münster, 2014.

Schmidt, Jeremy. *Melancholy and the Care of the Soul: Religion, Moral Philosophy and Madness in Early Modern England.* Aldershot, UK: Ashgate, 2007.

———. "Melancholy and the Therapeutic Language of Moral Philosophy in Seventeenth-Century Thought." *Journal of the History of Ideas* 65, no. 4 (2004): 583–601.

Schoenfeldt, Michael C. *Bodies and Selves in Early Modern England: Physiology and Inwardness in Spenser, Shakespeare, Herbert, and Milton.* Cambridge: Cambridge University Press, 1999.

————. "Reading Bodies." In *Reading, Society and Politics in Early Modern England*, edited by Kevin Sharpe and Steven N. Zwicker, 215–43. Cambridge: Cambridge University Press, 2003.

Schott, Heinz. "Paracelsus and Van Helmont on Imagination." In *Paracelsian Moments: Science, Medicine, & Astrology in Early Modern Europe*, edited by Gerhild Scholz Williams and Charles D. Gunnoe Jr., 135–47. Kirksville, MO: Truman State University Press, 2002.

Schwartz, Scott. "Take Small Bites!" Review of *The Anatomy of Melancholy* (New York Review Books Classics) (Paperback), June 16, 2008. http://www.amazon.com/review/R1EF6JHBOLQ98A/ref=cm_srch_res_rtr_alt_1.

Scodel, Joshua. *Excess and the Mean in Early Modern English Literature*. Princeton, NJ: Princeton University Press, 2002.

Shelly, John. "Rhythmical Prose in Latin and English." *Church Quarterly Review*, 1912.

Shirilan, Stephanie. "The Forbidden Pleasures of Style." *Prose Studies* 34, no. 2 (2012): 115–28.

Shuger, Debora. "Conceptions of Style." In *The Cambridge History of Literary Criticism*, edited by Glynn Norton, 3:181–6. Cambridge: Cambridge University Press, 1999.

————. "Foundations of Sacred Rhetoric." In *Rhetorical Invention and Religious Inquiry: New Perspectives*, edited by Walter Jost and Wendy Olmsted. New Haven, CT: Yale University Press, 2000.

————. *Sacred Rhetoric: The Christian Grand Style in the English Renaissance*. Princeton, NJ: Princeton University Press, 1988.

Shumaker, Wayne. *Natural Magic and Modern Science: Four Treatises, 1590–1657*. Binghamton: Center for Medieval and Early Renaissance Studies, State University of New York Press, 1989.

Solomon, Julie Robin. *Objectivity in the Making: Francis Bacon and the Politics of Inquiry*. Baltimore: Johns Hopkins University Press, 2002.

Speak, G. "An Odd Kind of Melancholy: Reflections on the Glass Delusion in Europe (1440–1680)." *History of Psychiatry* 1, no. 2 (1990): 191–206.

Spruit, Leen. *Species Intelligibilis: From Perception to Knowledge*. Vol. 2. Leiden: Brill, 1994.

Stachniewski, John. *The Persecutory Imagination: English Puritanism and the Literature of Religious Despair*. Oxford: Clarendon Press, 1991.

Strier, Richard. "Against the Rule of Reason: Praise of Passion from Petrarch to Luther to Shakespeare to Herbert." In *Reading the Early Modern Passions: Essays in the Cultural History of Emotion*, edited by Gail Kern Paster, Katherine Rowe, and Mary Floyd-Wilson, 23–42. Philadelphia: University of Pennsylvania Press, 2004.

————. *The Unrepentant Renaissance: From Petrarch to Shakespeare to Milton*. Chicago: University of Chicago Press, 2011.

Sutton, John. *Philosophy and Memory Traces: Descartes to Connectionism*. Cambridge: Cambridge University Press, 1998.

———. "Soul and Body in Seventeenth-Century British Philosophy." In *The Oxford Handbook of British Philosophy in the Seventeenth Century*, edited by Peter Anstey. Oxford: Oxford University Press, 2013.

———. "Spongy Brains and Material Memories." In *Environment and Embodiment in Early Modern England*, edited by Mary Floyd-Wilson and Garrett A. Sullivan Jr. New York: Palgrave Macmillan, 2007.

Swan, Claudia. "Eyes Wide Shut. Early Modern Imagination, Demonology, and the Visual Arts." *Zeitsprünge: Forschungen Zur Frühen Neuzeit* 7 (2003): 560–81.

Taubenhaus, Godfrey. *Echoes of Wisdom: Or, Talmudic Sayings with Classic, Especially Latin, Parallelisms*. Brooklyn, NY: Haedrich & Sons, 1900.

Taylor, C.C.W., ed. *The Atomists, Leucippus and Democritus: Fragments: A Text and Translation with a Commentary*. Toronto, ON: University of Toronto Press, 2010.

Tempest, Norbert. *The Rhythm of English Prose*. Cambridge: Cambridge University Press, 1930.

Thompson, Ann. *The Art of Suffering and the Impact of Seventeenth-Century Anti-Providential Thought*. Aldershot, UK: Ashgate, 2003.

Thorndike, Lynn. *A History of Magic and Experimental Science*. Vol. 1. New York: Macmillan, 1923.

Tilmouth, Christopher. "Burton's 'Turning Picture': Argument and Anxiety in *The Anatomy of Melancholy*." *The Review of English Studies* 56, no. 226 (2005): 524–49.

Todd, Margo. *Christian Humanism and the Puritan Social Order*. Cambridge: Cambridge University Press, 2002.

Tomlinson, Gary. *Music in Renaissance Magic: Toward a Historiography of Others*. Chicago: University of Chicago Press, 1993.

Trevor, Douglas. *The Poetics of Melancholy in Early Modern England*. Cambridge: Cambridge University Press, 2004.

Trevor-Roper, Hugh. *Catholics, Anglicans and Puritans: Seventeenth-Century Essays*. Chicago: Chicago University Press, 1987.

Tucker, Hugo. "Justus Lipsius and the *Cento* Form." In *(Un)masking the Realities of Power: Justus Lipsius and the Dynamics of Political Writing in Early Modern Europe*, 163–92. Leiden: Brill, 2010.

Turner, Victor W. *From Ritual to Theatre: The Human Seriousness of Play*. Vol. 1. Performance Studies Series. New York: Performing Arts Journal Publications, 1982.

Tylor, Sir Edward Burnett. *Researches into the Early History of Mankind and the Development of Civilization*. New York: Henry Holt, 1878.

van Eck, Caroline. *Translations of the Sublime: The Early Modern Reception and Dissemination of Longinus' Peri Hupsous in Rhetoric, the Visual Arts, Architecture and the Theatre*. Leiden: Brill, 2012.

Verbeke, Gérard. *L'évolution de la doctrine du Pneuma: du stoicisme à S. Augustin*. Paris: Desclée de Brouwer, 1945.

———. *The Presence of Stoicism in Medieval Thought*. Washington, DC: Catholic University of America Press, 1983.

Vermeir, Koen. "The 'Physical Prophet' and the Powers of the Imagination. Part I: A Case-Study on Prophecy, Vapours and the Imagination (1685–1710)." *Studies in History and Philosophy of Science Part C: Studies in History and Philosophy of Biological and Biomedical Sciences* 35, no. 4 (2004): 561–91.

Verweyen, Theodor, and Gunther Wittig. "The Cento: A Form of Intertextuality from Montage to Parody." In *Intertextuality*, edited by Heinrich F. Plett. Berlin: Walter de Gruyter, 1991.

Vicari, E. Patricia. *The View from Minerva's Tower: Learning and Imagination in "The Anatomy of Melancholy."* Toronto, ON: University of Toronto Press, 1989.

Vickers, Brian. "Analogy versus Identity: The Rejection of Occult Symbolism, 1580–1660." In *Occult and Scientific Mentalities*, edited by Brian Vickers. Cambridge: Cambridge University Press, 1986.

Wack, Mary Frances. *Lovesickness in the Middle Ages: The Viaticum and Its Commentaries*. Middle Ages Series. Philadelphia: University of Pennsylvania Press, 1990.

Waddington, Raymond. *Aretino's Satyr: Sexuality, Satire and Self-Projection in Sixteenth-Century Literature and Art*. Toronto, ON: University of Toronto Press, 2004.

Walker, D.P. "The Astral Body in Renaissance Medicine." *Journal of the Warburg and Courtauld Institutes* 21 (1958): 119–33.

———. "Ficino's Spiritus and Music." *Annales Musicologiques* 1 (1953): 131–50.

———. *Spiritual & Demonic Magic: From Ficino to Campanella*. University Park: Pennsylvania State University Press, 2000.

Warnke, Frank J. *Versions of Baroque: European Literature in the Seventeenth Century*. New Haven, CT: Yale University Press, 1972.

Webb, Ruth. *Ekphrasis, Imagination, and Persuasion in Ancient Rhetorical Theory and Practice*. Farnham, UK: Ashgate, 2009.

Webber, Joan. *The Eloquent "I": Style and Self in Seventeenth-Century Prose*. Madison: University of Wisconsin Press, 1968.

Webster, Charles. "Paracelsus: Medicine as Popular Protest." In *Medicine and the Reformation*, edited by Ole Peter Grell and Andrew Cunningham. London: Routledge, 1993.

Webster, John. *The Duchess of Malfi and Other Plays*. Edited by René Weis. Oxford: Oxford University Press, 2009.

Webster, Tom. "Writing to Redundancy: Approaches to Spiritual Journals and Early Modern Spirituality." *The Historical Journal* 39, no. 1 (1996): 33–56.

Weeks, Andrew. *Paracelsus: Speculative Theory and the Crisis of the Early Reformation*. Albany: State University of New York Press, 1997.

Weinberg, Bernard. *A History of Literary Criticism in the Italian Renaissance*. Chicago: University of Chicago Press, 1961.

Wells, Marion A. *The Secret Wound: Love-Melancholy and Early Modern Romance*. Stanford: Stanford University Press, 2007.

Wendell, Barrett. *Temper of the Seventeenth Century in English Literature.* New York: Scribner, 1904.

Westfall, Richard S. "Science and Technology during the Scientific Revolution: An Empirical Approach." In *Renaissance and Revolution: Humanists, Scholars, Craftsmen and Natural Philosophers in Early Modern Europe*, edited by Judith Veronica Field and Frank A.J.L. James, 63–72. Cambridge: Cambridge University Press, 1997.

White, Peter. "The Rise of Arminianism Reconsidered." *Past & Present* 101 (1983): 34–54.

Wilkerson, Robert Steve. "This Playing Labour: The Preface to Burton's *Anatomy of Melancholy* as a Satiric Apologia." PhD dissertation, Georgia State University, 1975.

Williams, G.D. "Cleombrotus of Ambracia: Interpretations of a Suicide from Callimachus to Agathias." *The Classical Quarterly* 45, no. 1 (1995): 154–69.

Williams, Robert Grant. "Disarticulating Fantasies: Figures of Speech, Vices, and the Blazon in Renaissance English Rhetoric." *RSQ* 29, no. 1 (1999): 43–54.

———. "Disfiguring the Body of Knowledge: Anatomical Discourse and Robert Burton's *The Anatomy of Melancholy*." *ELH* 68, no. 3 (2001): 593–613.

———. "Heterological Rhetoric: Textual Waste in *The Anatomy of Melancholy*." London, ON: University of Western Ontario, 1995.

Williamson, George. "Mutability, Decay, and Seventeenth-Century Melancholy." *ELH* 2, no. 2 (1935): 121–50.

———. *The Senecan Amble.* Chicago: University of Chicago Press, 1951.

Wind, Edgar. "The Christian Democritus." *Journal of the Warburg Institute* 1, no. 2 (1937): 180–82.

Winkler, Amanda Eubanks. *O Let Us Howle Some Heavy Note: Music for Witches, the Melancholic, and the Mad on the Seventeenth-Century English Stage.* Bloomington: Indiana University Press, 2006.

Woolf, D.R. "Hearing Renaissance England." In *Hearing History: A Reader*, edited by Mark M. Smith, 112–35. Athens: University of Georgia Press, 2004.

Index

Milton Keynes UK
Ingram Content Group UK Ltd.
UKHW040101071024
449327UK00019B/733